The Spectrum of Family Caregiving
for Adults and Elders with Chronic Illness

The Spectrum of Family Caregiving for Adults and Elders with Chronic Illness

EDITED BY **LOUIS D. BURGIO**

JOSEPH E. GAUGLER

AND

MICHELLE M. HILGEMAN

OXFORD
UNIVERSITY PRESS

OXFORD
UNIVERSITY PRESS

Oxford University Press is a department of the University of
Oxford. It furthers the University's objective of excellence in research,
scholarship, and education by publishing worldwide.

Oxford   New York
Auckland   Cape Town   Dar es Salaam   Hong Kong   Karachi
Kuala Lumpur   Madrid   Melbourne   Mexico City   Nairobi
New Delhi   Shanghai   Taipei   Toronto

With offices in
Argentina   Austria   Brazil   Chile   Czech Republic   France   Greece
Guatemala   Hungary   Italy   Japan   Poland   Portugal   Singapore
South Korea   Switzerland   Thailand   Turkey   Ukraine   Vietnam

Oxford is a registered trademark of Oxford University Press
in the UK and certain other countries.

Published in the United States of America by
Oxford University Press
198 Madison Avenue, New York, NY 10016

Cataloging-in-Publication data is on file at the Library of Congress

ISBN 978-0-19-982803-6

CONTENTS

PREFACE

While a member of the faculty at the University of Michigan, Ann Arbor, one of the coeditors (LDB) formed and chaired an interdisciplinary study group for faculty and students who shared an interest in dementia caregiving. The purpose of the group was to share ideas and information, facilitate research, and generate scholarly papers. Primarily as a result of the chair's research interests, the emphasis of the meetings was on interventions to ease the stress and burden of providing care. Attendance at these meetings began with a core of four to five dedicated faculty members. However, as word spread gradually across campus about the existence of the study group, attendance increased markedly, and the professional interests of the new members was noteworthy.

The first wave of new members, primarily nurses and social workers, were clinicians. As one would expect from demographic trends, these clinicians were encountering an ever-growing number of family caregivers seeking assistance in providing care to their loved ones. These clinicians attended the meetings to learn how to serve their caregiver clients better. Specifically, they sought information on how to help their clients become better caregivers and how to help them manage the stress and burden often associated with providing care. Also, a few of the clinicians had devised their own strategies for intervention. Most of these efforts were creative and potentially effective. Thus, their participation in the group was beneficial to both researchers and other clinicians.

The identity of the next wave of attendees came as a bit of a surprise. Our dementia caregiving study group began to draw attendance from faculty and students studying other types of chronic illnesses: cancer, stroke, HIV/AIDS, severe mental illness, musculoskeletal disorders associated with pain, and patients with multiple chronic illnesses who required palliative care. Thanks to a small grant from the Pfizer Medical Education Group (no. 025512), we were able to expand the scope of the study group to accommodate these researchers. Consequently, we changed the name of our study group to the *Caregiving for Chronic Illnesses Workgroup*.

This combination of researchers and clinicians discussing the needs of patients with various chronic illnesses became fertile ground for many scholarly efforts.

This volume is one outcome of these efforts. It became clear that some chronic illnesses (e.g., dementia, stroke, and cancer) had a sizable amount of research literatures on both caregivers and caregiver interventions. Other illnesses requiring chronic care had active caregiver research agendas, but the research literature was less extant (e.g., for palliative care/end-of-life care, caring for adult children with severe mental illness). As a result of improvements in medical treatments and the consequent increase in patient survival, some chronic illnesses identified caregiving as an area of emerging interest (e.g., severe cardiovascular conditions); however, relatively few papers focusing on caregiving had been published in these areas.

As the expanded workgroup began discussing various topics, it appeared as if caregiving researchers across various chronic illnesses were working from within isolated "academic silos." The majority of workgroup members were unaware of the vast literature on both the caregiving role and caregiver interventions available in some areas of chronic care. Moreover, reviews of the areas with extensive caregiving literature seemed to suggest that existing studies seldom referenced caregiving research done in other areas of chronic care.

Workgroup members discussed topics such as the similarities and differences in patients with different chronic illnesses and the resulting demands placed on their caregivers. We discovered that, although some empirical research was available that compared caregiving needs across different chronic illnesses (see Chapter 10), the number of available published papers was quite small. Last, considering the varying types of demands placed on caregivers, questions arose regarding the applicability of existing caregiver interventions to different chronic illnesses. Could evidence-based caregiver interventions developed in one area of chronic care be adapted easily to other areas? Were the demands on caregivers so different that new interventions were needed?

The goal of this edited volume is to review research on the caregiving role and interventions developed to assist family caregivers of older adults and elders with different chronic conditions. The selection of chronic illnesses included in this volume is based on our judgment that each area was supported by a sufficient caregiving database. Caregiving research has been conducted in other areas of chronic illness, such as diabetes (e.g., Langa et al., 2002), chronic obstructive pulmonary disease (Bergs, 2002), and end-stage renal disease (Wicks, Milstead, Hathaway, & Cetingok, 1997). These and other chronic conditions were not included because of the relatively limited number of published documents in these areas. We also decided to limit the scope of the volume to chronic illnesses in older adults and elders. Not included here is the extensive body of caregiving research on children and adolescents with chronic conditions such as intellectual disability (e.g., Hastings & Beck, 2004) and severe autism spectrum disorders (e.g., Schieve, Blumberg, Rice, Visser, & Boyle, 2007).

ORGANIZATION OF THE VOLUME
AND CHAPTER FORMAT

There are eight disease-specific caregiving chapters in this volume (Chapters 2–9) written by experts in these areas. The coeditors have contributed two chapters (Chapters 1 and 10). Chapter 1 sets the stage for the disease-specific chapters, with discussions of definitions, demographics, and theoretical models of caregiving in chronic illness; and introduces the topic of translating research findings to real-world settings. Chapter 10 is divided into three sections. In the first two sections we summarize the state of the science on caregiving roles and caregiver interventions. In the third section we discuss the most relevant challenges and barriers faced by today's caregivers and caregiver advocates. We discuss in some detail the necessity of implementing caregiver interventions in clinics and other community settings (i.e., the "real world") where they are most likely to affect the lives of caregivers and care recipients. We conclude the chapter with a peek into the future of caregiving for the chronically ill, discuss emerging issues, and offer some suggestions for addressing the pressing challenges to come.

The authors of the disease-specific chapters were asked to format their chapters to provide information that would be useful for both researchers and clinicians. Most of the chapters in this volume are divided in to two discrete sections: The Caregiving Role and Caregiver Interventions. The Caregiving Role section includes a thorough review of the literature on the characteristics of caregivers and care recipients, including related care needs, issues, and challenges unique to the chronic illness discussed in the chapter. The latter section reviews the available published literature on caregiver interventions, including descriptions of the interventions and evidence of efficacy.

Because the definitions of *evidence-based* and *evidence-informed* interventions are still under intense debate in the research community, the authors provide an evidence table so that the reader can judge more easily the level of available evidence. The tables summarize the types of interventions, study sample, racial/cultural factors, study design, outcomes, and evaluative comments on study quality.

If available, authors were asked to include discussions of positive aspects of caregiving, which was neglected historically by researchers but is now recognized as a critical variable in understanding caregiving and in developing new interventions. Also, any efforts to translate and implement interventions in community settings were to be included. Last, to increase the utility of the volume for clinicians, each chapter includes two case studies describing common problems encountered by caregivers, along with descriptions of interventions used to address these problems.

Our small study group was formed to provide an opportunity for like-minded researchers to share ideas on how to provide better care for dementia caregivers. Although we had no intention of expanding our interests beyond our initial narrow scope of interest, our group evolved in a way that we now see as inevitable. Our new members provided the perspective that dementia was only one of many chronic illnesses. As a result of advances in medical science and demographic trends, the number of individuals with chronic illness is increasing exponentially. Each chronic illness presents family members who care for an affected loved one with a unique set of challenges. This volume is an attempt to characterize the needs of individuals with different chronic illnesses and the challenges faced by their caregivers. Most important, it provides the reader—both clinicians and researchers—with an array of evidence-based interventions developed to reduce caregiver stress and burden, and to help caregivers become more effective in their role.

—Louis D. Burgio

REFERENCES

Bergs, D. (2002). The hidden client: Women caring for husbands with COPD: Their experience of quality of life. *Journal of Clinical Nursing, 11*(5), 613–621.

Hastings, R. P, & Beck, A. (2004). Practitioner review: Stress intervention for parents of children with intellectual disabilities. *Journal of Child Psychology and Psychiatry, 45*(8), 1338–1349.

Langa, K. M., Vijan, S., Hayward, R. A., Chernew, M. E., Blaum, C. S., Kabeto, M. U., et al. (2002). Informal caregiving for diabetes and diabetic complications among elderly Americans. *Journals of Gerontology: Series B Psychological Sciences and Social Sciences, 57*(3), 177–186.

Schieve, L. A., Blumberg, S. J., Rice, C., Visser, S. N., & Boyle, C. (2007). The relationship between autism and parenting stress. *Pediatrics, 119*(S1), S114–S121.

Wicks, M. N., Milstead, E. J., Hathaway, D. K., & Cetingok, M. (1997). Family caregivers' burden, quality of life, and health following patients' renal transplantation. *American Nephrology Nurses' Association, 24*(5), 527–528, 531–538.

Louis D. Burgio, PhD, is founder and director of Burgio Geriatric Consulting. During a career that spans more than three decades, Dr. Burgio has held several full-time academic leadership positions. Most recently he was the Harold R. Johnson Endowed Chair of Gerontology in the School of Social Work, University of Michigan. Prior to that, he was University Distinguished Professor and Founding Director of The Center for Mental Health and Aging, University of Alabama. His research, which appears in more than 175 peer-reviewed publications, has focused on the development of social–behavioral interventions to improve the quality of care and quality of life of patients with dementia and their caregivers. In recognition of the impact of his research in the field of applied gerontology, Dr. Burgio was awarded the M. Powell Lawton Awards from both the Gerontological Society of America (GSA) and the American Psychological Association (APA), the Rosalynn Carter Institute Award for Excellence in Caregiving Research, and the Outstanding Research Award, Psychologists in Long-Term Care, also from the APA. Dr. Burgio has been the Principle Investigator on numerous research grants awarded by the National Institutes of Health (NIH). He has served on several national advisory committees, including the National Advisory Council of the National Institute for Nursing Research (NIH), and has served on 11 journal editorial boards.

Joseph E. Gaugler, PhD, is a Professor in the School of Nursing and Center on Aging at the University of Minnesota. Dr. Gaugler's research examines the sources and effectiveness of long-term care for chronically disabled older adults. A developmental psychologist with an interdisciplinary research focus, Dr. Gaugler's interests include Alzheimer's disease and long-term care, the longitudinal ramifications of family care for disabled adults, and the effectiveness of community-based and psychosocial services for chronically ill adults and their caregiving families. Underpinning these substantive areas, Dr. Gaugler also has interests in longitudinal and mixed methods.

Dr. Gaugler currently serves as Editor-in-Chief for the *Journal of Applied Gerontology* and on the editorial boards of *Journals of Gerontology: Psychological*

Sciences, Journals of Gerontology: Social Sciences, and *Psychology and Aging.*
He was awarded the 2003 Springer Early Career Achievement Award in Adult
Development and Aging Research, the 2011 M. Powell Lawton Distinguished
Contribution Award for Applied Gerontology from the APA (Division 20: Adult
Development and Aging), and 2011 Dean's Award from the University of
Minnesota School of Nursing. He is a Fellow of the Gerontological Society of
America and the APA, and the 2016 Gordon Streib Distinguished Academic
Gerontologist Award from the Southern Gerontological Society.

Michelle M. Hilgeman, PhD, is a licensed Clinical Research Psychologist in the
Research & Development Service at the Tuscaloosa Veterans Affairs (VA) Medical
Center. Dr. Hilgeman is an Adjunct Professor in the University of Alabama's
Department of Psychology and the University of Alabama at Birmingham's
Department of Medicine; she is also a Faculty Affiliate of the Alabama Research
Institute on Aging, and an Investigator at the Tuscaloosa Research Education
and Advancement Corporation. Dr. Hilgeman's clinical and research interests
are in geriatric mental health, including the behavioral and psychological symptoms of dementia, enhancement of quality of life for those with chronic physical or mental illnesses, medical decision making and advance care planning,
and family caregiving. Dr. Hilgeman established a Telephone-Assisted Dementia
Outreach clinic in 2012 with support from the VA Office of Rural Health. This
clinical demonstration provides evidence-based interventions to rural veterans
with dementia and their family caregivers. Her other current work on optimizing the delivery of family interventions in dementia and the assessment of
pain in dementia is funded by the VA Rehabilitation Research & Development
Service and the VA Health Services Research & Development Service, respectively. Dr. Hilgeman has been published in numerous scientific journals and was
recognized with a New Investigator Award in 2012. This award was renewed
in 2015. She is a member of the Gerontological Society of America, the APA,
and the American Telemedicine Association. She also serves as the Continuing
Education Committee Chair for the Society for Clinical Geropsychology (APA
Division 12, Section 2).

CONTRIBUTORS

Rebecca S. Allen, PhD
Alabama Research Institute on Aging
The University of Alabama

Lisa N. Beck, MS
Department of Psychology
The University of Alabama

Louis D. Burgio, PhD
Burgio Geriatric Consulting
Department of Psychology, University
  of Alabama
Department of Psychology, Western
  Michigan University

Lisa Dixon, MD, MPH
Columbia University Medical Center
Center for Practice Innovations
New York State Psychiatric Institute

Timothy R. Elliott, PhD, ABPP
Department of Educational
  Psychology
Texas A&M University

James Friedman, RN, PHN, CHPN
School of Nursing
University of Minnesota-Twin Cities

Joseph E. Gaugler, PhD
Center for Aging, School of Nursing
University of Minnesota

Barbara A. Given, PhD, RN, FAAN
College of Nursing
Michigan State University

Charles W. Given, PhD
Research Institute for Health
  Care Studies
Department of Family Medicine
College of Human Medicine
Michigan State University

Michelle M. Hilgeman, PhD
Research & Development Service
Tuscaloosa Veterans Affairs
  Medical Center

Miyeon Jung, PhD, MSN, RN
School of Nursing
University of Michigan

Helen M. Land, PhD, MSW
School of Social Work
University of Southern California

Brooklyn Levine, PhD, MSW
School of Social Work
University of Southern California

Hyunjin Noh, PhD
School of Social Work
The University of Alabama

Klaus Pfeiffer
Robert-Bosch-Hospital
Stuttgart, Germany

Karl Pillemer, PhD
Departments of Human Development
  and Human Ecology
Cornell University

Julia M. P. Poritz
Department of Educational
   Psychology
Texas A&M University

Susan J. Pressler, PhD, RN,
   FAAN, FAHA
Department of Acute, Critical, and
   Long-term Care
University of Michigan School of
   Nursing

Cary Reid, MD, PhD
Division of Geriatric Medicine
Weill Cornell Medical College

Catherine Riffin, MA
Department of Human Development
Cornell University

Laura Jane Smith, BS
Department of Psychology
The University of Alabama

Helle Thorning, PhD, LCSW
Center for Practice Innovations
Columbia University
Division of Mental Health Services
   and Policy Research
New York State Psychiatric Institute

The Spectrum of Family Caregiving
for Adults and Elders with Chronic Illness

Caregiving for Family Members with Chronic Illness

LOUIS D. BURGIO AND JOSEPH E. GAUGLER ■

At the turn of the 20th century, the major causes of death and disease were acute conditions such as tuberculosis, diarrhea, and similar transmitted diseases. Today, deaths from infectious diseases have been far surpassed by chronic illnesses such as heart disease and stroke, cancer, and Alzheimer's disease (National Association of Chronic Disease, 2011). However, deaths alone do not convey the full impact of chronic disease. By definition, chronic illnesses that affect older adults and elders are manageable but not curable. Often, these conditions can span several decades, with the patient becoming increasingly debilitated throughout the course of the disease. Although American taxpayers and businesses experience a significant economic impact, the family members caring for these patients bear the brunt of emotional, physical, and economic burdens associated with giving care.

A sampling of data from recent reports provides some perspective on the enormity of the problem (e.g., Federal Interagency Forum on Aging-Related Statistics, 2012; National Association of Chronic Disease, 2011; Thies, Bleiler, & Alzheimer's Association, 2013):

- More than 133 million Americans live with at least one chronic condition.
- An estimated 5.2 million Americans have Alzheimer's disease.
- Chronic musculoskeletal conditions, including arthritis, are the number one cause of disability, affecting nearly one of every three adults.
- Stroke has left 1 million Americans with disabilities; many can no longer perform daily tasks, such as walking or bathing, without help.
- A total of 18.9%, or 43.5 million, Americans care for someone 50 years of age or older.

- More than 75% of all our healthcare costs relate to chronic diseases—or more than $2 trillion in 2005.

Almost every family is affected adversely by chronic illness in one way or another—family members with long-term illness, disability, or a compromised quality of life; or by the huge personal financial burden wrought by these diseases. Given healthcare budget constraints and the epidemic of chronic illnesses, it is perhaps not surprising that we continue to see a chasm between what patients need and what health systems can provide. Simply put, many patients need more support than they can expect to receive from formal systems of care, and no one fix to healthcare payment or system design can address the daunting array of patients' problems (Piette, Rosland, Silveira, Kabeto, & Langa, 2010). Family caregivers play essential roles in filling the gaps in services found in most formal healthcare systems by providing assistance with transportation, medication refilling, emotional support, activities of daily living (ADLs), and a host of other vital tasks. For many chronically ill patients, sharing their burden with intimate others makes living with their disease not only possible physically, but also worthwhile emotionally and spiritually (Rosland & Piette, 2010).

In Chapters 2 through 9 in this book we see there are evidence-based "interventions" (i.e., programs and/or services) available to assist caregivers in managing the tasks of caregiving and the stress and burden associated with the caregiving role. It is a tragic fact that very few healthcare professionals are aware of these resources, and few caregivers receive training in how to fulfill their critical role. This introductory chapter to *The Spectrum of Family Caregiving for Adults and Elders with Chronic Illness* provides some background information on family caregiving as an issue of scientific relevance and public health import.

DEFINING FAMILY CAREGIVING

What is *caregiving*? As becomes evident fairly quickly when reviewing the literature on family care in chronic disease contexts, there is no universally accepted definition of caregiving. This problem was identified quite early in caregiving research (Gaugler, Kane, & Kane, 2002), but has yet to be resolved. Many researchers rely heavily on an individual's own subjective perception of herself or himself as a "caregiver" to another relative. Some researchers have developed definitions that differentiate caregiving based on the reasons why such help is provided. Relying on this approach, one definition of caregiving is that it "reflects extraordinary care that exceeds the bounds of what is considered normative for others" (Schulz & Quittner, 1998, p. 107). The latter component of this definition is critical. When identifying a caregiver, one must be certain the care provided is different qualitatively and quantitatively from what is provided routinely/normatively within the context of a relationship (Gaugler, 2013). Other definitions of caregiving are more objective or discrete in nature. For example, caregiving is often operationalized as the provision of assistance with one or more ADLs, such as bathing, dressing, and transferring (Gaugler et al., 2002; Schulz & Quittner, 1998). In various disease contexts, ADL assistance often extends into symptom-specific domains such as the management of behavioral disruptions or memory loss, as seen in patients with Alzheimer's disease. If a more task-based definition of family caregiving is used, however, it is important to note the wide range of activities that can be considered "caregiving." In addition to providing in-person assistance in ADLs, family caregiving can include provision of skilled health care, such as injections or medication management; financial support (Gitlin & Schulz, 2012); monitoring of patients for safety; or long-distance assistance (e.g., coordination with healthcare providers).

A final issue to consider when defining caregiving is one of labeling. Much of the literature has adopted the term *informal* care to refer to the unpaid assistance that is often provided by family caregivers (*formal* refers to paid care). However, some advocacy organizations prefer not to use the term *informal* when describing family caregivers. This is understandable, because the term *informal* appears to refer not only to unpaid assistance but also to care that is not as complex as formal or paid care. As noted earlier and throughout the caregiving literature (Gitlin & Schulz, 2012), the assistance families provide is often multidimensional, complex, and long term in nature. In this regard, the term *informal care*, although used widely in epidemiological and health economics research, describes the multifaceted and complex tasks required of many family caregivers inadequately (Gaugler, 2013; Gaugler, Potter, & Pruinelli, 2014). Box 1.1 summarizes some of the recommendations scientists and others should consider when establishing criteria for who is or who is not a "caregiver."

WHO WITHIN THE FAMILY PROVIDES CARE?

Similar to caregiving definitions, there is a fair amount of heterogeneity in terms of who within the family actually provides care. According to a recent national survey, family caregivers are on average 48 years of age and are predominantly female (66%). The typical recipient of care is also female (62%) and averages 61 years of age (National Alliance for Caregiving and American Association of Retired Persons, 2009). Seventy-two percent of family caregivers in the United States are white, 13% are African American, 2% are Hispanic, and 2% are Asian American. Nearly all family caregivers live within close proximity to care recipients, with more than 90% living within 30 minutes from the care recipient. Seventy-eight percent of older adults and elders who require help receive it from family members only, with most care occurring in the caregiver's home

Box 1.1

KEY CONSIDERATIONS WHEN DEFINING FAMILY CAREGIVING
(GAUGLER, KANE, & KANE, 2002).

Considerations
1. **What "counts" as family caregiving?** The tasks that are considered caregiving should be described carefully when measuring the amount of family care.
2. **What characteristics of the care recipient are necessary?** Although disease-specific studies are usually clear on this issue (e.g., the care recipient must have a diagnosis of Alzheimer's disease), indicators of care-recipient need that qualify them as needing care are required.
3. **Care that is provided because of a health need should be differentiated from care that is provided because of a care recipient's disability and illness.** This becomes critical when determining the amount of family care for dimensions such as instrumental activities of daily living (e.g., shopping, transportation, arrangement of financial matters or appointments, housework, and so on).
4. **Duration of care, or when family caregiving help was provided because the care recipient needed it, is necessary.** See Gaugler (2010).

(National Alliance for Caregiving and American Association of Retired Persons, 2009; Wolff & Kasper, 2006).

An important issue in the study of family caregiving is the focus on the "primary caregiver." The primary caregiver is usually defined as the one person most responsible for the assistance provided to a care recipient. His or her importance derives from the fact that nearly all the existing research on family caregiving comes from samples of "primary caregivers," whose determination or identification often derives from self-identification. This practice has led to the findings of caregiving studies overrepresenting white and middle- to high-income individuals who are much more facile in identifying a primary caregiver. When caregivers from other economic strata or ethnically/racially diverse backgrounds are considered, this primary caregiving structure is not as readily apparent (Dilworth-Anderson, 2001; Dilworth-Anderson, Williams, & Copper, 1999). A second reason for the focus on primary caregivers is that it presents fewer complications during statistical analysis of data. Focusing on more complex family systems requires more advanced statistical techniques that extend beyond the expertise of many caregiving researchers (Gaugler et al., 2014).

WHAT DO FAMILY CAREGIVERS DO?

Individuals with chronic illnesses receive a range of assistance from family caregivers. A sizable proportion of chronically ill family members require assistance with ADLs (e.g., bathing, dressing, getting in and out of bed, ambulation, transferring). A little more than 20% of care recipients receive help with one to two ADLs whereas 10% need assistance with three to four ADLs. Approximately 15% of adults in the United States are receiving family help with five to six ADLs. The remaining adults receive help with instrumental ADLs (e.g., shopping, transportation, arranging appointments, housework)only. Even requiring help for one ADL can represent substantial caregiver burden. The 15% of individuals with considerable impairment (needing help with five to six ADLs) rely solely on relatives for this extensive care (Gaugler et al., 2014; National Alliance for Caregiving and American Association of Retired Persons, 2009).

Family caregivers provide an average of 20.4 hours a week of caregiving, and this hourly commitment often depends on the disease status of the care recipient. Caring for a person with more progressive, chronic diseases such as dementia can result in families providing even more frequent care (Fisher et al., 2011; Gaugler, 2013; Thies, Bleiler, & Alzheimer's Association, 2013).

Recent national data indicate that most family caregivers provide assistance to a single care recipient (roughly two thirds of all family caregivers). However, a little more than 20% are providing care to two care recipients and around 10% are providing care to three or more care recipients. Just as primary caregivers are overrepresented in caregiving research, family members providing care to multiple family members are rarely included in research studies. This again suggests that current caregiving literature might mask the reality of more complex caregiving relationships within certain families (Gaugler, 2013; Gaugler et al., 2014; National Alliance for Caregiving and American Association of Retired Persons, 2009).

The type of care families provide routinely extends well beyond ADLs to include communicating and negotiating with others regarding care decisions; providing socioemotional support and companionship; arranging and coordinating health care from primary or other care providers; conducting nursing-related tasks such as injections, wound care, and medication management; and making complex decisions (Gitlin & Schulz, 2012). The reader will glean from Chapters 2 through 9 that the specific disease context strongly influences the type of family care provided and, consequently, how it is measured. For example, family care for neurologically based chronic diseases may focus not only on the help provided for ADLs but also on assistance related to behavior or cognitive management. Alternatively, family care for cancer patients may focus on assisting the care recipient in managing the negative sequelae of chemotherapy, surgery, or disease recurrence.

DURATION OF FAMILY CAREGIVING

As reported in the 2009 National Alliance for Caregiving and American Association of Retired Persons national survey, 7 of 10 family caregivers were currently providing assistance, with 3 of 10 providing care during the past 12 months. Roughly one third (32%) had been providing care for less than a year. Another 34% had been providing assistance from between 1 year and 4 years, and 32% had been providing assistance for 5 years or more. It is important to note that such statistics do not take into account individuals who are entering and exiting family care responsibilities as a result of the healthcare needs of the care recipient (e.g., recurrent cancer) (Gaugler et al., 2014).

Although family caregiving can last for long periods of time, when does it begin? Family assistance is often provided before the formal diagnosis of a chronic disease or during the early emergence of disease symptoms. As a chronic disease progresses, family care becomes more intensive and focused on meeting the health needs of the care recipient (Gitlin & Schulz, 2012; Seltzer & Li, 1996). The transition to family caregiving onset may be almost imperceptible for some family members (Reinardy, Kane, Penrod, & Huck, 1999). Yet, how family caregivers initiate their caregiving responsibilities can have important implications for caregiving duration. For example, researchers have found that dementia caregivers who provided assistance before a diagnosis were more likely to delay institutionalization. Moreover, these "gradual" caregivers experienced less emotional distress than individuals who reported entering the caregiving role at the time of diagnosis (Gaugler, Zarit, & Pearlin, 2003). The current understanding of onset of the caregiving role is based on the assumption that family care continues until the caregiver "exits" her or his role (e.g., because of the death of the care recipient). However, caregiving can be episodic in chronic illnesses such as cancer and HIV/AIDS, when patients can experience cycles of remission and reemergence of symptoms. Few studies report whether family caregivers are currently in an initial or subsequent episode of care (Gaugler et al., 2002).

For examining key issues such a duration or onset of the caregiving role, longitudinal studies are critical. As a result of the varied trajectories of chronic illnesses, a host of health-related transitions are possible: discharge from hospital to home, fluctuating needs for assistance in instrumental ADLs and ADLs, multiple hospitalizations, and consideration of community-based or residential long-term care services (Gaugler, 2010; Gitlin & Schulz, 2012). The challenges and complications that emerge from these various transitions can influence how family caregivers adapt to the caregiving role. These demands can affect caregivers across multiple domains—emotional, psychological, social, physiological, as well as financial. Although caregiving in some chronic illnesses has been examined longitudinally (e.g., cancer and Alzheimer's disease), the dearth of prospective, long-term analyses of family care in most areas of chronic illness remains a glaring gap in the state of the science (Gaugler, 2010).

THEORIES OF CAREGIVING

In the previous sections of this chapter, we provided the reader with a generic description of various characteristics and situational factors that affect family members who care for individuals with chronic illness. We discussed definitions of caregiving and examined who within the family provides care, types of care, the length of time devoted to caring. A number of theoretical models have been generated by researchers that attempt to synthesize these factors. In a sense, these models try to impose structure on what often appears to be a swirl of factors and characteristics that influence the quality of life of caregivers and the individuals to whom they provide care. To the extent that these models explain the sources of caregiver stress and burden, how stress and burden are perceived by the caregiver, and how stress and burden affect their well-being, theoretical models can facilitate our efforts to develop interventions to improve caregivers' quality of life.

A sampling of the more prominent theoretical models is described next. These models differ primarily with regard to the perspective or context from which the caregiver–care-recipient dyad is viewed. Each theory examines the caregiving prism from a different facet of that prism (Clair & Allman, 2000). For example, social ecology theory (Kahana, Kahana, Johnson, Hammond, & Kercher, 1994) views the caregiving dyad from the various social contexts in which it operates. Dyad quality of life is the function of factors within family relationships, and the dyad relationship with other members of the community who provide different types of care (e.g., healthcare workers, neighbors). Life course theory (Marks & Lambert, 1997) focuses on a different facet of the caregiving prism. Here, caregiving is seen as a life course role that has discrete entry, exit, and transition points. This theory places emphasis on how caregivers' other life roles as well as their sociohistorical context (i.e., their cohort) influence the caregiving experience. Other theories emphasize the caregiver's sense of identity (Montgomery & Kwak, 2008), and the experience of loss (Hall & Buckwalter, 1987), whereas several theories have focused on the temporal nature of the illness, symptoms, and symptom management (Corbin, 1998; Henly, Kallas, Klatt, & Swenson, 2003; Verbrugge & Jette, 1994).

A conceptual model that has been used across many chronic illnesses to understand caregivers and to develop interventions to improve their quality of life is Pearlin's stress process model (Pearlin, Mullan, Semple, & Skaff, 1990) and more recently Susan Folkman's revised stress process model (Folkman, 2008). Pearlin's stress process model is derived from classic models of stress and coping (Lazarus & Folkman, 1984) to help describe how caregivers experience, appraise, and cope with care demands; and how this process can influence negative, global outcomes (Figure 1.1). The model first identifies primary stressors, which are defined as challenges or problems that are embedded in the caregiving situation and are a direct result of the care recipient's illness or disability. Primary objective stressors refer to care recipient functional and health status, such as type

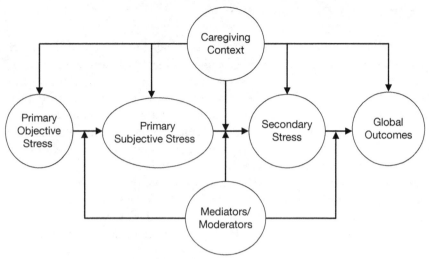

Figure 1.1 Pearlin's Stress Process Model.
SOURCE: Pearlin, L. I., Mullan, J. T., Semple, S. J., & Skaff, M. M. (1990). Caregiving and the stress process: An overview of concepts and their measures. *The Gerontologist, 30,* 583–594. New York: Oxford University Press. Reprinted with kind permission from Oxford University Press, USA.

and severity of the disease and behavioral disturbances. Caregivers' emotional reactions to these demands are primary subjective stressors. These stressors represent the degree to which caregivers perceive care demands as exhausting, confining, or distressing (Aneshensel, Pearlin, Mullan, Zarit, & Whitlatch, 1995; Pearlin et al., 1990). Stress in life domains outside the sphere of caregiving, such as work or family conflict, are considered secondary stressors.

The cumulative effects of these stressors are then postulated to influence family caregiver and care-recipient outcomes. Outcomes refer to indices of caregiver global health, e.g., aspects of psychological well-being such as depressive symptoms, subjective ratings of physical health, etc. The stress process model also includes resources that may potentially reduce stress. These resources include support provided to the family caregiver by other relatives, feelings of emotional connectedness with members in the social network, and coping strategies (Aneshensel et al., 1995). The mechanism underlying the stress process model is guided by the concept of "proliferation," or the spread of stress, strain, and conflict from the actual provision of care (primary stressors) to other life domains (secondary stressors). As caregiving stress proliferates, global outcomes are likely affected.

Folkman's revised stress process model (Folkman, 1997) places more emphasis on caregiver stress-coping mechanisms than Pearlin's original conceptualization. The revised model posits that individuals appraise their transactions with their environment constantly (Figure 1.2). Transactions that are appraised as stressful (e.g., patient behavioral disturbances, concurrent job or family responsibilities) require coping to regulate distress. Coping responses can be adaptive

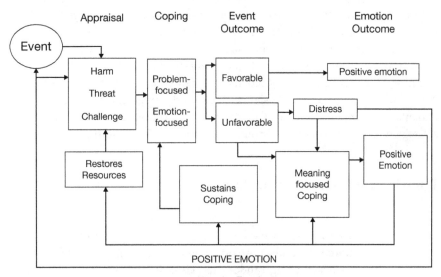

Figure 1.2 Folkman's Revised Stress Process Model.
SOURCE: Folkman, S. (2008). The case for positive emotions in the stress process. *Anxiety Stress Coping, 21*(1), 3–14. Reprinted with kind permission from Taylor & Francis Ltd, http://www.tandfonline.com.

(e.g., problem-focused coping) or nonadaptive (e.g., avoidance coping). Coping processes lead to an event outcome (e.g., favorable resolution, unfavorable resolution, or no resolution). Emotion is generated through the process of appraisal, coping, and event outcomes. A favorable outcome is likely to lead to positive emotions during the caregiving experience. Unsatisfactory outcomes (e.g., an unfavorable or no resolution) lead to additional distress and, ideally, additional coping. Significantly, Folkman incorporated into the model meaning-based coping (e.g., positive reappraisal, spiritual beliefs, and caregivers' perceptions of positive aspects of caregiving) as mediators of the impact of negative event outcomes.

Meaning-based coping strategies have accumulated a good deal of empirical support and have been incorporated into many caregiver support interventions. An entire issue of *Aging and Mental Health* was dedicated to a single meaning-based coping mechanism: caregivers' perception of positive aspects of caregiving (PAC) (Zarit, 2012). PAC is typically defined as the rewards and satisfaction derived from the caregiving relationship. In one study researchers asked dementia caregivers if they could identify and describe at least one positive aspect of their caregiving relationship (Cohen, Colantonio, & Vernich, 2002). Results showed that 73% of the caregivers could identify at least one PAC, mentioning a range of positive experiences from feeling fulfilled, important, and responsible; to finding a sense of companionship and meaning within the relationship. Moreover, levels of depression, burden, and even subjective health were significantly lower in individuals high in PAC.

Intervention researchers have begun to harness meaning-based coping strategies such as PAC and benefit finding, and are combining them with more traditional treatment components such as problem solving. There are published reports of successful use of interventions that combine traditional and meaning-based treatment components with dementia caregivers (Hebert et al., 2003; Judge, Yarry, & Orsulic-Jeras, 2014) and caregivers of palliative care patients (Allen et al., 2014; see Chapter 6 in this volume). Applications of this strategy to caregivers of other chronic conditions are forthcoming.

THE CHRONIC CARE MODEL: A GUIDE FOR THE FUTURE?

The aforementioned theories have helped researchers understand the caregiving experience more fully and to provide guidance in developing interventions tested for initial efficacy using randomized clinical trials or other traditional experimental designs. As we discuss in greater detail in our concluding chapter, very few of these evidence-based caregiver intervention programs have been implemented in the "real world" (Maslow, 2012). Although not a caregiving model per se, it is our belief that Wagner's chronic care model (CCM) offers much potential for developing caregiver interventions that are both feasible and sustainable in real-world settings (Bodenheimer, Wagner, & Grumbach, 2002; Wagner, 1998). The CCM is an integrative approach to care delivery developed to provide optimal care for adults with chronic conditions (Robert Wood Johnson Foundation, 2006). The model focuses on producing effective behavior change across all aspects of care delivery, along with coordination from within and outside the healthcare system.

As shown in Figure 1.3, the CCM includes six areas of health care that can serve as targets of chronic care improvement efforts. The first four areas are considered practice strategies and include *organizational support* (system leadership and practice culture; ideally, appropriate management of chronic disease and quality improvement in chronic disease practice is emphasized by committed leadership), *clinical information systems* (the provision of relevant health information about individual patients and patient populations that can also yield tailored recommendations and care plans), *delivery system design* (team-based care approaches, innovative delivery approaches including group visits), and *decision support* (increasing access of healthcare providers to evidence-based guidelines and specialists to guide service delivery). The final two components of the CCM are person centered. *Self-management support* involves interventions that empower patients, when possible, and their caregivers to manage their own care plan in partnership with the care team. The care plans (interventions) focus on problem solving, decision making, and enhancing resource use. The sixth area of care focuses on *community resources*, such as enhancing connections with community-based care providers.

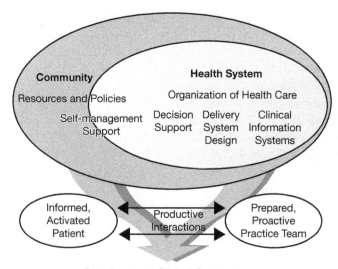

Functional and Clinical Outcomes

Figure 1.3 The Chronic Care Model.
SOURCE: Wagner, E. H. (1998). Chronic disease management: What will it take to improve care for chronic illness? *Effective Clinical Practice*, 1, 1–4. Reproduced with permission of American College of Physicians.

CONCLUSION

As a result of advances in medical science and demographic trends, the number of individuals with chronic illness is increasing rapidly. Each chronic illness presents family caregivers with a unique set of challenges. In this chapter we provided generic characteristics of caregivers. The chapters that follow characterize the needs of individuals with different chronic illnesses, as well as the challenges faced by their caregivers. Most important, subsequent chapters discuss an array of evidence-based interventions developed to reduce caregiver stress and burden, and to help caregivers become more effective in their role.

Many of the interventions discussed in the following chapters are at the stage of establishing initial efficacy of the treatment package. Very few were developed through partnerships with critical stakeholders such as caregivers, care recipients, social workers, nurses and primary care physicians, community health organizations, and/or healthcare systems. Input from these stakeholders on acceptability and feasibility of caregiver interventions is necessary for implementation and dissemination in real-world settings (Wethington & Burgio, 2015). Without this integration of effort across the process of care delivery for patients with chronic illness and their caregivers, efforts to develop caregiver interventions will remain in the domain of experimental trials and will stay within the pages of academic journals describing these trials.

In the chapters that follow the reader will find discussions of a myriad of issues affecting caregiving, specialized terminology, and over 200 interventions developed to assist caregivers helping individuals with a number of prevalent, costly chronic conditions. To assist the reader in a search of more information on any of these topics we have included a section at the end of the text titled "Additional Resources on Caregiving and Interventions." The section is divided into five subsections: (a) general caregiving, (b) selected disease-specific resources for caregivers, (c) tools for translation and intervention research, and (d) caregiving and intervention-focused glossaries of terms. Each subsection contains links to several websites where additional information can be located easily.

REFERENCES

Allen, R. S., Harris, G. M., Burgio, L. D., Azuero, C. B., Miller, L. A., Shin, H. J., Eichorst, M. K., Csikai, E. L., DeCoster, J., Dunn, L. L., Kvale, E., & Parmelee, P. (2014). Can senior volunteers deliver reminiscence and creative activity interventions? Results of the Legacy Intervention Family Enactment randomized controlled trial. *Journal of Pain and Symptom Management, 48*(4), 590–601.

Aneshensel, C. S., Pearlin, L. I., Mullan, J. T., Zarit, S. H., & Whitlatch, C. J. (1995). *Profiles in caregiving: The unexpected career.* San Diego: Academic Press.

Bodenheimer, T. S., Wagner, E. H., & Grumbach, K. (2002). Improving primary care for patients with chronic illness: The chronic care model, part 2. *Journal of the American Medical Association, 288*(15), 1775–1779.

Clair, J., & Allman, R. (Eds.). (2000). *The gerontological prism: Developing interdisciplinary research and priorities.* Society in aging series. Amityville, NY: Baywood Publishing.

Cohen, C. A., Colantonio, A., & Vernich, L. (2002). Positive aspects of caregiving: Rounding out the caregiver experience. *International Journal of Geriatric Psychiatry, 17*, 184–188.

Corbin, J. M. (1998). The Corbin and Strauss chronic illness trajectory model: An update. *Scholarly Inquiry for Nursing Practice, 12*(1), 33–41.

Dilworth-Anderson, P. (2001). Family issues and the care of persons with Alzheimer's disease. *Aging & Mental Health, 5*(S1), S49–S51.

Dilworth-Anderson, P., Williams, S. W., & Copper, T. (1999). Family caregiving to elderly African-Americans: Caregiver types and structures. *Journal of Gerontology: Social Sciences, 54*(4), S237–S241.

Federal Interagency Forum on Aging-Related Statistics. (2012). *Older Americans 2012: Key Indicators of Well-being.* Washington, DC: U.S. Government Printing Office. Also, [Online]. Available: http://www.agingstats.gov.

Fisher, G. G., Franks, M. M., Plassman, B. L., Brown, S. L., Potter, G. G., Llewellyn, D., Rogers, M. A., & Langa, K. M. (2011). Caring for individuals with dementia and cognitive impairment, not dementia: Findings from the Aging, Demographics, and Memory Study. *Journal of the American Geriatrics Society, 59*(3), 488–494.

Folkman, S. (2008). The case for positive emotions in the stress process. *Anxiety Stress Coping, 21*(1), 3–14.

Gaugler, J. E. (2010). The longitudinal ramifications of stroke caregiving: A systematic review. *Rehabilitation Psychology, 55*(2), 108–125.

Gaugler, J. E. (2013). *Informal care supports: The basics* [Online]. Available: https://
netfiles.umn.edu/sph/hpm/Magec/GEM%20Modules/Gaugler%20Informal%20
Care%20Support%20Basics/Gaugler%20Basics%20module%207.htm.

Gaugler, J. E., Kane, R. L., & Kane, R. A. (2002). Family care for older adults with disabilities: Toward more targeted and interpretable research. *International Journal of
Aging & Human Development, 54*(3), 205–231.

Gaugler, J. E., Potter, T., & Pruinelli, L. (2014). Partnering with caregivers. *Clinics in
Geriatric Medicine, 30*(3), 493–515.

Gaugler, J. E., Zarit, S. H., & Pearlin, L. I. (2003). The onset of dementia caregiving and
its longitudinal implications. *Psychology and Aging, 18*, 171–180.

Gitlin, L. N., & Schulz, R. (2012). Family caregiving of older adults. In T. R. Prohaska,
L. A. Anderson & R. H. Binsotck (Eds.), *Public health for an aging society.*
(pp. 181–204). Baltimore, MD: The Johns Hopkins University Press. Also [Online].

Hall, G. R., & Buckwalter, K. C. (1987). Progressively lowered stress threshold: A conceptual model for care of adults with Alzheimer's disease. *Archives of Psychiatric
Nursing, 1*(6), 399–406.

Hebert, R., Levesque, L., Vezina, J., Lavoie, J., Ducharme, F., Gendron, C., Preville,
M., Voyer, L., & Dubois, M. (2003). Efficacy of a psychoeducative group program
for caregivers of demented persons living at home: A Randomized controlled trial.
Journal of Gerontology Series B: Social Sciences, 58(1), S58–S67.

Henly, S. J., Kallas, K. D., Klatt, C. M., & Swenson, K. K. (2003). The notion of time in
symptom experiences. *Nursing Research, 52*(6), 410–417.

Judge, K. S., Yarry, S. J., & Orsulic-Jeras, S. (2014). Acceptability and feasibility results
of a strength-based skills training program for dementia caregiving dyads. *The
Gerontologist, 50*(3), 408–417.

Kahana, E., Kahana, B., Johnson, J. R., Hammond, R. J., & Kercher, K. (1994).
Developmental challenges and family caregiving. In E. Kahana, D. E. Biegel & M.
L. Wykle (Eds.), *Family caregiving across the lifespan* (pp. 3–41). Thousand Oaks,
CA: Sage Publications.

Lazarus, R. S., & Folkman, S. (1984). *Stress, appraisal, and coping.* New York: Springer.

Marks, N. F., & Lambert, J. D. (1997). *Family caregiving: Contemporary trends and issues.*
No. NSFH working paper no. 78. Madison, WI: University of Wisconsin-Madison,
Child of Family Studies.

Maslow, K. (2012). *Translating innovation to impact: Evidence-based interventions
to support people with Alzheimer's disease and their caregivers at home and in the
community.* Washington, D.C.: Administration on Aging.

Montgomery, R., & Kwak, J. (2008). TCARE: Tailored caregiver assessment and referral. *The American Journal of Nursing, 108*(9 Suppl), 54–57; quiz 57.

National Alliance for Caregiving and American Association of Retired Persons. (2009).
Caregiving in the U.S. Bethesda, MD: National Alliance of Caregiving.

National Association of Chronic Disease. (2011). *Chronic disease prevention and control: A wise investment [Online].* National Association of Chronic Disease Directors.
Available: http://c.ymcdn.com/sites/www.chronicdisease.org/resource/resmgr/
white_papers/a_wise_investment_2011.pdf.

Pearlin, L. I., Mullan, J. T., Semple, S. J., & Skaff, M. M. (1990). Caregiving and the
stress process: An overview of concepts and their measures. *The Gerontologist, 30*,
583–594.

Piette, J. D., Rosland, A. M., Silveira, M., Kabeto, M., & Langa, K. M. (2010). Chronic illness. *Support of Older Adults with Chronic Illness, 6*(1), 34–45.

Reinardy J., Kane, R. A., Penrod, J. D., & Huck, S. (1999). After the hospitalization is over: A different perspective on family care. *Journal of Gerontological Social Work, 31*(1–2), 119–141.

Robert Wood Johnson Foundation. (2006). *Improving chronic illness care* [Online]. Available: http://www.improvingchroniccare.org/index.php?p=Model_Elements&s=18.

Rosland, A. M., & Piette, J. D. (2010). Emerging models for mobilizing family support for chronic disease management: A structured review. *Chronic Illness, 6*(1), 7–21.

Schulz, R., & Quittner, A. L. (1998). Caregiving for children and adults with chronic conditions: Introduction to the special issue. *Health Psychology, 17*(2), 107–111.

Seltzer, M. M., & Li, L. W. (1996). The transitions of caregiving: Subjective and objective definitions. *The Gerontologist, 36*(5), 614–626.

Thies, W., Bleiler, L., & Alzheimer's Association. (2013). 2013 Alzheimer's disease facts and figures. *Alzheimer's & Dementia: The Journal of the Alzheimer's Association, 9*(2), 208–245.

Verbrugge, L. M., & Jette, A. M. (1994). The disablement process. *Social Science & Medicine, 38*(1), 1–14.

Wagner, E. H. (1998). Chronic disease management: What will it take to improve care for chronic illness? *Effective Clinical Practice, 1*, 1–4.

Wethington, E., & Burgio, L. D. (2015). Translational research on caregiving: Missing links in the translation process. In J. E. Gaugler & R. L. Kane (Eds.), *Family caregiving in the new normal* (pp. 193–210). San Diego, CA: Academic press.

Wolff, J. L., & Kasper, J. D. (2006). Caregivers of frail elders: Updating a national profile. *The Gerontologist. 46*(3), 344–356.

Zarit, S. H. (2012). Positive aspects of caregiving: More than looking on the bright side. *Aging & Mental Health, 16*(6), 673–674.

2

Caregiving for Individuals with Alzheimer's Disease and Related Disorders

JOSEPH E. GAUGLER AND LOUIS D. BURGIO ■

Alzheimer's disease (AD) is a progressive, and ultimately fatal, neurological disorder. Alzheimer's disease impairs an individual's cognition and other mental abilities to the extent that one's capacity to carry out basic activities of daily living (ADLs) is threatened. As highlighted in the 2014 *Alzheimer's Disease Facts and Figures* report (Alzheimer's Association, 2014):

- Alzheimer's disease is the most common cause of dementia, or, an "overall term for diseases and conditions characterized by a decline in memory or other thinking skills that affects a person's ability to perform everyday activities."
- Although there are multiple types of dementia that include different pathological processes, the accumulation of beta-amyloid plaques and neurofibrillary tangles that are the classic hallmarks of AD represent the most common type of dementia, accounting for 60% to 80% of all cases.
- AD is currently the sixth leading cause of death in the United States, and is the fifth leading cause for persons 65 years of age or older in the United States.
- AD has contributed more to poor health and disability than other chronic diseases during the past decade, and total healthcare costs for people with AD are three times greater than those without AD who are older than the age of 65.
- In instances of co-occurring chronic conditions (or, when an individual has more than one chronic disease), the presence of AD or a related dementia (ADRD) appears to increase costs significantly among those

with co-occurring chronic conditions who are already extensive users of healthcare services.

The costs and challenges of ADRD extend well beyond the individuals who have these disorders. In 2013 there were more than 15 million unpaid people who provided 17.7 billion hours of care to persons with AD. Most of these individuals (85%) in the United States are family members; (Alzheimer's Association, 2014; Gitlin & Schulz, 2012). Health economists in the United States often "value" family caregiving by estimating the costs to society of replacing available family caregivers with home healthcare aides or similar professional care providers; this led to a value of AD family care of $220 billion in 2013 (Alzheimer's Association, 2014). To place such a value in perspective, if the 2013 value of AD family caregiving was considered revenue, AD family caregiving would have been a top-five Fortune 500 company in 2013 (Fortune, 2013).

Although the public health importance of AD caregiving is significant simply because of its prevalence, the challenges of providing family care to a person with AD are substantial. In this chapter, we provide an overview of the various emotional, psychological, and health-related challenges for family caregivers, and then synthesize available research on programs that support family caregivers of persons with AD (often called *interventions*) with the objective of highlighting the various types of interventions that have been tested. We then conclude with a summary of efforts to implement, or translate, these interventions into various community settings along with a consideration of the successes and challenges of such efforts. When compared with other disease contexts, the volume of descriptive and intervention research on family caregiving for persons with AD is more extensive, and a number of systematic literature reviews and meta-analyses on intervention efficacy have already been conducted (see the next section and Table 2.1). This chapter thus focuses on synthesizing these existing efforts to summarize the literature on efficacy and effectiveness of AD caregiving interventions, and then to explore the link between promising evidence-based AD caregiver interventions and their associated translational efforts in various community and clinical contexts.

THE PUBLIC HEALTH RAMIFICATIONS OF AD

Much of the following information is based on the extensive data provided in The Alzheimer's Association 2014 *Alzheimer's Disease Facts and Figures* report (Dr. Gaugler is a contributor to this annual report); interested readers are urged to review this compendium for more in-depth information regarding the burden AD poses to U.S. citizens and the healthcare system. In 2014, 5.2 million persons in the United States had AD (Alzheimer's Association, 2014). Most (5 million) were 65 years of age and older. Because they live longer and age is a principal risk factor of AD, two thirds of women have AD. Although the degree of difference varies across reports, it appears that older blacks and Hispanics are more likely than older whites to have AD, although there are more white persons overall currently living with AD in the United States. Some studies suggest that blacks are more than twice as likely to have AD; Hispanics are 1.5 times as likely to have AD (Alzheimer's Association, 2014). Duration of AD, or at least duration of time lived with an AD diagnosis (this is an important qualification; many people may have or exhibit AD symptomatology but do not receive a formal diagnosis until later in the disease trajectory) is approximately 4 to 8 years on average, with some individuals living with AD as long as two decades. Persons with AD spend most of their time with this disease in the later, more severe stages.

The disability of AD, which comes in the form of impaired cognition, impaired functional dependence, and exacerbated behavioral and psychiatric challenges, has grown more significantly when compared with other chronic diseases in the United States. Cost analyses further suggest that AD is associated with considerably greater healthcare use, including hospital costs, medical services, and long-term care (Alzheimer's Association, 2014). Taken together, these results emphasize that AD poses a significant threat to the public health of the United States, and with the aging of the U.S. population, the burden of AD is likely to increase significantly absent therapies that can prevent or delay significantly the insidious progression of this disease (which do not exist at present).

THE ALZHEIMER'S DISEASE CAREGIVING ROLE

The demographic profile of caregivers of persons with ADRD in the United States is as follows. Close to two thirds of all ADRD caregivers in the United States are women, and more than one third are older than 65 years of age (Alzheimer's Association, 2014; Bouldin & Andresen, 2010; Kasper, Freedman, & Spillman, 2014). Another two thirds of caregivers are either married or in a long-term/committed relationship (Alzheimer's Association, 2014; Kasper et al., 2014). Approximately two thirds of ADRD caregivers are white, 10% are black, 8% are Hispanic, and 5% are Asian (Alzheimer's Association, 2014; Kasper et al., 2014). Less than half of ADRD caregivers have a college degree or greater education (40%) (Alzheimer's Association, 2014; Kasper et al., 2014). Similarly, 41% of ADRD caregivers report an annual household income of more than $50,000 per year (Alzheimer's Association, 2014). The majority (55%) of family caregivers live with persons with ADRD who also consider themselves the "primary" caregiver, or person most responsible in providing help to the relative with ADRD (Fisher et al., 2011). Family caregivers tend to live with the person with ADRD or live within 20 minutes traveling distance (27% and 46%, respectively [Alzheimer's Association, 2014]).

There are important racial and cultural variations regarding how family care for persons with ADRD is delivered. More than half of white caregivers

Table 2.1. SYNTHESIS OF FAMILY CAREGIVER INTERVENTIONS FOR PERSONS WITH ALZHEIMER'S DISEASE OR RELATED DEMENTIAS

Author (Year)	Sample (Baseline)[a]	Racial/Cultural Factors			Design	Interventions	Results	Evaluation
		Diversity of Study Sample	Cultural Diversity Training Received?	Comparisons of Racial/Cultural Factors				
SYSTEMATIC REVIEWS AND META-ANALYSES								
Acton and Kang (2001)	24 studies, N = 1,254	NR	NR	NR	RCTs, controlled, pretest/ posttest design, meta-analysis	• Support group • Education • Psychoeducation • Counseling • Respite • Multicomponent	Only multicomponent interventions reduced burden significantly ($n = 3$, $d = 0.46$).	Because of its imprecise content, burden may be difficult to modify via CG intervention; more specific measures are needed.
Boots et al. (2014)	12 studies, N = 1,458	NR	NR	NR	RCT, controlled, mixed methods, formative evaluation, systematic review	• Internet-based interventions	Six of 12 interventions appeared to influence caregiver well-being positively, particularly if they were multicomponent and tailored.	Intervention design and quality was diverse. More RCTs are needed.
Brodaty et al. (2003)	30 studies, N = 2,040	NR	NR	NR	RCTs, controlled studies, meta-analysis	• Counseling • Education • Family counseling/extended family involvement • Patient involvement • Support group/program • Stress management/training	Overall, psychosocial interventions improved psychological morbidity modestly but significantly (weighted average effect size, .31), but not CG burden. Small but significant effects were found for CG knowledge and CR mood (.68 and .51, respectively); four of seven studies delayed CR institutionalization.	There was significant heterogeneity in reported empirical effects. Involvement of CG and CG in intervention, ongoing provision of support, a combination of interventions, and flexibility/tailoring of intervention content seemed linked to delayed CR institutionalization along with other CG outcomes.

Brodaty, et al. (2012)	23 studies,	N = 3,279	NR	NR	NR	RCTs, controlled studies, meta-analysis	• Skills training • Education • Activity planning/environmental redesign • Enhancing support • Self-care techniques • Multicomponent • Other	Nonpharmacological CG interventions were associated with modestly reduced CR symptom outcomes (SMD = .34) and CG reactions to dementia symptoms (SMD = .15). No adverse effects were reported.	Multicomponent CG interventions appeared to reduce CR behavioral and psychiatric symptoms and how CG's manage these issues significantly.
Cooke, et al. (2001)	40 studies,	N = 7,353	NR	NR	NR	RCTs, controlled studies, pretest/ posttest, systematic review	• Social skills training • Social support • Social activities • Cognitive problem solving • Cognitive therapy • Cognitive skills • Practical caregiving skills • Record keeping • Relaxation • Psychotherapy and counseling • Respite • Other	Two thirds of the studies included showed no improvement in any outcomes. Interventions that included social support (n = 15 interventions) and problem solving (n = 21 controlled studies) were more effective.	Interventions with social components appeared more effective in improving psychological well-being for dementia CGs. The review was hindered by heterogeneous study design and outcome measurement quality.
Cooper et al. (2007)	24 studies,	N = 1,558	NR	NR	NR	RCTs, controlled, systematic review	• Group CBT • BMT • IT • Exercise therapy • Additional support • Respite • Relaxation and yoga • Individual CBT • Group psychotherapy • Full-time care for CG	One of three group CBTs showed reduction in anxiety. BMT, IT, exercise, respite, and additional support did not show efficacy for CG anxiety.	Interventions considered were not effective in reducing anxiety in CGs, with the exception of only one evaluation of CBT.
Corbett et al. (2012)	13 studies		NR	NR	NR	RCTs, meta-analysis	• Information provision	Meta-analyses indicated that two of three studies showed an effect on quality of life, five of six studies showed effects on neuropsychiatric symptoms (WMD = 1.48), and no effect on burden was noted in three studies.	Interpretation was difficult because many interventions provided more than information. The evidence supports information and advice as part of a multicomponent intervention strategy.

(continued)

Table 2.1. CONTINUED

Author (Year)	Sample (Baseline)[a]	Racial/Cultural Factors			Design	Interventions	Results	Evaluation
		Diversity of Study Sample	Cultural Diversity Training Received?	Comparisons of Racial/Cultural Factors				
Egan et al. (2010)	13 studies, $N = 315$	NR	NR	NR	RCT, controlled, pretest/ posttest, cohort, single subject, systematic review	Interventions to improve communication between CGs (formal and informal) and CRs: • Memory books • Training programs • Activity	Memory aids ($n = 8$) appeared to improve CRs focused communication with CGs in some studies. Other intervention approaches yielded mixed results.	The lack of high-quality research featured in this review greatly complicates any conclusions or inferences of efficacy or lack of effect.
Elvish, et al. (2013)	20 studies, $N = 4616$[b]	NR	NR	NR	RCTs, two qualitative studies, systematic review	• Psychoeducation • Psychotherapy/counseling • Multicomponent • Technology based	Psychoeducation can influence CG well-being (seven of eight studies). Multicomponent interventions show not only maintenance but also improvement in outcomes ($n = 6$).	Interventions that combine individual and group components are most effective. Tailored interventions for individuals or group-based interventions focused on a single issue also appear most effective.
Flint (1995)	4 studies, $N = 762$	NR	NR	NR	Controlled, systematic review	• Overnight, institutional, in-home respite • Adult day services	Respite had no effect on CG stress, and psychological or physical health, or CR institutionalization.	The small number of studies included and their lack of rigor make any conclusion related to lack of efficacy tentative at best.

Author (year)	Sample			Design	Interventions	Findings	Conclusions
Gitlin and Hodgson (2015)	24 reviews (7 meta-analyses), 15 studies, N = 1,879	NR	NR	NR	RCTs, controlled, systematic review	• Professional support • Psychoeducation • Behavior management/skills training • Counseling/psychotherapy • Self-care/relaxation training • Multicomponent	Multicomponent interventions had the largest effects on burden. Psychoeducation was most likely to improve knowledge; relaxation training showed the largest benefit for anxiety. Multicomponent interventions had the largest effects on CR institutionalization.	Sufficient evidence exists for CG intervention efficacy. Interventions are of low risk and tend to target CGs of CRs in moderate or late stages of dementia. Extending the conceptual focus beyond the stress process is needed. Intervention characteristics and mechanisms need to be specified; measurement and scalability are additional concerns.
Godwin et al. (2013)	8 studies representing 4 interventions, N = 772	NR	NR	NR	RCTs, systematic review	• Technology-driven interventions that used the computer • Internet-based technology-driven interventions • Excluded: decision aids, telephone only, videotape only, or CD interventions	Each study reported positive findings; four studies reported reductions in depression and two reported reductions in anxiety.	Overall, the evidence base is emerging and inconclusive. There is considerable diversity in study design and measurement.
Goy et al. (2010)	30 studies, N = 13,458[b]	Subgroup effects noted	NR	NR	RCTs, systematic review	• Multicomponent • Exercise training • Case management interventions • Behavior management training • Individual skills training • Group skills training • Individual group and combined individual/group support CG counseling	Multicomponent interventions were included that were tailored individually for reducing depression and burden, and for enhancing well-being and confidence (n = 5). Case management had some effect on CG outcomes (n = 5). Behavior management training, individual skills training, and group skills training effects were inconsistent (n = 22). Combined counseling interventions were clearly effective in reducing depression, improving mood, and delaying CR institutionalization (n = 7).	Multicomponent and combined interventions that were provided over time and tailored appeared most effective.

(continued)

Table 2.1. CONTINUED

| Author (Year) | Sample (Baseline)[a] | Racial/Cultural Factors | | | Design | Interventions | Results | Evaluation |
		Diversity of Study Sample	Cultural Diversity Training Received?	Comparisons of Racial/ Cultural Factors				
Griffin et al. (2013)	29 studies, $N = 4,631$	19% of participant were not white	NR	NR	RCTs, systematic review	• Training to manage CR behaviors • Support or counseling and training to manage symptoms/behaviors of CR • Unique interventions	Few studies reported statistically significant effects on CR outcomes. Suggestive findings indicated that targeted interventions were more effective than general ones; 5 of 11 showed significant improvement in symptom control.	Targeted family interventions were most effective. It is not clear whether reducing CG stress can improve CR outcomes. Study quality must be improved.
Jensen et al. (2015)	7 studies, $N = 764$	NR (samples' country of origin identified)	NR	NR	RCTs, meta-analysis	• Educational programs/ psychoeducation	Moderate effect on burden ($n = 5$; SMD $= -.52$), small effect on depression ($n = 2$; SMD $= -.37$), and no effect on transitions to residential long-term care for CRs were noted.	The effects of educational programs were moderate to small. Longer follow-up to determine effects on CR long-term measurement as well as standardized measurement will advance the field.
Jones et al. (2012)	12 studies	NR	NR	NR	RCTs, controlled studies, other; systematic review	• Intervention studies with costs reported for outcomes (pharmacological, psychosocial, services)	Four of 12 studies reported significant differences in CG outcomes (burden, competence, coping, and knowledge). One of three studies found that CG intervention was less costly than the control.	Few studies provided sufficient detail on costs. Joint collection of CG and CR data are needed to examine cost effectiveness of interventions.

Knight et al. (1993)	20 studies, N = 1138	NR	NR	NR	Controlled studies, meta-analysis	• Psychosocial intervention • Respite/care planning	Moderately strong effects were noted for individual psychosocial interventions and for respite care when the treatment group received more respite than the control (d = .63 for three studies with control groups). Group psychosocial interventions showed small, positive effects on caregiver distress (p. 243).	Reports of ineffectiveness of CG interventions at the time were exaggerated. There is a need to determine which interventions work best and the mechanisms of effect.
Lingler et al. (2005)	17 studies, N = 3,002	NR	NR	NR	RCTs, meta-analysis	• Studies of cholinesterase inhibitors or N-methyl-D-aspartate receptor modulator drugs	There was a small, statistically significant reduction in burden (d = .18) and CG time (d = .15) among CGs whose CRs received cholinesterase inhibitors. Heterogeneity was not significant.	Cholinesterase inhibitor effects were small but beneficial for CGs.
Llanque and Enriquez (2012)	10 studies, N = 1,881[b]	Yes; all interventions included a Latino sample	Yes	Yes	RCTs, pretest/posttest, systematic review	• Multicomponent • Coping • Psychoeducation • Computer and telephone support • Family therapy • Community collaboration	Empirical results were not synthesized. Various interventions appeared to reduce CG depression and similar outcomes.	A greater focus on rural Latinos and Latinos from different countries of origin, and use of participatory approaches considering acculturation, are areas that require greater attention in future research.

(continued)

Table 2.1. Continued

Author (Year)	Sample (Baseline)[a]	Racial/Cultural Factors			Design	Interventions	Results	Evaluation
		Diversity of Study Sample	Cultural Diversity Training Received?	Comparisons of Racial/ Cultural Factors				
Maayan et al. (2012)	4 studies, $N = 753$	One study included AI/ AN sample	NR	NR	RCTs, meta-analysis	• Respite	No significant effect of respite on any CG outcome was noted.	Evidence quality was low. No benefits or adverse effects of respite for CGs were demonstrated. Well-designed trials are needed to obtain more valid conclusions.
Martin-Carrasco et al. (2014)	35 studies, $N = 3,729$[b]	NR	NR	NR	RCTs, systematic review	• Nonprofessional support/ support groups • Counseling • Psychoeducation	A total of 51.4% of studies reported benefits for at least depression, anxiety, or burden. Psychoeducational interventions appeared most consistent in their effects.	Concerns remain regarding methodological quality of CG interventions, although evidence suggests they are appropriate for reducing negative CG outcomes.
Mason et al. (2007)	22 studies, $N = 1,593$ CGs of CRs with dementia	NR	NR	NR	RCTs, controlled, systematic review	• Adult day services • Host family • In-home respite • Institutional respite • Video respite	Respite does not influence institutionalization nor adversely affect CRs. Effects on CGs and CRs were generally small; better controlled studies found modest benefits in some subgroups. CG satisfaction was high. Respite was associated with greater costs and either no or slight benefit.	Respite may have a small effect on CGs' burden and mental health. A greater understanding of the process of respite and objectives, improved measurement, and adequate samples are needed via rigorous trials.

McKechnie et al. (2014)	14 studies, $N = 1{,}165$	NR	NR	NR	RCT, controlled, single-group pretest/posttest, systematic review	• Computer-mediated interventions (DVD, CD-ROM, Internet, or computer delivered) that offered therapy, professional/peer support, or education/information • Excluded: telephone-only CG interventions	Medium to higher quality interventions were associated with reductions in burden ($n = 5$) and depression ($n = 4$). Two studies that were also high quality were associated with reduced anxiety. Positive CG outcomes were also increased. Effects on social support were mixed, and there was no effect on the physical aspects of care provision.	Computer-mediated interventions appear to offer a wide range of positive, albeit mixed, benefits. Methodological quality was mixed.
Napoles et al. (2010)	18 studies, $N = 4{,}142^{b}$	Yes	Yes: interventions including African Americans ($n = 10$), Latinos ($n = 11$), and Chinese Americans ($n = 1$)	RCTs, pretest/posttest, meta-analyses, systematic review	• Multicomponent • Skills training • Telephone support • Ecosystems therapy • Psychoeducation • Behavioral management • Cognitive behavioral therapy • Home occupational therapy/skill visits • Yoga/meditation	Only 11 of 18 studies addressed cultural tailoring, such as familism, language, bilingual/bicultural staff, and literacy.	Most interventions were associated with one multisite trial (REACH). More research is needed.
Olazarán et al. (2010)	3 studies	NR	NR	3 RCTs, systematic review	• Multicomponent interventions	Multicomponent interventions were associated with a lower likelihood of CR institutionalization (relative risk, .67).	Multicomponent interventions that offered education and support delayed CR institutionalization, with comparatively fewer resources used.

(continued)

Table 2.1. CONTINUED

| Author (Year) | Sample (Baseline)[a] | Racial/Cultural Factors | | | Design | Interventions | Results | Evaluation |
		Diversity of Study Sample	Cultural Diversity Training Received?	Comparisons of Racial/ Cultural Factors				
Orgeta and Miranda-Castillo (2014)	4 studies	NR	NR	NR	RCTs, systematic review	• Home-based supervised aerobic exercise or endurance training of low/moderate intensity	Two of four RCTs demonstrated reduced CG burden (SMD = −.43).	Higher quality trials are needed. No adverse effects of exercise were noted. Future interventions that can identify type, duration, and intensity of exercise that is most effective for particular CGs is needed.
Parker et al. (2008)	40 studies	NR	NR	NR	34 RCTs, 6 meta-analyses/ reviews, meta-analysis	• Psychoeducational • Support • Multicomponent • Other	Psychoeducation interventions showed small but significant effects on depression (n = 4; WMD = −1.93) and subjective well-being (n = 5; SMD = −.16). Support showed small, significant effect on burden (n = 2; SMD = −.41). Ten of 12 multicomponent interventions showed positive effects, but meta-analysis was not possible.	Involving both the CG and the CR is important. Active participation in educational interventions is ideal; individualized, ongoing support is optimal.
Peacock and Forbes (2003)	36 studies, N = 19,303[b]	NR	NR	NR	RCTs, controlled studies, pretest/ posttest, systematic review	• Education • Case management • Psychotherapy • Computer networking	Few significant effects found. Case management increased support service use (n = 4); education decreased depression (n = 4). Psychotherapy/ multicomponent delayed CR institutionalization (n = 2). Computer networking improved decision making (n = 1).	Positive findings appeared to have clinical significance. More controlled designs are needed. Individualized interventions appeared most successful.

Study	Sample				Design	Interventions	Findings	Conclusions
Pinquart and Sörensen (2006)	127 studies, $N = 5,930$	NR	NR	NR	RCTs, controlled, meta-analysis	• Psychoeducation • CBT • Counseling • Support • Training of CR • Respite • Multicomponent	Overall effects were small but significant ($d = -.24$ to .46). Psychoeducation had significant effects on burden, depression, well-being, knowledge, and symptoms of CR. CBT was associated with decreases in burden but no other outcomes. Counseling reduced burden; support interventions increased well-being. Respite reduced burden and depression, and increased well-being. Multicomponent interventions were associated only with delayed CR institutionalization.	"Active" psychoeducational interventions were more effective than information-only interventions. Structured protocols, multicomponent interventions were more effective than unstructured interventions.
Powell et al. (2008)	15 studies across 5 interventions	NR	NR	NR	RCTs, controlled, pretest/ posttest, cohort, systematic review	• Networked technologies allowed transfer of digital information across geographic locations • Excluded: telephone-only interventions	Interventions were multifaceted and featured small samples. Intervention use was low. Networked technologies may have moderate effects on burden and depression ($n = 5$ interventions).	Treatment effects were diverse and influenced different CGs in various ways. Because of multiple subgroup analyses, interpretations of effectiveness are tentative at best.
Schoenmakers et al. (2009)	7 studies, $N = 3,424$	NR	NR	NR	RCTs, controlled, meta-analysis	Psychotropic drugs delivered to CRs: • Neuroleptics • Ant-psychotics • Antidepressants • Cognitive enhancement	Small, significant benefits on burden for CRs who received antipsychotics ($SMD = .27$) or cholinesterase inhibitors ($SMD = .23$). Cholinesterase inhibitors also reduced CG time ($SMD = 41.65$ min/day). No heterogeneity was apparent.	Pharmacological treatments for CRs appeared to reduce CG burden to a modest extent. Offering CGs skills to manage CR behavior problems was emphasized.

(continued)

Table 2.1. CONTINUED

Author (Year)	Sample (Baseline)[a]	Racial/Cultural Factors — Diversity of Study Sample	Racial/Cultural Factors — Cultural Diversity Training Received?	Racial/Cultural Factors — Comparisons of Racial/Cultural Factors	Design	Interventions	Results	Evaluation
Schoenmakers et al. (2010)	22 of 29 studies, N = 8,873 in 22 studies included in meta-analysis	NR	NR	NR	RCTs, pretest/ posttest, meta-analysis	• Psychosocial intervention • Telephone support • Case management • Respite care	Psychosocial, telephone support, and case management intervention had no effect on CG depression. Respite increased burden; psychosocial intervention had no effect.	Significant heterogeneity for psychosocial and case management interventions were apparent. Current evidence base is weak for home interventions, although these programs are valued by CGs.
Selwood et al. (2007)	62 studies, N = 5,061[b]	NR	NR	NR	RCTs, controlled studies, pretest/ posttest, systematic review	• Educational interventions • Dementia-specific therapies • Group coping strategies • Individual coping strategies • iBMT • iBMT of six or more sessions • Supportive therapy	Consistent evidence that iBMTs of six or more sessions is effective over short- and long-term intervals (n = 11). Coping strategies can reduce depression and distress over the short term (n = 16). Education alone and supportive therapies were not effective (n = 25).	Often unclear which intervention was evaluated. Quality evidence is lacking. The cost implications of delivering intensive iBMT requires greater attention.
Shaw et al. (2009)	104 studies (16 RCTs), N = est. more than 25,000 dementia CGs monitored[b]	NR	NR	NR	RCTs, controlled, pretest/posttest; observational, longitudinal, and cross-sectional studies; meta-analysis	• Interventions designed to provide the CG with respite/ time off from care provision	CG burden was reduced over 2 to 6 months in single-sample studies but not RCTs. Depression decreased in RCTs for home care, but not adult day services. Longer interventions had more positive effects. No effect on anxiety, but positive effects on morale, anger, and hostility were noted. Institutionalization of CRs increased and CG quality of life was worse in single-group studies.	Some evidence suggests the positive effects of respite on CG outcomes, but study quality is low. Existing studies lack cost analyses or descriptions of intervention processes.

Author	Sample	% nonwhite		Design	Intervention types	Findings	Conclusions
Smits et al. (2007)	25 studies, N = 4,686	NR	NR	NR	RCTs, controlled, pretest/posttest, systematic review	• Multicomponent/"combined" programs	Effects on CG depression and competence were mixed. Three of four studies showed significant mental health benefits; two of three studies found no effects on well-being. Most studies did not find any effect on burden. Eight of 12 studies found that multicomponent interventions delayed CR institutionalization.	Multicomponent interventions had mixed effects for most CG and CR outcomes, although influence on delaying CR institutionalization is more consistent.
Sörensen et al. (2002)	78 studies (48 dementia specific), 4–2,268 participants (*Mean* (*M*) = 24) in treatment condition	14% nonwhite	NR	NR	Controlled studies, meta-analysis	• Psychoeducation • Supportive • Psychotherapy • Respite • Training of care recipient • Multicomponent • Other	In RCTs, psychotherapy was effective in improving all outcomes (CG stress and depression, ability/knowledge, CR symptoms; n = up to 12; ES = –.19 to .42). Psychoeducation was effective for all but CG well-being and CR symptoms (n = up to 33; ES = –.43 to .53). Multicomponent was effective in improving CG burden, well-being, and ability/knowledge (n = up to 7; ES = –.62 to .86). Supportive interventions were effective for improving CG burden and ability/knowledge only (n = 5 and 2; ES = –.35 and .17, respectively). Respite was not effective. Dementia-specific interventions tended to have reduced benefit across all CG outcomes except improved symptoms of CR (weighted B, –.06 to –.33).	Psychotherapy, psychoeducation, and multicomponent interventions had broad positive effects, whereas supportive interventions were more targeted in their benefits.

(*continued*)

Table 2.1. CONTINUED

Author (Year)	Sample (Baseline)[a]	Racial/Cultural Factors			Design	Interventions	Results	Evaluation
		Diversity of Study Sample	Cultural Diversity Training Received?	Comparisons of Racial/ Cultural Factors				
Spijker et al. (2008)	13 studies, $N = 9,303$	NR	NR	NR	RCTs, controlled, meta-analysis	• Home-based or outpatient multicomponent interventions	Nonpharmacological, multicomponent interventions reduced CR institutionalization ($n = 10$, OR = .66) and time to placement ($n = 10$, SMD = 1.44). High-quality studies have a significant benefit on odds of placement (OR = .60) but not time to placement.	Significant study heterogeneity was apparent. Programs that emphasized CG involvement and choice appeared most likely to reduce CR institutionalization.
Thompson et al., 2007	44 studies, $N = 1,205$	NR	NR	NR	RCTs, meta-analysis	Psychoeducational: • Technology based • Individual • Group based	Group psychoeducational interventions only had positive effects on caregiver depression (WMD = –.71).	Overall study quality was poor. Clinical significance of effects was unclear. Outcomes included were heterogeneous.
Van't Leven et al. (2013)	41 studies	NR	NR	NR	RCTs	Dyadic • Information • Case management • Skills training • Support • Psychoeducation • Physical activity • Coping strategies • Multicomponent	Only two of nine studies showed improvement in mood; others demonstrated efficacy in later intervals. Twelve of 17 studies showed improvements in burden and competence; 7 of 10 studies showed quality-of-life improvements.	A dyadic intervention strategy is a potentially effective one, but more clinical attention is needed to match the needs of the CG and CR in such intervention modalities.
Vernooij-Dassen et al. 2011	11 studies, $N = 1,392$	NR	NR	NR	RCTs	• Group or individual cognitive reframing interventions (changing CGs' beliefs and interpretations of care)	Cognitive reframing was effective in reducing psychological morbidity and distress, but was not effective for coping or efficacy, burden, or CR institutionalization.	Cognitive reframing is a good candidate for a supplement intervention as part of larger, individualized CG intervention protocols.

RECENT INDIVIDUAL STUDIES (9/1/14–PRESENT)

Study					Design	Intervention	Results	Conclusion
Araki et al. (2014)	$N = 37$	NR	NR	NR	RCT/CE	• Donepezil and memantine • Donepezil only	CGs in the combination group indicated less burden ($F = 14.77$).	Memantine reduced blood flow in the prefrontal area of the brain for CRs, reducing symptoms and thus potentially reducing CG burden. The small-scale nature of this trial makes further interpretation or extrapolations tenuous.
Barnes et al. (2015)	$N = 10$	82% white	NR	NR	Controlled	• Procedural memory training for basic movements, mindful body awareness, and social connection for CRs in an adult day program	Nonsignificant results, but moderate effect sizes for decrease in caregiver burden was noted (standard deviation = .49).	Integrative exercise for CRs may benefit CGs as well, but larger RCTs are required.
Blom et al. (2015)	$N = 251$	98.7% Dutch national	NR	NR	RCT	• Internet intervention, "Mastery over Dementia"	Significantly fewer symptoms of depression and anxiety were noted. ESs were small (.26) and moderate (.48).	The results suggest the potential efficacy of Internet-delivered psychoeducational content for CGs, particularly as more CGs become comfortable using such technology.
Cheng et al. (2014)	$N = 25$	Chinese sample	NR	NR	RCT/CE	• Benefit finding • Psychoeducation	CGs who received benefit finding reported decreases in depressive symptoms that approached significance ($p = .07$). Both groups indicated reductions in role overload.	Benefit finding may alleviate CG depression and is feasible, but larger samples and trials are needed to establish this approach.
Chiu et al. (2015)	$N = 56$	UA	UA	UA	RCT	• Problem-solving therapy	CGs reported improved mastery, coping, and competence; and reduced stress ($p < .01$ to $p < .001$)	Problem-solving therapy appeared to enhance CG coping and capacity significantly, but demonstration of longer term effects of this approach on other outcomes are necessary.

(continued)

Table 2.1. CONTINUED

Author (Year)	Sample (Baseline)[a]	Racial/Cultural Factors			Design	Interventions	Results	Evaluation
		Diversity of Study Sample	Cultural Diversity Training Received?	Comparisons of Racial/ Cultural Factors				
Chodosh et al. (2015)	$N = 151$	78% Latino	Yes	Yes	RCT/CE	• Comparison of a telephone-only with a telephone and in-person dementia care coordination program	Costs for the in-person version of the intervention were greater ($142 more per month). Outcomes did not differ across the two groups. Care quality improved significantly in both groups (number of quality indicators doubled compared with baseline).	Dementia care management in general proved to enhance care quality regardless of delivery mechanism. Differences in costs or effectiveness were either not apparent or small.
Cove et al. (2014)	$N = 68$	9.5% Black Caribbean	NR	NR	RCT	• CST for CR plus CG training • CST only	No significant differences were reported.	More intensive CG training, along with more frequent CST, may be required to influence key outcomes.
Döpp et al. (2014)	$N = 71$	NR	NR	NR	RCT	• Community occupational therapy program that included a course, training, outreach visits, meetings, and a reporting system for occupational therapists	No differences in CG outcomes were found.	It is possible that delivering this program solely through providers is not sufficient to alleviating CG distress or other outcomes, and that such intervention should occur directly.
Ducharme et al. (2015)	$N = 60$	NR	NR	NR	RCT	• An educational intervention to facilitate the diagnosis transition for CGs • The educational program plus a booster session	Preparedness for care was increased after the booster session (55%, vs. 41% without the booster, and 28% for control). No effects for the booster were found on other outcomes.	The booster session was broad and it was recommended that future booster sessions focus on program components that CGs needed to review (i.e., tailoring).

	N	Sample			Design	Intervention	Results	Implications
Gallagher-Thompson et al. (2015)	N = 110	Latino sample	Yes	Yes	RCT	• A pictorial tool, or FN, to offer psychoeducation and appropriate service use	CGs who received the FN reported greater decreases in depression and found the FN more helpful than traditional educational materials.	The FN, which is tailored to the cultural needs of Latino CGs, may help to overcome accessing needed resources.
Gaugler et al. (2015)	N = 107	More than 95% sample white	NR	NR	RCT	• Multicomponent	Significant linear declines in negative reactions to CR disruptive behaviors (B, –3.23 to –.134) and overall negative reactions to behavior problems ($B = -2.16$) occurred. No other effects were found.	Long-term, multicomponent consultation may benefit adult child CGs over time, although attrition and sample size were limitations of this study.
Gonzalez et al. (2014)	N = 102	Stratified by race (57% African American)	NR	NR	RCT	• Group resourcefulness training	Small to medium effects were shown on resourcefulness (.36, .54), anxiety (.23, .44), and preparedness (.26, .41). No effects were found for other outcomes.	CGs can be taught resourcefulness via small-group sessions; however, larger scale evaluations are needed.
Logsdon et al. (2015)	N = 187	75% white sample	NR	NR	Controlled	• Specialized dementia wellness services provided in adult day programs	CGs indicated significantly less distress resulting from CR behavior problems ($p = .01–.02$)	Enhancing routine adult day service care with specialized dementia programming may benefit CRs and CGs. More rigorous designs are needed to establish the efficacy of such an approach.
Morgan et al. (2015)	N = 434	NR	NR	NR	Controlled	• Telephone-based care coordination and support	Intervention participants reported statistically similar changes in costs when compared with controls when controlling for prebaseline and baseline covariates.	The provision of telephone-based care coordination appears cost-effective, given the previously reported results of this intervention in reducing unmet CG needs and improving other outcomes.

(continued)

Table 2.1. Continued

Author (Year)[a]	Sample (Baseline)[a]	Racial/Cultural Factors			Design	Interventions	Results	Evaluation
		Diversity of Study Sample	Cultural Diversity Training Received?	Comparisons of Racial/Cultural Factors				
Remington et al. (2015)	N = 106	NR	NR	NR	RCT	• Nutritional intervention for CR	CGs reported nonsignificant improvements in CR neuropsychiatric symptoms.	Targeting CR symptoms directly with nutritional intervention may benefit CGs, but larger trials are needed.
Tanner et al. (2014)	N = 289	27% of sample was black	NR	NR	RCT	• Multicomponent care coordination intervention	No differences were apparent.	Providing care coordination by nonclinical community workers that focused on referral and linkage, and care planning—and not direct counseling—may have attenuated the clinical impact of this intervention.
Thivierge et al. (2014)	N = 20	NR	NR	NR	Controlled	• Memory rehabilitation to relearn instrumental activities of daily living for CRs	No effects on caregiver outcomes.	Although the intervention required CGs to practice with CRs, more direct intervention tailored to CG needs may be necessary to improve CG outcomes.

NOTE. AI/AN = American Indian/Alaskan native; BMT, behavior management techniques; CBT, cognitive–behavioral therapy; CE, comparative effectiveness; CG, caregiver; CR, care recipient; CST, cognitive stimulation training; d, Cohen's d; ES, effect size; FN, fotonovela; iBMT, Individual behavioral management techniques; IT, information technology; NR, not reported; OR, odds ratio; RCT, randomized controlled trial; SMD, standardized mean difference; B, unstandardized regression coefficient; UA, information was unavailable to Dr. Gaugler; WMD, weighted mean difference; REACH = Resources for Enhancing Alzheimer Caregiver Health.

[a]Estimates may be subject to error as a result of manual calculation by Dr. Gaugler.

[b]Participants double counted across some data sources/interventions.

help parents (54%) when compared with other racial and ethnic groups (38%). In addition, Hispanic and black caregivers spend more time per week on average assisting relatives with ADRD (~30 hours per week) than either white or Asian American caregivers (20 hours/week and 16 hours/week, respectively). Paralleling this time involvement, black and Hispanic caregivers are more likely to report a greater burden from their care responsibilities compared with white or Asian American caregivers (45%, 57%, 33%, and 30%, respectively) (Alzheimer's Association, 2014; National Alliance for Caregiving and American Association of Retired Persons, 2009).

Care Provision

As with other chronic disease contexts, family caregivers provide a wide range of assistance, including activity of daily living (ADL) and instrumental activity of daily living (IADL) help, management of disease-specific symptoms, care coordination, supervision, and a range of other activities. However, as a result of the long duration of ADRD and the demands posed by cognitive decline, functional impairments, and behavioral/psychiatric symptoms often wrought by the neuropathological complications of AD, family care to relatives with ADRD is more extensive than other disease contexts. For example, family caregivers of persons with ADRD are more likely to provide assistance with ADLs overall and specific ADL tasks than other family caregivers (Alzheimer's Association, 2014; National Alliance for Caregiving/AARP, 2009). Recent data from the National Survey of Caregiving (2011) found that 14% and 11% more of caregivers of people with ADRD offer assistance with self-care/mobility and health/medical care, respectively (Kasper et al., 2014; Spillman, Wolff, Freedman, & Kasper, 2014). More persons with ADRD rely on multiple caregivers; 9% more of persons with ADRD rely on three or more individuals to provide help compared with persons without ADRD (Kasper et al., 2014).

Because of the long disease trajectory of AD and associated disorders, family caregivers of persons with these conditions also tend to provide help for longer periods of time. Ten percent more caregivers of persons with ADRD provided assistance for 1 to 4 years compared with family caregivers of persons without ADRD, whereas 4% more ADRD caregivers offered help for 5 years or more when compared with nondementia caregivers (National Alliance for Caregiving/ AARP, 2009). Family caregivers of persons with ADRD offer an average of 27 hours more per month than non-ADRD caregivers; the extent of daily care provision is even more pronounced for primary ADRD caregivers (approximately 9 hours per day [Fisher et al., 2011; Kasper et al., 2014]).

There is a large body of descriptive literature that emphasizes the negative emotional, social, psychological, and physical health ramifications of providing assistance to someone with ADRD over time (Brodaty et al., 2014; Mausbach, 2014). Family caregivers of persons with ADRD are more likely to report greater emotional stress and burden resulting from care provision (Alzheimer's

Association, 2014; Kasper et al., 2014; National Alliance for Caregiving/AARP, 2009). Close to half of ADRD caregivers (47%) indicate considerable strain resulting from financial issues (Alzheimer's Association, 2014). Five to 17% of noncaregivers in the U.S. population have depression whereas 40% of ADRD caregivers do. Depressive symptoms exacerbate as the severity of dementia becomes more pronounced (Baumgarten et al., 1992; Epstein-Lubow et al., 2012; Kessler, Chiu, Demler, Merikangas, & Walters, 2005; Mausbach, Chattillion, Roepke, Patterson, & Grant, 2013; Pinquart & Sörensen, 2003; Schulz, O'Brien, Bookwala, & Fleissner, 1995; Seeher, Low, Reppermund, & Brodaty, 2013). The accumulation of stress and the other negative ramifications of caregiving can also expedite nursing home admission for the person with ADRD (Gaugler, Yu, Krichbaum, & Wyman, 2009). It is important to note that ADRD caregiving is not a wholly negative experience; many family caregivers report a great sense of reward and accomplishment in providing ongoing assistance to a relative in need (and such positive dimensions are often important to identify and build on in any type of intervention model). However, the accumulation of descriptive research evidence suggests that ADRD family care can also be overwhelming for many individuals.

The accumulation and exacerbation of family care for persons with ADRD may also result in health complications for caregivers. Although the effects of ADRD caregiving on mortality are mixed, the provision of ADRD care appears to influence cellular and physiological mechanisms negatively in family caregivers. This suggest that the emotional/psychosocial ramifications of family care for persons with ADRD are intertwined with the physiological effects of negative stress appraisal, which may influence a number of health complications for family caregivers (Alzheimer's Association, 2014).

Conceptual or theoretical models of caregiving stress (see Chapter 1) often emphasize how the immediate challenges posed by family caregivers of persons with ADRD can proliferate, or spill over, to other life domains of the caregiver. One such domain is employment. Almost 1 in 10 ADRD caregivers had to leave their job entirely because of care provision. More than half (54%) had disruptions to work schedules resulting from ADRD family caregiving (National Alliance for Caregiving/AARP, 2009).

CAREGIVING INTERVENTION RESEARCH

As noted earlier, there have been multiple reviews conducted on the efficacy of AD caregiving interventions for an array of outcomes, including caregiver stress, caregiver psychological well-being, and care-recipient outcomes (Gitlin & Hodgson, 2015). Thus, the focus of this section is to synthesize existing reviews of the AD caregiver intervention literature to ascertain the overall efficacy and effectiveness of these approaches. Additional randomized controlled trials (RCTs) and controlled evaluations of interventions not included in the most recent syntheses of the literature are highlighted as well.

Using the Population, Intervention, Comparison, Outcomes (PICO) frame-work, the following search parameters were developed:

- *Population*: Family caregivers of persons with ADRD
- *Intervention*: Nonpharmacological (e.g., education, support groups, training, therapy/counseling, respite) services or support for family caregivers
- *Comparison*: Those receiving "usual" care
- *Outcomes*: Caregiver stress, caregiver depression, or similar measures of caregiver distress and care recipient nursing home admission

The PICO framework and elements noted earlier resulted in the following search question: *Do family caregivers of persons with dementia who receive nonphar-macological intervention (psychosocial or community-based services) experience improved well-being and delay nursing home admission of care recipients when compared with those who receive "usual care?"*

Systematic reviews and meta-analyses were identified on the Cochrane library and by using the PubMed clinical queries Systematic Reviews search tool. Recent, single RCTs not included in the most up-to-date systematic reviews or meta-analyses were searched using the PubMed database. Combinations of the keywords *dementia/Alzheimer's disease* and *caregiver/caregiving* were used. In addition, cross-referencing of a current library of articles Dr. Gaugler is currently assembling for a meta-analysis of clinical interventions to prevent or delay nurs-ing home admission was conducted to identify additional reviews of interest.

Using this search method, 40 systematic reviews and meta-analyses were identified. All identified reports reviewed solely the efficacy/effectiveness of care-giver interventions for persons with ADRD, with the exception of three reports (Mason et al., 2007; Shaw et al., 2009; Sörensen, Pinquart, & Duberstein, 2002). These three reports were included because they featured a sizable number of ADRD caregiver studies in their review. One additional report of respite was excluded for this reason (McNally, Ben-Shlomo, & Newman, 1999). Purely nar-rative reviews that did not include an overview of the search method (i.e., non-systematic reviews) were also excluded. An additional 17 individual studies since August 31, 2014, were identified (the end search date of the most recent review [Gitlin & Hodgson, 2015]). Table 2.1 features key extracted information from included reviews and individual studies.

A quick scan of the retrieved reviews and individual studies resulted in the following impressions: (a) there remains a lack of high-quality evidence to derive conclusions of efficacy (e.g., RCTs, blinding), although recent research has improved in this regard; (b) it is difficult to classify the "type" of intervention delivered, particularly because many interventions tend to combine treatments to maximize effect; (c) there exist considerable variations in study design and sampling; (d) outcome measures tend to be heterogeneous and not necessar-ily comparable, even within the same domains (e.g., "stress"); (e) the statistical power of some trials are suspect; and (f) the inclusion/exclusion criteria in trials are often not well justified. Overall ADRD caregiver intervention efficacy for a range of domains tends to be moderately positive at best.

The typology used to summarize caregiver interventions across existing systematic reviews and meta-analyses was derived from the framework of Sörensen et al. (2002), which was later updated and expanded (Pinquart & Sörensen, 2006). The following caregiver intervention types are identified (Sörensen, Pinquart, Habil, & Duberstein, 2002, pp. 357–358):

- *Psychoeducation* involves structured programs that offer information about the disease, resources, and services. Psychoeducational interventions may also include training caregivers to manage problems.
- *Supportive interventions* include professional or peer-led support groups that focus on exchange of feelings, ideas, and problems/successes.
- *Respite* includes services designed to give caregivers "time off" from responsibilities; respite is either at-home or site-specific.
- *Psychotherapy* involves the establishment of a therapeutic relationship between the caregiver and a professional (see Case Study 1).
- *Multicomponent interventions* include those protocols that combine various intervention elements, such as education, therapy, support, and respite (see Case Study 2).

As shown in Table 2.1, multiple meta-analyses and systematic reviews have concluded that psychoeducational interventions are effective. For example, meta-analyses have found that group-based supportive interventions based on a psychoeducational framework were effective in reducing psychological morbidity, and that psychoeducational interventions had consistent, short-term benefits on several caregiver outcomes including caregiver burden, depression, and well-being (Sörensen et al., 2002; Thompson et al., 2007). In several systematic reviews, psychoeducational interventions emerged as consistent in their positive effects on caregiver outcomes. In addition, individual strategies were more effective than group or education-based approaches, although teaching coping strategies in group or individual settings seemed to provide short-term psychological benefits. However, combining social support and problem-solving approaches also appeared effective, and providing brief education intervention appeared to reduce caregiver depression (Cooke, McNally, Mulligan, Harrison, & Newman, 2001; Jensen, Agbata, Canavan, & McCarthy, 2015; Martin-Carrasco, Ballesteros-Rodriguez, Dominguez-Panchon, Munoz-Hermoso, & Gonzalez-Fraile, 2014; Peacock & Forbes, 2003; Selwood, Johnston, Katona, Lyketsos, & Livingston, 2007). A more recent systematic review of 20 RCTs found that seven of the eight of the psychoeducational/skills-building interventions reviewed offered a range of benefits to dementia caregivers, including reductions in depressive symptoms and improvements in quality of life (Elvish, Lever, Johnstone, Cawley, & Keady, 2013). Parker and colleagues also found small, significant effects of psychoeducational interventions on caregiver depression, but not other outcomes (Parker, Mills, & Abbey, 2008).

A more recent review of Internet-delivered interventions for dementia caregivers suggested that education or information interventions delivered online were less efficacious (Boots, de Vugt, van Knippenberg, Kempen, & Verhey, 2014). Similarly, interventions that primarily provide information or advice to persons with dementia and their caregivers were not found to reduce caregiver distress significantly (Corbett et al., 2012). In a review of 50 dyadic psychosocial interventions (many of them offering psychoeducation and all RCTs), Van't Leven and colleagues reported that close to 70% of the studies reviewed reported improvements in quality of life and reductions in burden, with fewer positively influencing caregivers' mood (Van't Leven et al., 2013).

Additional meta-analyses and systematic reviews suggest that supportive interventions are, at best, modestly effective. An early review indicated that supportive interventions exerted small but positive effects on dementia caregivers' distress (Knight, Lutzky, & Macofsky-Urban, 1993). Only when social support and problem-solving approaches were combined did supportive interventions emerge as effective (Cooke et al., 2001). In a meta-analysis, supportive interventions had some effect on burden and ability/knowledge, but not on other outcomes (Sörensen et al., 2002). A systematic review indicated that individual strategies were more effective than group or education-based approaches in alleviating dementia caregivers' distress (Selwood et al., 2007).

Respite is often viewed as a critical component of long-term care services and supports in communities, but available evaluations have yielded little evidence of efficacy for dementia caregivers. Respite had some effect on burden, depression, and well-being of caregivers in one meta-analysis and an earlier review (Knight et al., 1993; Sörensen et al., 2002). In a comprehensive systematic review respite appeared to reduce burden and depression in some studies; however, this trend tended to occur among lower quality studies (Shaw et al., 2009). A more common finding was that respite was not beneficial for family caregivers of persons with ADRD (Flint, 1995). In several meta-analyses of all controlled trials, respite showed modest benefits for subgroups only and no benefit for nursing home admission, although caregiver satisfaction was high (Mason et al., 2007; see also Jones, Edwards, & Hounsome, 2012; Schoenmakers, Buntinx, & DeLepeleire, 2010). In a systematic review of respite interventions for caregivers, no consistent or enduring effects were found, and respite appeared ineffective in reducing caregiver anxiety (Cooper, Balamurali, Selwood, & Livingston, 2007). A Cochrane meta-analysis of RCTs found there were no benefits (or risks) associated with respite use for older adults with cognitive impairment or their family caregivers (Maayan, Soares-Weiser, & Lee, 2014), but a review by Shaw et al. (2009) suggested that institutionalization rates increased for older respite users.

Psychotherapy for ADRD caregivers, such as cognitive–behavioral therapy, has demonstrated fairly consistent, positive effects on family caregiver outcomes, perhaps as a result of the intensive, long-term delivery of clinical content common in such strategies. In an earlier meta-analysis, psychotherapy had an effect on all outcome variables (Sörensen et al., 2002), whereas in a systematic review cognitive–behavioral therapy (along with relaxation-based therapy) appeared effective in reducing caregiver anxiety (Cooper et al., 2007). Similarly, another systematic review demonstrated that individual strategies, such as multisession behavior management therapy, were effective (Selwood et al., 2007). A psychotherapy study appeared to delay nursing home admission in another systematic review (Peacock & Forbes, 2003). There is some inconsistency in the conclusions reported in reviews of the literature (perhaps a result of how interventions are categorized across reviews); "individual-based" interventions were not effective when compared with group-based approaches in one meta-analysis (Thompson et al., 2007). A more recent meta-analysis examined 11 RCTs of cognitive reframing for ADRD caregivers and found that these approaches had beneficial effects for caregivers' anxiety, depression, and subjective stress whereas caregiver burden, care-recipient institutionalization, and other outcomes were not influenced (Vernooij-Dassen, Draskovic, McCleery, & Downs, 2011).

Perhaps the most consistent findings of efficacy are demonstrated for multicomponent ADRD caregiver interventions. A meta-analysis found that only multicomponent interventions were effective among the various intervention types considered (Acton & Kang, 2001). Parker and colleagues found that multicomponent interventions had small but significant effects on caregiver depression only (Parker et al., 2008). Although another meta-analysis found moderate benefits for all psychosocial interventions considered, multicomponent, continuous, flexible support appeared linked to delayed institutionalization along with other caregiver outcomes (Brodaty, Green, & Koschera, 2003; Goy, Freeman, & Kansagara, 2010; Spijker et al., 2008). A systematic review of "combined" interventions for dementia caregivers found these approaches were most effective in improving caregiver mental health and delaying nursing home admission of care recipients (Smits et al., 2007). A meta-analysis of grade A and grade B recommendations (high-quality and low-quality RCTs, respectively) found that multicomponent interventions for dementia caregivers were effective in delaying institutionalization and improving an array of caregiver outcomes (Olazarán et al., 2010); similar results were apparent in a more recent meta-analysis (Brodaty & Arasaratnam, 2012) as well as reviews of Internet-delivered interventions for dementia caregivers (Boots et al., 2014; McKechnie, Barker, & Stott, 2014). Elvish and colleagues found that all six randomized, controlled evaluations of multicomponent interventions in their review exerted positive effects on caregiver depression, well-being, and social support (Elvish et al., 2013). In an earlier meta-analysis, intervention effects for multicomponent strategies were powerful for select outcomes (e.g., caregiver burden, well-being, ability/knowledge), but at the time few such studies existed (Sörensen et al., 2002; see also Pinquart & Sörensen [2006]). A more recent review and meta-analysis (synthesizing research through the year 2014) suggested that multicomponent interventions were most consistently effective across a range of caregiver outcomes, as well as delayed care-recipient institutionalization and improved caregivers' competence, preparedness, and mastery via traditional face-to-face, telephone, and videophone delivery (Gitlin & Hodgson, 2015; for an exception to these review findings, see Griffin et al. [2013]).

Several other reviews and meta-analyses were identified and are of note, although they did not fit into the caregiving intervention typology used earlier. A review of technology-based interventions for dementia caregivers indicated some positive effects on caregiver outcomes, but also considerable heterogeneity in study design and quality (Godwin, Mills, Anderson, & Kunik, 2013). One meta-analysis found that acetylcholinesterase inhibitors had moderate effects in reducing time spent on caregiving and burden for ADRD caregivers (Lingler, Martire, & Schulz, 2005; Schoenmakers, Buntinx, & De Lepeleire, 2009). Lower level evidence suggests that exercise is not effective, although some studies available at the time supported the use of yoga and relaxation techniques (systematic review of Cooper et al. [2007]). A more recent review through 2014 indicated several pilot trials of caregiver stress reduction using meditation techniques, which suggest these modalities as a promising avenue for larger scale evaluation among ADRD caregivers (Gitlin & Hodgson, 2015). Another recent meta-analysis suggests that physical activity for dementia caregivers can reduce burden, but was not as effective in alleviating other negative outcomes on the part of caregivers (Orgeta & Miranda-Castillo, 2014). A systematic review found that the use of memory aids along with caregiver training can help communication between dementia caregivers and care recipients in a small number of studies of limited methodological rigor (Egan, Berube, Racine, Leonard, & Rochon, 2010). Psychosocial interventions delivered at home were found to be beneficial in a nonsignificant way on caregivers' burden and depression, although respite was responsible for an increase in burden (Schoenmakers et al., 2010). Computer networked peer support appeared to have moderate effects on improving dementia caregiver stress and depression, as well (Powell, Chiu, & Eysenbach, 2008).

Overall, existing reviews imply that the efficacy of ADRD caregiver interventions remains questionable, although more recent evaluations appear stronger both in design, inferential quality, and outcomes. Psychosocial interventions that are more intensive, flexible, and individualized appear most effective at meeting the multifaceted needs of caregivers.

A review of recent single studies reveals results that do not depart significantly from the synthesis of existing reviews or meta-analyses. However, several trends illustrate how ADRD caregiver interventions are evolving. One is the inclusion of caregiver outcomes alongside the person with ADRD in various pharmacological and nonpharmacological trials. Although recent studies have not revealed consistent or large benefits of such interventions (Araki et al., 2014; Barnes et al., 2015; Cove et al., 2014; Remington et al., 2015; Thivierge, Jean, & Simard, 2014), such a trend does imply that AD clinical trials are incorporating caregiver outcomes more consistently. Other interventions have evaluated the cost implications of their interventions or have evaluated the efficacy of a given intervention in different populations or clinical settings (Gaugler, Reese, & Mittelman, 2015; Logsdon, Pike, Korte, & Goehring, 2014; Morgan et al., 2015), although only one published study to date has used a rigorous comparative effectiveness design

(Chodosh et al., 2015). The increasing availability and use of the Internet or other networked technologies have led to the evaluation of ADRD caregiver interventions using these delivery platforms—and with promising results (see Blom, Zarit, Groot Zwaaftink, Cuijpers, & Pot, 2015). Last, in addition to the inclusion of more ethnically and racially diverse subsamples than prior evaluations, more recent interventions have begun to develop and test, with great promise, culturally tailored interventions to facilitate access to services and education for heretofore underserved ADRD caregiving populations (Gallagher-Thompson et al., 2015). These developments are heartening; in addition to demonstrating efficacy, this new generation of ADRD caregiver interventions has addressed some of the limitations of prior evidence with an eye toward their eventual implementation and adoption as routine options for clinical treatment of ADRD (see "Translation of Interventions to Community Settings" in this chapter).

Implications

As this synthesis implies, the large number of interventions for AD caregivers (as well as interventions for persons with AD that track caregiver outcomes) has evolved considerably during the past 30 years. Researchers have distilled five key characteristics that appear to define effective interventions (Gitlin & Hodgson, 2015; Zarit & Femia, 2008):

1. "Active involvement of family caregivers in the intervention process rather than a didactic, prescriptive approach
2. Tailoring to specific needs identified by caregivers
3. Addressing multiple areas of need
4. Longer interventions or episodic (i.e., booster) support over time or duration of caregiving
5. Adjusting dose, intensity, and specific focus of an intervention based on a caregiver's risk or need profile" (Gitlin & Hodgson, 2015; p. 339)

As we and others have noted in appraisals of the family caregiving literature (Gaugler & Kane, 2015; Gitlin & Hodgson, 2015), the lack of consistency in overall effects of AD family caregiver interventions suggest several strategies for future research to consider. One consideration is the heterogeneity in samples and, specifically, diversity in disease stage of care recipients. To maximize sample sizes in a population that is often difficult to recruit, many studies tend to include persons with ADRD that are in various stages of disease severity (e.g., early, middle, late). It is possible the clinical mechanisms of certain interventions operate differently in care scenarios that vary by dementia severity. The persistence of short-term follow-ups is a further complicating factor. Although this is not entirely surprising as the costs of longitudinal, randomized, controlled evaluations can be high, using follow-up periods of less than a year may obscure the effects of ADRD caregiver interventions on key outcomes such as residential long-term care admission (we have recommended a 3-year follow-up period in the context of ADRD to document effects on nursing home admission [Gaugler et al., 2009]). The overwhelming majority of ADRD caregiver interventions often target a select set of domains (albeit with wildly diverse measures) such as burden or depression. With the emergence of person-centered outcomes and comparative effectiveness research, selecting measures that are of the greatest relevance to caregivers themselves, such as family conflict, work–life balance, and quality of relationship with the care recipient, may not only result in findings that are of the greatest meaning to caregiving families, but also could demonstrate broader efficacy on the part of ADRD caregiver interventions (use of approaches such as Goal Attainment Scaling may also facilitate such efforts; see Rockwood et al., 2006). As noted earlier and related to the issue of outcome selection, most descriptive and intervention studies of ADRD caregiving approach this phenomena from a deficit perspective, in which the experience of ADRD caregiving is viewed as entirely negative. Ascertaining how positive domains can inform outcome measurement as well as clinical content may further advance the state of the science of ADRD caregiver intervention research (Gitlin & Hodgson, 2015).

Similar to the issue of outcome selection is that many caregiver interventions in ADRD (or perhaps other disease contexts as well) have not aligned their outcomes effectively with those that are reimbursable by entities such as Medicare or Medicaid (e.g., prevention of hospitalizations on the part of the person with ADRD). Because of this omission, almost all ADRD caregiver interventions are not necessarily viewed as integral to care management or treatment efforts. Positioning ADRD caregiver interventions so they are in concert with third-payer reimbursement streams may help to facilitate the implementation and translation of interventions (see "Translation of Interventions to Community Settings"), and one way this is possible is to conduct high-quality, rigorous scientific trials with reimbursable outcomes at the core of such evaluations.

A common criticism that was raised in many of the systematic reviews and meta-analyses presented in Table 2.1 was the lack of information provided to allow for a determination of mechanisms of benefit. In other words, intervention reports often do not conduct analyses to ascertain why a given protocol "works." In instances of complex, multicomponent interventions, this is particularly problematic because avoiding processes or mechanisms of clinical benefit makes it difficult to ascertain whether one component works better than another, or whether one component is more important than another when delivering a given intervention. As the synthesis of reviews noted here seems to suggest, interventions that are delivered over time and with sufficient intensity seem to exert the greatest benefits for ADRD caregivers and their care recipients, but how frequently and for how long do such intense, long-term interventions need to be implemented to achieve long-lasting benefits? By not examining clinical processes of benefit in more detail, the state of the science of ADRD caregiver interventions is hampered because subsequent researchers are left to wonder which intervention components are integral to incorporate into new protocols and strategies (e.g., using intervention principles in new modes of delivery, such as embedding an existing psychoeducational intervention into an online, social media platform).

Whether findings are applicable across various ADRD caregivers and care recipients, times, and environments is an ongoing concern. With some notable exceptions—such as the Medicare Alzheimer's Disease Demonstration Evaluation and the Resources for Enhancing Alzheimer's Caregiver Health (REACH) I and II trials (Belle et al., 2006; Newcomer et al., 1999; Schulz et al., 2003)—most ADRD caregiver interventions are conducted in specialized settings with little generalizability potential. Several reviews noted issues with the selection of outcome measures, and perhaps a more important issue is whether the statistical effects reported in many ADRD caregiver interventions are clinically meaningful. It is not apparent in many interventions that when a key caregiving outcome is changed with the delivery of a given intervention that this change results in clinically relevant improvement (Schulz et al., 2002).

Cultural Considerations

As shown in Table 2.1, prior reviews and meta-analyses have often not considered the cultural applicability and relevance of current ADRD caregiver interventions for families of diverse racial and ethnic background. However, ADRD caregiving intervention research has emerged in this area during the past 20 years. The recent promising work of Gallagher-Thompson and colleagues in evaluating a *fotonovela* intervention for Latino caregivers is evidence of such advances (Gallagher-Thompson et al., 2015). Prior reviews have found that, although a number of descriptive quantitative and qualitative studies on diverse ADRD caregiving intervention populations exist, there are fewer evaluations of interventions for these families. Most high-quality evaluations for diverse ADRD family caregivers were derived from the multisite REACH I and II trials (Llanque & Enriquez, 2012). As noted by Llanque and Enriquez (2012), a greater focus on rural Latinos and Latinos from different countries of origin, use of participatory approaches, and consideration of acculturation are all areas that require greater attention in future ADRD caregiver intervention research. As Napoles and colleagues also suggest in a 2010 systematic review of ADRD caregiver interventions for black, Latino, and Chinese American samples, most of the existing work on cultural tailoring is derived from the REACH I and II trials (Napoles, Chadiha, Eversley, & Moreno-John, 2010). Although REACH I and II represented a significant achievement in demonstrating how the cultural tailoring of interventions can result in improved psychosocial outcomes for caregivers, increased attention on familism, language, bilingual/bicultural staff, and literacy must continue to situate ADRD caregiver interventions better in culturally, racially, and geographically diverse contexts (Napoles et al., 2010; for a recent exception, see Chodosh et al., 2015).

TRANSLATION OF INTERVENTIONS
TO COMMUNITY SETTINGS

As we discussed earlier, meta-analyses of dementia caregiver interventions have shown, at best, moderate effect sizes. Many have not been replicated nor has efficacy been shown in diverse populations. Clearly, more work needs to be done to improve the evidence base. Thus, one can rightly question whether it is premature to invest time and money in translating caregiving interventions into real-world settings. It is our view that despite these limitations, evidence is accumulating that social and behaviorally based caregiver intervention programs show promise for translation to the community. This view is based on the following. As Covinsky and Johnston (2006) stated in editorial comments that accompanied the publication of the REACH II randomized controlled trial (Belle et al., 2006) in the *Annals of Internal Medicine*:

> [Although work is needed to strengthen these interventions,] we shouldn't let the perfect be the enemy of the good. If these [i.e., caregiver] interventions were drugs, it is hard to believe that they would not be on the fast track to approval. The magnitude of benefit and quality of evidence supporting these interventions considerably exceed those of currently approved pharmacologic therapies for dementia (Covinsky & Johnston, 2006; p. 780).

Moreover, considering the ever-growing number of caregivers in need of assistance, withholding interventions with known, albeit small to moderate positive effects, risks doing harm to those who might benefit from them. In addition, although most caregiving interventions currently require more work before they achieve maximal effectiveness and efficiency, our argument in this chapter is that social and behavioral scientists should plan for dissemination and implementation in the real world as they test and refine their interventions under study. Forward-looking planning, "designing with the outcome in mind," will help future efforts at translation to succeed.

Translational efforts in caregiving have been summarized in one recently published paper (Gitlin et al., 2015) and a chapter we currently published (Wethington & Burgio, 2015). Although somewhat different in focus, these sources offered similar conclusions. Funding for translational research has been provided by various federal agencies, although the overall amount of funding has been very modest. By far, the biggest funder of translational efforts has been the Administration on Aging (AoA) through the congressionally mandated Alzheimer's Disease Supportive Services Program (Administration for Community Living, 2014). An AoA review group published a white paper that identified 44 caregiver intervention programs that had been funded as translation trials from 2002 to 2012 (Maslow, 2012). Augmenting the white paper, Gitlin and colleagues (2015) used a rapid review process and identified only 16 publications that describe translational efforts of proven dementia caregiver interventions. Moreover, only six of the more than 200 dementia caregiver interventions developed throughout the years have been submitted to the translational process: REACH II, Skills Care, The New York University Caregiver Intervention, Savvy Caregiver Program, Reducing Disability in Alzheimer's Disease, and Staff Training in Assisted Living Residences-Caregiver (see Table 2.1 for descriptions). It is noteworthy, however, that 13 (of 16) published papers that reported outcomes were positive.

Translational researchers have recommended a series of steps necessary for successful translation of caregiver support programs (Burgio et al., 2009; Gitlin et al., 2015). In an action guide for implementing community-based programs for dementia caregivers, developed by L. Burgio in collaboration with the Centers for Disease Control and Prevention (University of Michigan's Institute of Gerontology & the National Association of Chronic Disease Directors, 2009), the following actions were suggested: (a) translate intervention programs that have detailed training manuals available; (b) assess the setting's readiness and available resources to support program implementation; (c) form a stakeholder advisory board to assess acceptability, enhance "buy-in," and recommend possible adaptation of the intervention to the specific setting; (d) train the interventionists in how to deliver the intervention to an established criterion, using a certification process if possible; (e) designate a "supervisor" (i.e., an individual with particular expertise with the intervention) who the interventionist can contact if questions arise (the supervisor can also train new personnel for program sustainability); (f) assess treatment fidelity periodically and understand that this assessment is an ongoing process; and (g) maintain vigilance for program sustainability, both in terms of funding and knowledge transfer (see (e)).

Thus, we have established that there is a critical need for caregiver support programs in the community, a half-dozen evidence-based interventions have been translated successfully, and we even have a degree of consensus regarding the necessary steps for successful translation. Yet, translation into community action has been very slow. What are the barriers to translation and how can they be overcome? Succinctly stated, there is a lack of funding and there is a lack of consensus from the fledgling translational sciences on the best design and methods for transfer, implementation, and dissemination of caregiver interventions.

The barriers to funding are twofold. First, although some states have limited work-arounds for reimbursement through Medicare, we are currently lacking federal policies that provide reimbursement for health service providers who provide support services for dementia caregivers. Second, research funding for translation science from federal and private funding agencies is extremely limited. Gitlin et al. (2015) recommended creating a central repository for proven programs from which to access training information and intervention details, and revamping reimbursement policies or bundling programs and payment structures to incentivize providers to offer proven programs. Wethington and Burgio (2015) propose that the scientific barriers would be overcome by the development, or perhaps it would be more accurate to say acceptance, of designs and procedures that allow researchers to adapt evidence-based interventions while they are being implemented in different clinical settings and for different patient populations. Although there is consensus that stakeholder input is critical in translational research, there is as yet no consensus about how and to what extent community stakeholders should be involved in the process of design and implementation. We lack basic information about whether stakeholder involvement results in improved research translation that meets rigorous scientific standards.

A number of adaptive approaches have been developed in recent years (Wethington & Burgio, 2015), and when combined with mixed-methods approaches, the critical voice of community stakeholders can be incorporated into decisions regarding adaptation (e.g., see the Explore Values, Operationalize and Learn, and eValuate Efficacy [EVOLVE] process developed by Peterson et al., 2013). Gaugler and Kane (2015) offer a convincing argument that our current caregiving crisis, if left unchecked, is quickly heading toward a "perfect storm." Still, we do not believe that this is cause for despair. Just as crises lead to opportunities, we believe that current and future exigencies will lead to solutions.

CONCLUSION

Among chronic care illnesses in the United States, dementia and dementia caregiving have the most negative impact on public health (National Alliance for Caregiving and American Association of Retired Persons, 2009). However, this area also has the richest research literature on the caregiving experience, caregiving interventions, and translation of these interventions to community settings. As we discussed in Chapter 1, and as is articulated further in subsequent chapters, each chronic illness presents family caregivers with a unique set of challenges. Despite these unique challenges, it is our belief that it would benefit researchers across chronic illnesses to familiarize themselves with the dementia caregiving literature. Much can be learned from the roads taken by dementia caregiving researchers, and both researcher time and money can be conserved by becoming aware of the many "dead ends" hit by dementia researchers over several decades of research.

CASE STUDIES

Case Study 1: "Providing Psychotherapy Using the NYUCI Intervention"

Mrs. L was the primary caregiver for her husband of 42 years. Mr. L had formerly been a controlling and domineering leader of his family, commanding submission from his wife because of his intimidating manner. Moderate AD exacerbated Mr. L's aggressive and demanding style, so that

Mrs. L feared for her physical safety if she were to attempt to restrict Mr. L's access to the car or to the household finances. Despite the fact that Mr. L was clearly incapable of driving or managing financial matters (his mismanagement had already cost the family devastating losses), Mrs. L felt helpless in controlling her husband's behavior. The L's son, Jonathan, had gradually taken the reins of the family business and could not understand why his mother could not do the same at home. Feeling helpless and invalidated, Mrs. L appeared depressed and anxious, and reported suffering from debilitating gastrointestinal problems. She ceased all social interactions because of her fear of leaving Mr. L alone, and he refused any substitute companion. Mrs. L's relationship with her son was strained as a result of her frequent complaints about Mr. L (often in the form of desperate telephone calls) and the son's minimization of the problem.

The NYUCI Intervention: NYUCI involves six, 1 to 2 hour-long therapeutic sessions (sometimes more depending on family need) spread over a 4-month period. The initial and final session include the primary caregiver only, but the other four sessions include the primary caregiver and other family members involved in offering help to the relative with AD. In this case, the sessions took place in the home, but they can occur in private practice or clinic settings. *Assessment*: An assessment battery is administered at the end of sessions 1 and 6, and includes assessments of burden, depression, caregiver self-reported health, reaction to problem behaviors, and satisfaction with social support. *Intervention*: NYUCI focuses directly on the mediators of caregiver depression and burden by improving family support of the primary caregiver, reducing negative family interactions, and helping the caregiver and family to understand and react more effectively to the behavior of the person with dementia via the guidance of a professional counselor (often a master's-level licensed clinical social worker or similar expert). NYUCI requires that both caregiver and family or friends participate in at least half of the initial counseling sessions. NYUCI tailors both the content and the style of counseling to the needs of the caregiver/family, based initially on the intake assessment and modified in response to the needs and desires of the primary caregiver and family, as revealed in the counseling sessions. Ad hoc phone contact with the therapist plays an important role in this intervention. *Application to Mrs. L*: During the early sessions, the therapist determined that Mrs. L's low status in her family's hierarchy was a central problem and contracted with Mrs. L to work on enhancing her effectiveness at managing Mr. L's behavior and gaining respect and support from her son. The therapist recognized that Jonathan would be a valuable member of the family leadership structure and aimed to facilitate an alliance between Mrs. L and her son. However, Mrs. L was reluctant because she believed that Jonathan lacked perspective on the difficulties of caring for an AD patient. The therapist recognized an opportunity for change when Mrs. L reported that her son was going to take Mr. L on a business trip. The trip had an eye-opening impact on Jonathan's perspective regarding Mr. L's level of functioning. With 5 days of constant contact, he was able to experience his father's difficulties in managing his own care, his disorientation, and his insistence that he could be self-reliant. Mrs. L gained tremendous satisfaction from her son's acknowledgment of her daily struggle, and Jonathan began attending therapy sessions. He was appreciative of the therapist's expression of sympathy regarding his experiences on the business trip. To reinforce the mother–son alliance, the therapist guided mother and son while they worked together to generate a solution to the problem of Mr. L's driving (the son would take the car keys and they would tell Mr. L that the car was being repaired). The issue of household finances was more challenging because the son's solution was to take over their management, whereas Mrs. L wanted to be more involved. The therapist was encouraged by the assertive manner in which Mrs. L expressed her desire to participate in this leadership function. She guided mother and son in creating a list of finance tasks and divided up some short-term tasks. All tasks generated during therapy were monitored by the therapist in subsequent sessions. By session 6, Jonathan accepted the role of "financial advisor" to his mother whereas Mrs. L established a routine for paying bills. Mrs. L hired a housekeeper who she could trust to watch over Mr. L, freeing her to make social contacts and to maintain regular attendance in a support group. Mrs. L's contacts with her son were also more positive and he visited more regularly. As Mr. L's dementia began to progress, his behaviors became less disruptive and aggressive, but also began to influence his functional capacity negatively. Mrs. L contacted the NYUCI counselor by phone 4 months later to discuss his situation and to solicit advice regarding whether it was time to begin consideration of residential long-term care. The NYUCI counselor instead provided alternative, community-based long-term care options, including a visiting home health aide, whom Mrs. L began to use—reluctantly at first. However, the home health aide had prior experience working with persons with AD and was able to build a strong rapport with Mr. L. The improved relationship between Mrs. L and her son, and the provision of community-based support allowed Mrs. L to continue providing help to Mr. L at home for longer than she had imagined.

Case Study 2: "Using the REACH OUT Multicomponent Intervention"

Mr. S was the primary caregiver of his wife of 30 years who had later stage AD. Mr. S was fiercely protective of Mrs. S. During the first in-home session, the therapist was moved by Mr. S's tender and constant attention to Mrs. S. Although she could not respond and seemed completely oblivious to the content of the conversation, Mr. S. attempted to include her in the discourse and whispered protectively when speaking with the therapist about his concerns for Mrs. S's health.

Mr. S's devotion to his wife came at the expense of considerable personal sacrifice. He was with her constantly and had completely cut off a normally active social life as a result of Mrs. S's increased infirmity. Mr. S. would not entrust his wife to the care of an aide, and he left the house only to run brief errands while a trusted neighbor sat with Mrs. S. Mr. S had also failed to attend to his own health needs, having gone years without a checkup, and was showing visible signs of poor health.

Mr. S was isolated from most of his family. He had become so immersed in his caregiving duties that he had distanced himself from three of his four children, although he was closer to their daughter Marie, who lived nearby and visited occasionally. The consequences of Mr. S's negligence of his own health care was evident. He appeared physically exhausted, possibly depressed, and mentioned that at times his "ticker" would flutter.

The Resources for Enhancing Alzhiemer's Caregiver Health: Offering Useful Treatments (REACH OUT) Intervention: REACH OUT involves six hour-long therapeutic sessions spread over a 6-month period. In this case, the sessions took place in the home, but these meetings can occur in private practice or clinic settings. As many as two of the six sessions can be conducted by phone if scheduling problems are confronted. *Assessment*: An assessment battery is administered at the end of sessions 1 and 6, and it includes brief screens for caregiver burden, reaction to problem behaviors, depression, self-reported health, and perception of care-recipient health. *Intervention*: The goal of the intervention is to engage the primary caregiver in joint problem solving, with the objective of creating a written action plan that targets specific caregiving problems. Special emphasis is placed on the context in which the target problem occurs, and problem solving is used as a dynamic guiding strategy so that action plans are modified as necessary during the 6-month intervention period. *Application to Mr. S*: During session 1, and in tandem with the clinical interview, the therapist completes the standardized Risk Appraisal Measure (Czaja et al., 2009) that focuses on identifying problems with caregiver physical health, emotional well-being, stress level, and social isolation; dangers in the physical environment; and care-recipient problem behaviors. The therapist and Mr. S agreed that the problems to be addressed during intervention were physical health, emotional well-being, and social isolation. Mr. S was asked to prioritize the problems on the basis of severity, and his ranking determined the order in which the problems were addressed. *Action plan 1*: The therapist helped Mr. S recognize that not seeing a physician regarding his own health, and assuming responsibility for essentially all caregiving tasks, were undermining his own mental and physical health as well as his ability to sustain long-term caregiving. Elements of his written action plan included identifying an available physician, scheduling an appointment, ensuring that either his daughter or neighbor were available to watch over Mrs. S while he was at his appointment or during possible medical tests, filling prescriptions, and attending follow-up appointments. During each session, Mr. S committed to completing certain tasks in the action plan, which were monitored by the therapist at the next session or by a follow-up phone call. Mr. S's physician identified cardiac arrhythmia and depression, for which he prescribed medication and continued monitoring. *Action Plan 2*: The therapist helped Mr. S understand that his diminished emotional well-being and social isolation were closely intertwined. He explained that eliminating all pleasant social and solitary activities from one's life can, and often does, result in negative emotional (depression) and even physiological sequelae (compromised immune system). The second action plan involved the steps of pleasant events training—identifying pleasant events that Mr. S could do on his own and some he could do with Mrs. S, scheduling these events formally into his day, and finding respite care for Mrs. S to ensure he had time for these events. In addition to scheduling time for visiting the movie theater and bowling once a week, Mr. S decided that it was time to try to reestablish a relationship with his three semiestranged children. With the assistance of his daughter Marie, he set up a monthly informal dinner for the family. Although they were rarely all in attendance, scheduling this monthly dinner ensured increased contact with his children. An added positive effect was that the children saw firsthand the pressures of caregiving for their mother; consequently, they became more involved in providing Mr. S with emotional and physical support.

REFERENCES

Acton, G. J., & Kang, J. (2001). Interventions to reduce the burden of caregiving for an adult with dementia: A meta-analysis. *Research in Nursing & Health, 24,* 349–360.

Administration for Community Living (2014). Administration on Aging (AoA): Alzheimer's Disease Supportive Services Program. Retrieved from http://www.aoa.acl.gov/AoA_Programs/HPW/Alz_Grants/index.aspx.

Alzheimer's Association. (2014). 2014 Alzheimer's disease facts and figures. *Alzheimer's & Dementia, 10,* e47–e92.

Araki, T., Wake, R., Miyaoka, T., Kawakami, K., Nagahama, M., Furuya, M., et al. (2014). The effects of combined treatment of memantine and donepezil on Alzheimer's disease patients and its relationship with cerebral blood flow in the prefrontal area. *International Journal of Geriatric Psychiatry, 29,* 881–889.

Barnes, D. E., Mehling, W., Wu, E., Beristianos, M., Yaffe, K., Skultety, K., et al. (2015). Preventing loss of independence through exercise (PLIE): A pilot clinical trial in older adults with dementia. *PLoS One, 10,* e0113367.

Baumgarten, M., Battista, R. N., Infante-Rivard, C., Hanley, J. A., Becker, R., & Gauthier, S. (1992). The psychological and physical health of family members caring for an elderly person with dementia. *Journal of Clinical Epidemiology, 45,* 61–70.

Belle, S. H., Burgio, L., Burns, R., Coon, D., Czaja, S. J., Gallagher-Thompson, D., et al. (2006). Enhancing the quality of life of dementia caregivers from different ethnic or racial groups: A randomized, controlled trial. *Annals of Internal Medicine, 145,* 727–738.

Blom, M. M., Zarit, S. H., Groot Zwaaftink, R. B., Cuijpers, P., & Pot, A. M. (2015). Effectiveness of an Internet intervention for family caregivers of people with dementia: Results of a randomized controlled trial. *PLoS One, 10,* e0116622.

Boots, L. M., de Vugt, M. E., van Knippenberg, R. J., Kempen, G. I., & Verhey, F. R. (2014). A systematic review of Internet-based supportive interventions for caregivers of patients with dementia. *International Journal of Geriatric Psychiatry, 29,* 331–344.

Bouldin, E. D., & Andresen, E. (2010). *Caregiving across the United States: Caregivers of persons with Alzheimer's disease or dementia in 8 states and the District of Columbia: Data from the 2009 & 2010 Behavioral Risk Factor Surveillance System.* Chicago, IL: Alzheimer's Association.

Brodaty, H., & Arasaratnam, C. (2012). Meta-analysis of nonpharmacological interventions for neuropsychiatric symptoms of dementia. *The American Journal of Psychiatry, 169,* 946–953.

Brodaty, H., Green, A., & Koschera, A. (2003). Meta-analysis of psychosocial interventions for caregivers of people with dementia. *Journal of the American Geriatrics Society, 51,* 657–664.

Brodaty, H., Woodward, M., Boundy, K., Ames, D., Balshaw, R., & PRIME Study Group. (2014). Prevalence and predictors of burden in caregivers of people with dementia. *The American Journal of Geriatric Psychiatry, 22,* 756–765.

Burgio, L. D., Collins, I. B., Schmid, B., Wharton, T., McCallum, D., & Decoster, J. (2009). Translating the REACH caregiver intervention for use by area agency on aging personnel: The REACH OUT program. *The Gerontologist, 49,* 103–116.

Cheng, S. T., Lau, R. W., Mak, E. P., Ng, N. S., & Lam, L. C. (2014). Benefit-finding intervention for Alzheimer caregivers: Conceptual framework, implementation issues, and preliminary efficacy. *The Gerontologist, 54,* 1049–1058.

Chiu, M., Pauley, T., Wesson, V., Pushpakumar, D., & Sadavoy, J. (2015). Evaluation of a problem-solving (PS) techniques-based intervention for informal carers of patients with dementia receiving in-home care. *International Psychogeriatrics, 27,* 937–948.

Chodosh, J., Colaiaco, B. A., Connor, K. I., Cope, D. W., Liu, H., Ganz, D. A., et al. (2015). Dementia care management in an underserved community: The comparative effectiveness of two different approaches. *Journal of Aging and Health.* Still E-Pub ahead of print.

Cooke, D. D., McNally, L., Mulligan, K. T., Harrison, M. J., & Newman, S. P. (2001). Psychosocial interventions for caregivers of people with dementia: A systematic review. *Aging & Mental Health, 5,* 120–135.

Cooper, C., Balamurali, T. B., Selwood, A., & Livingston, G. (2007). A systematic review of intervention studies about anxiety in caregivers of people with dementia. *International Journal of Geriatric Psychiatry, 22,* 181–188.

Corbett, A., Stevens, J., Aarsland, D., Day, S., Moniz-Cook, E., Woods, R., et al. (2012). Systematic review of services providing information and/or advice to people with dementia and/or their caregivers. *International Journal of Geriatric Psychiatry, 27,* 628–636.

Cove, J., Jacobi, N., Donovan, H., Orrell, M., Stott, J., & Spector, A. (2014). Effectiveness of weekly cognitive stimulation therapy for people with dementia and the additional impact of enhancing cognitive stimulation therapy with a carer training program. *Clinical Interventions in Aging, 9,* 2143–2150.

Covinsky, K. E., & Johnston, C. B. (2006). Envisioning better approaches for dementia care. *Annals of Internal Medicine, 145,* 780–781.

Czaja, S. J., Gitlin, L. N., Schulz, R., Zhang, S., Burgio, L. D., Stevens, A. B., ... Gallagher-Thompson, D. (2009). Development of the Risk Appraisal Measure: A brief screen to identify risk areas and guide interventions for dementia caregivers. *Journal of the American Geriatrics Society, 57,* 1064–1072.

Döpp, C. M., Graff, M. J., Teerenstra, S., Olde Rikkert, M. G., Nijhuis-van der Sanden, M. W., & Vernooij-Dassen, M. J. (2014). Effectiveness of a training package for implementing a community-based occupational therapy program in dementia: A cluster randomized controlled trial. *Clinical Rehabilitation.* e-Pub ahead of print.

Ducharme, F., Lachance, L., Levesque, L., Zarit, S. H., & Kergoat, M. J. (2015). Maintaining the potential of a psycho-educational program: Efficacy of a booster session after an intervention offered family caregivers at disclosure of a relative's dementia diagnosis. *Aging & Mental Health, 19,* 207–216.

Egan, M., Berube, D., Racine, G., Leonard, C., & Rochon, E. (2010). Methods to enhance verbal communication between individuals with Alzheimer's disease and their formal and informal caregivers: A systematic review. *International Journal of Alzheimer's Disease, 2010.* See http://www.ncbi.nlm.nih.gov/pmc/articles/PMC2925413/

Elvish, R., Lever, S., Johnstone, J., Cawley, R., & Keady, J. (2013). Psychological interventions for carers of people with dementia: A systematic review of quantitative and qualitative evidence. *Counselling and Psychotherapy Research, 13,* 106–125.

Epstein-Lubow, G., Gaudiano, B., Darling, E., Hinckley, M., Tremont, G., Kohn, R., et al. (2012). Differences in depression severity in family caregivers of hospitalized individuals with dementia and family caregivers of outpatients with dementia. *The American Journal of Geriatric Psychiatry, 20,* 815–819.

Fisher, G. G., Franks, M. M., Plassman, B. L., Brown, S. L., Potter, G. G., Llewellyn, D., et al. (2011). Caring for individuals with dementia and cognitive impairment, not dementia: Findings from the Aging, Demographics, and Memory Study. *Journal of the American Geriatrics Society, 59*(3), 488–494.

Flint, A. J. (1995). Effects of respite care on patients with dementia and their caregivers. *International Psychogeriatrics, 7*(4), 505–517.

Fortune (2013). *Fortune 500 2013.* Retrieved from http://fortune.com/fortune500/2013/.

Gallagher-Thompson, D., Tzuang, M., Hinton, L., Alvarez, P., Rengifo, J., Valverde, I., et al. (2015). Effectiveness of a fotonovela for reducing depression and stress in Latino dementia family caregivers. *Alzheimer Disease and Associated Disorders, 29,* 146–153.

Gaugler, J. E., & Kane, R. L. (2015). The perfect storm? The future of family caregiving. In J. E. Gaugler, & R. L. Kane (Eds.), *Family caregiving in the new normal.* (pp. 357–380). San Diego, CA: Elsevier.

Gaugler, J. E., Reese, M., & Mittelman, M. S. (2015). Effects of the Minnesota adaptation of the NYU Caregiver Intervention on primary subjective stress of adult child caregivers of persons with dementia. *The Gerontologist.* E-Pub ahead of print.

Gaugler, J. E., Yu, F., Krichbaum, K., & Wyman, J. F. (2009). Predictors of nursing home admission for persons with dementia. *Medical Care, 47*(2), 191–198.

Gitlin, L. N., & Hodgson, N. (2015). Caregivers as therapeutic agents in dementia care: The evidence-base for interventions supporting their role. In J. E. Gaugler, &

R. L. Kane (Eds.), *Family caregiving in the new normal* (pp. 305–356). Philadelphia, PA: Elsevier.

Gitlin, L. N., Marx, K., Stanley, I. H., & Hodgson, N. (2015). Translating evidence-based dementia caregiving interventions into practice: State-of-the-science and next steps. *The Gerontologist, 55*(2), 210–226.

Gitlin, L. N., & Schulz, R. (2012). Family caregiving of older adults. In T. R. Prohaska, L. A. Anderson & R. H. Binsotck (Eds.), *Public health for an aging society.* (pp. 181–204). Baltimore, MD: Johns Hopkins University Press.

Godwin, K. M., Mills, W. L., Anderson, J. A., & Kunik, M. E. (2013). Technology-driven interventions for caregivers of persons with dementia: A systematic review. *American Journal of Alzheimer's Disease and Other Dementias, 28*(3), 216–222.

Gonzalez, E. W., Polansky, M., Lippa, C. F., Gitlin, L. N., & Zauszniewski, J. A. (2014). Enhancing resourcefulness to improve outcomes in family caregivers and persons with Alzheimer's disease: A pilot randomized trial. *International Journal of Alzheimer's Disease.* See http://www.ncbi.nlm.nih.gov/pmc/articles/PMC4195254/

Goy, E., Freeman, M., & Kansagara, D. (2010). *A systematic evidence review of interventions for nonprofessional caregivers of individuals with dementia.* VA-ESP project #05-225. Portland, OR: Portland VA Medical Center.

Griffin, J. M., Meis, L., Greer, N., Jensen, A., MacDonald, R., Rutks, I., et al. (2013). *Effectiveness of family and caregiver interventions on patient outcomes among adults with cancer or memory-related disorders: A systematic review.* Washington, DC: Department of Veterans Affairs.

Jensen, M., Agbata, I. N., Canavan, M., & McCarthy, G. (2015). Effectiveness of educational interventions for informal caregivers of individuals with dementia residing in the community: Systematic review and meta-analysis of randomised controlled trials. *International Journal of Geriatric Psychiatry, 30*, 130–143.

Jones, C., Edwards, R. T., & Hounsome, B. (2012). A systematic review of the cost-effectiveness of interventions for supporting informal caregivers of people with dementia residing in the community. *International Psychogeriatrics, 24*, 6–18.

Kasper, J. D., Freedman, V. A., & Spillman, B. C. (2014). *Disability and care needs of older Americans by dementia status: An analysis of the 2011 National Health and Aging Trends Study.* Washington, DC: U.S. Department of Health and Human Services, Assistant Secretary for Planning and Evaluation, Office of Disability, Aging, and Long-Term Care Policy.

Kessler, R. C., Chiu, W. T., Demler, O., Merikangas, K. R., & Walters, E. E. (2005). Prevalence, severity, and comorbidity of 12-month DSM-IV disorders in the National Comorbidity Survey replication. *Archives of General Psychiatry, 62*, 617–627.

Knight, B. G., Lutzky, S. M., & Macofsky-Urban, F. (1993). A meta-analytic review of interventions for caregiver distress: Recommendations for future research. *The Gerontologist, 33*, 240–248.

Lingler, J. H., Martire, L. M., & Schulz, R. (2005). Caregiver-specific outcomes in anti-dementia clinical drug trials: A systematic review and meta-analysis. *Journal of the American Geriatrics Society, 53*(6), 983–990.

Llanque, S. M., & Enriquez, M. (2012). Interventions for Hispanic caregivers of patients with dementia: A review of the literature. *American Journal of Alzheimer's Disease and Other Dementias, 27*, 23–32.

Logsdon, R. G., Pike, K. C., Korte, L., & Goehring, C. (2014). Memory care and wellness services: Efficacy of specialized dementia care in adult day services. *The Gerontologist.* E-Pub ahead of print.

Maayan, N., Soares-Weiser, K., & Lee, H. (2014). Respite care for people with dementia and their carers. *The Cochrane Database of Systematic Reviews, 1,* CD004396.

Martin-Carrasco, M., Ballesteros-Rodriguez, J., Dominguez-Panchon, A. I., Munoz-Hermoso, P., & Gonzalez-Fraile, E. (2014). Interventions for caregivers of patients with dementia. *Actas Espanolas De Psiquiatria, 42*(6), 300–314.

Maslow, K. (2012). *Translating innovation to impact: Evidence-based interventions to support people with Alzheimer's disease and their caregiver at home and in the community.* Washington, D.C.: Administration on Aging.

Mason, A., Weatherly, H., Spilsbury, K., Arksey, H., Golder, S., Adamson, J., et al. (2007). A systematic review of the effectiveness and cost-effectiveness of different models of community-based respite care for frail older people and their carers. *Health Technology Assessment, 11,* 1–157, iii.

Mausbach, B. T. (2014). Caregiving. *The American Journal of Geriatric Psychiatry, 22,* 743–745.

Mausbach, B. T., Chattillion, E. A., Roepke, S. K., Patterson, T. L., & Grant, I. (2013). A comparison of psychosocial outcomes in elderly Alzheimer caregivers and non-caregivers. *The American Journal of Geriatric Psychiatry, 21,* 5–13.

McKechnie, V., Barker, C., & Stott, J. (2014). Effectiveness of computer-mediated interventions for informal carers of people with dementia: A systematic review. *International Psychogeriatrics, 26,* 1619–1637.

McNally, S., Ben-Shlomo, Y., & Newman, S. (1999). The effects of respite care on informal carers' well-being: A systematic review. *Disability and Rehabilitation, 21,* 1–14.

Morgan, R. O., Bass, D. M., Judge, K. S., Liu, C. F., Wilson, N., Snow, A. L., et al. (2015). A break-even analysis for dementia care collaboration: Partners in Dementia Care. *Journal of General Internal Medicine, 30,* 804–809.

Napoles, A. M., Chadiha, L., Eversley, R., & Moreno-John, G. (2010). Reviews: Developing culturally sensitive dementia caregiver interventions: Are we there yet? *American Journal of Alzheimer's Disease & Other Dementias, 25,* 389–406.

National Alliance for Caregiving and American Association of Retired Persons. (2009). *Caregiving in the U.S. 2009.* Bethesda, MD: National Alliance of Caregiving.

National Alliance for Caregiving/AARP. (2009). *Caregiving in the U.S.: Unpublished data analyzed under contract for the Alzheimer's Association.* Chicago, IL: The Alzheimer's Association.

Newcomer, R., Spitalny, M., Fox, P., & Yordi, C. (1999). Effects of the Medicare Alzheimer's Disease Demonstration Evaluation on the use of community-based services. *Health Services Research, 34,* 645–667.

Olazarán, J., Reisberg, B., Clare, L., Cruz, I., Pena-Casanova, J., Del Ser, T., et al. (2010). Nonpharmacological therapies in Alzheimer's disease: A systematic review of efficacy. *Dementia & Geriatric Cognitive Disorders, 30,* 161–178.

Orgeta, V., & Miranda-Castillo, C. (2014). Does physical activity reduce burden in carers of people with dementia? A literature review. *International Journal of Geriatric Psychiatry, 29,* 771–783.

Parker, D., Mills, S., & Abbey, J. (2008). Effectiveness of interventions that assist care-givers to support people with dementia living in the community: A systematic review. *International Journal of Evidence-Based Healthcare, 6*, 137–172.

Peacock, S. C., & Forbes, D. A. (2003). Interventions for caregivers of persons with dementia: A systematic review. *Canadian Journal of Nursing Research, 35*, 88–107.

Peterson, J. C., Czajkowski, S., Charlson, M. E., Link, A. R., Wells, M. T., Isen, A. M., … Jobe, J. B. (2013). Translating basic behavioral and social science research to clini-cal application: The EVOLVE mixed methods approach. *Journal of Consulting and Clinical Psychology, 81*(2), 217–230.

Pinquart, M., & Sörensen, S. (2003). Associations of stressors and uplifts of caregiv-ing with caregiver burden and depressive mood: A meta-analysis. *The Journals of Gerontology Series B, Psychological Sciences and Social Sciences, 58*, P112–P128.

Pinquart, M., & Sörensen, S. (2006). Helping caregivers of persons with demen-tia: Which interventions work and how large are their effects? *International Psychogeriatrics, 18*, 577–595.

Powell, J., Chiu, T., & Eysenbach, G. (2008). A systematic review of networked tech-nologies supporting carers of people with dementia. *Journal of Telemedicine and Telecare, 14*, 154–156.

Remington, R., Bechtel, C., Larsen, D., Samar, A., Doshanjh, L., Fishman, P., et al. (2015). A phase II randomized clinical trial of a nutritional formulation for cogni-tion and mood in Alzheimer's disease. *Journal of Alzheimer's Disease, 45*, 395–405.

Rockwood, K., Fay, S., Song, X., MacKnight, C., & Gorman, M. (2006). Attainment of treatment goals by people with Alzheimer's disease receiving galantamine: A ran-domized controlled trial. *Canadian Medical Association Journal, 174*, 1099–1105. doi:10.1503/cmaj.051432

Schoenmakers, B., Buntinx, F., & De Lepeleire, J. (2009). Can pharmacological treat-ment of behavioural disturbances in elderly patients with dementia lower the bur-den of their family caregiver? *Family Practice, 26*, 279–286.

Schoenmakers, B., Buntinx, F., & DeLepeleire, J. (2010). Supporting the dementia fam-ily caregiver: The effect of home care intervention on general well-being. *Aging & Mental Health, 14*, 44–56.

Schulz, R., Burgio, L., Burns, R., Eisdorfer, C., Gallagher-Thompson, D., Gitlin, L. N., et al. (2003). Resources for Enhancing Alzheimer's Caregiver Health (REACH): Overview, site-specific outcomes, and future directions. *The Gerontologist, 43*(4), 514–520.

Schulz, R., O'Brien, A. T., Bookwala, J., & Fleissner, K. (1995). Psychiatric and physi-cal morbidity effects of dementia caregiving: Prevalence, correlates, and causes. *The Gerontologist, 35*, 771–791.

Schulz, R., O'Brien, A., Czaja, S., Ory, M., Norris, R., Martire, L. M., et al. (2002). Dementia caregiver intervention research: In search of clinical significance. *Gerontologist, 42*, 589–602.

Seeher, K., Low, L. F., Reppermund, S., & Brodaty, H. (2013). Predictors and outcomes for caregivers of people with mild cognitive impairment: A systematic literature review. *Alzheimer's & Dementia, 9*, 346–355.

Selwood, A., Johnston, K., Katona, C., Lyketsos, C., & Livingston, G. (2007). Systematic review of the effect of psychological interventions on family caregivers of people with dementia. *Journal of Affective Disorders, 101*, 75–89.

Shaw, C., McNamara, R., Abrams, K., Cannings-John, R., Hood, K., Longo, M., et al. (2009). Systematic review of respite care in the frail elderly. *Health Technology Assessment, 13*, 1–224.

Smits, C. H., de Lange, J., Droes, R. M., Meiland, F., Vernooij-Dassen, M., & Pot, A. M. (2007). Effects of combined intervention programmes for people with dementia living at home and their caregivers: A systematic review. *International Journal of Geriatric Psychiatry, 22*, 1181–1193.

Sörensen, S., Pinquart, M., & Duberstein, P. (2002). How effective are interventions with caregivers? An updated meta-analysis. *Gerontologist, 42*(3), 356–372.

Spijker, A., Vernooij-Dassen, M., Vasse, E., Adang, E., Wollersheim, H., Grol, R., et al. (2008). Effectiveness of nonpharmacological interventions in delaying the institutionalization of patients with dementia: A meta-analysis. *Journal of the American Geriatrics Society, 56*, 1116–1128.

Spillman, B., Wolff, J., Freedman, V., & Kasper, J. D. (2014). *Informal caregiving for older Americans: An analysis of the 2011 National Health and Aging Trends Study.* Washington, DC: Office of the Secretary for Planning and Evaluation, Department of Health and Human Services.

Tanner, J. A., Black, B. S., Johnston, D., Hess, E., Leoutsakos, J. M., Gitlin, L. N., et al. (2014). A randomized controlled trial of a community-based dementia care coordination intervention: Effects of MIND at home on caregiver outcomes. *The American Journal of Geriatric Psychiatry, 23*, 391–402.

Thivierge, S., Jean, L., & Simard, M. (2014). A randomized cross-over controlled study on cognitive rehabilitation of instrumental activities of daily living in Alzheimer disease. *The American Journal of Geriatric Psychiatry, 22*, 1188–1199.

Thompson, C. A., Spilsbury, K., Hall, J., Birks, Y., Barnes, C., & Adamson, J. (2007). Systematic review of information and support interventions for caregivers of people with dementia. *BMC Geriatrics, 7*, 18.

University of Michigan's Institute of Gerontology & the National Association of Chronic Disease Directors. (2009). *Implementing a Community-Based Program for Dementia Caregivers: An Action Guide using REACH OUT.* National Association of Chronic Disease Directors, Atlanta, GA.

Van't Leven, N., Prick, A. E., Groenewoud, J. G., Roelofs, P. D., de Lange, J., & Pot, A. M. (2013). Dyadic interventions for community-dwelling people with dementia and their family caregivers: A systematic review. *International Psychogeriatrics, 25*, 1581–1603.

Vernooij-Dassen, M., Draskovic, I., McCleery, J., & Downs, M. (2011). Cognitive reframing for carers of people with dementia. *The Cochrane Database of Systematic Reviews, Nov. 9 (11)*, CD005318.

Wethington, E., & Burgio, L. D. (2015). Translational research on caregiving: Missing links in the translation process. In J. E. Gaugler, & R. L. Kane (Eds.), *Family caregiving in the new normal.* (pp. 193-210). Philadelphia, PA: Elsevier.

Zarit, S., & Femia, E. (2008). Behavioral and psychosocial interventions for family caregivers. *American Journal of Nursing, 108*(9 Suppl.), 47–53.

3

Family Caregivers of Stroke Survivors

JULIA M. P. PORITZ, TIMOTHY R. ELLIOTT,
AND KLAUS PFEIFFER ■

Stroke is one of the leading causes of disability in the United States (Rosamond et al., 2007). Many stroke survivors subsequently experience persistent impairments that can include cognitive and neuromuscular dysfunction (ranging from memory problems to paralysis, hemiplegia, and weakness), vision problems, communication deficits (e.g., aphasia), emotional lability, and depression (Hackett, Yapa, Parag, & Anderson, 2005; Lai, Studenski, Duncan, & Perera, 2002), making them dependent on care and help in their daily living. Family members provide the majority of care and assistance received by stroke survivors. The burden and distress experienced by many of these caregivers has been recognized for some time. A sizeable amount of literature documents many of the problems experienced by these caregivers and the characteristics of those who are at risk for depression, distress, and poor health.

In this chapter we provide an overview of the issues and problems encountered by many caregivers of stroke survivors, and we describe some of their unique needs and challenges. We then review studies of caregiver interventions that appeared in the peer-reviewed literature from 2000 to 2013. We also attend to existing, major reviews of the intervention literature that were published during this time frame. We consider these interventions from the perspective of a chronic care model, evaluating the implementation and effectiveness of community and home-based programs. We close with brief case studies that illustrate elements of evidence-based practice.

STROKE CAREGIVER NEEDS, ISSUES, AND CHALLENGES

Consistent with caregivers for other health conditions, women are more likely than men to assume the role of caregiver after a stroke by a family member; wives of men who incur stroke are the most common (King & Semik, 2006; White, Mayo, Hanley, & Wood-Dauphinee, 2003). Although distress after stroke is a common and understandable occurrence among caregivers, caregiver adjustment is best understood as a dynamic process over time. Despite this understanding, only a few studies have examined the adjustment of family caregivers of stroke survivors beyond the initial year of caregiving (Gaugler, 2010). For our purposes, it is helpful to consider the varying caregiver needs that occur in five phases following stroke: (a) event/diagnosis, (b) stabilization during acute care, (c) preparation during acute care and in-patient rehabilitation, (d) implementation during the first few months after the patient returns home ("learning the ropes"), and (e) long-lasting adaptation in the home and community (Cameron & Gignac, 2008). Much of the extant literature concerns the issues and needs family caregivers face during acute and postacute care, during rehabilitation, and upon return to the community. These are critical periods during which family members assume a caregiver role while simultaneously having considerable interaction with health and rehabilitation staff as they provide prescribed services.

Event, Diagnosis, Stabilization, and Rehabilitation

For many stroke caregivers, hospitalization and the first few months after hospitalization are the most difficult time during in the first 2 years of caregiving. Early stroke caregiving stress often consists of uncertainty, new responsibilities, and dealing with the stroke survivor's impairments and emotions. Information about the patient's health is very important to stroke caregivers during the acute rehabilitation phase, perhaps more so than during the postacute rehabilitation phase (King & Semik, 2006). Stroke caregivers need information, support, and accessibility to the patient and the healthcare professional. Stroke caregivers need healthcare professionals to take the time to answer their questions honestly; having consistent access to a specific "contact" person is also valued (i.e., it is important to talk to the same nurse each time [Hafsteinsdóttir, Vergunst, Lindeman, & Schuurmans, 2011]). In the acute and postacute setting, caregivers want information about stroke in general, as well as resources that provide information on preventing recurrent strokes, communicating problems, coping with problems, preventing the physical and emotional deterioration of the stroke survivor, and handling the stroke survivor's changing moods.

Unmet psychosocial needs often concern issues with the healthcare team. In one study, a majority of caregivers wanted written information about stroke, its concomitants, and caregiving while their care recipient was hospitalized, but of those caregivers studied, less than half received any written information (Hoffman, McKenna, Worrall, & Read, 2004). Family members report they were inadequately prepared for caregiving and their role as a caregiver was taken for granted by healthcare staff regardless of their age, health, and other characteristics (Smith, Lawrence, Kerr, Langhorne, & Lees, 2004). One study found that stroke caregivers experienced difficulties speaking with the healthcare team when needed and were concerned that their input was not considered by the healthcare team. However, 90% of stroke caregivers reported being satisfied with the support they received from family and friends. The emotional needs of stroke caregivers included dealing with stress and anxiety, sadness and grief, and fear of another stroke. Practical needs consisted of caring for the stroke survivor and changing their usual routine and lifestyle (MacIsaac, Harrison, Buchanan, & Hopman, 2011). Stroke caregivers may be more satisfied with their community network support and their familial support during the postacute rehabilitation phase than they are during the acute rehabilitation phase (Kim & Moon, 2007).

Caregivers' needs vary with treatment settings. A South Korean study found that caregivers whose stroke survivors are being treated in inpatient facilities find health information more important than caregivers whose stroke survivors are being treated in outpatient clinics or in a geriatric day hospital (Kim & Moon, 2007). Caregivers whose stroke survivors are being treated in a geriatric day hospital report greater satisfaction with health information, emotional information, instrumental information, professional information, community network support, and familial support than caregivers whose stroke survivors are being treated in inpatient facilities or outpatient clinics (Kim & Moon, 2007).

Studies relying on a liberal indicator of depression suggest that more than one third of family caregivers may be at risk for major depression disorder within days of discharge from rehabilitation (Grant, Bartolucci, Elliott, & Giger, 2000; Grant, Weaver, Elliott, Bartolucci, & Giger, 2004b). Depression observed during hospitalization and rehabilitation may be the best single indicator of caregiver depression 6 months and 18 months after discharge (Berg, Palomaki, Lonnqvist, & Kaste, 2005).

Return to the Community and Initial Adjustment

For most caregivers, the first month after hospital discharge is the most stressful period as the limitations of the stroke survivor become salient at home (Grant, Glandon, Elliott, Giger, & Weaver, 2004a). The main issues and challenges that stroke caregivers face during the first month after hospital discharge are concerns about safety of the stroke care recipient (e.g., potential for falling as a result of stroke survivor impulsivity, weakness, dizziness), functional deficits of the stroke care recipient (e.g., dressing, bathing, walking, transferring), and managing cognitive, behavioral, and emotional changes in the stroke care recipient (Grant et al., 2004a). These three issues and challenges continue to be salient throughout the second and third months after hospital discharge. It is important to note that caregivers have reported experiencing improvements in these areas by the end of the second month and into the third month (Grant, Glandon, Elliott, Giger, & Weaver, 2006b).

A systematic review of educational needs after hospitalization found that stroke caregivers wanted information about preventing future strokes, dealing with communication problems, coping with problems, preventing the physical and emotional deterioration of the stroke survivor, and handling the stroke survivor's changing moods. Other needs included information about preventing falls, maintaining adequate nutrition, staying active, managing stress, and dealing with emotions and mood changes (Hafsteinsdóttir et al., 2011). Qualitative research has found that, during this time, caregivers experience an array of problems with a care recipient, including dealing with interpersonal issues, managing mood and behavioral disturbances, and assisting with activities of daily living (e.g., bowel incontinence [Grant et al., 2004a; Haley et al., 2009; King, Ainsworth, Ronen, & Hartke, 2010]). Despite the well-known difficulties caregivers have with these problems, caregivers in the study conducted by Smith and colleagues (2004) believed healthcare staff often choose to ignore these issues during hospitalization.

After the return to the community, a substantial percentage of caregivers are unable to maintain employment outside the home (Ko, Aycock, & Clark, 2007). Those lacking in social support who also possess a pessimistic view of solving problems are more likely to have more depressive symptoms during the first 13 weeks postdischarge (Grant, Elliott, Weaver, Glandon, & Giger, 2006a). However, the same study also found that a more optimistic approach to solving problems was associated with positive changes in personal health during this period. Indeed, in a review of the available literature concerning stroke caregiver adjustment over time, Gaugler (2010) observed that few studies actually examine changes in adjustment over an extended time period, and there may be unique characteristics of those who do and do not experience adjustment problems over time. Research concerning positive adjustment over time is lacking, but those at risk for increased burden, stress, and poor adjustment should be identified as early as possible before discharge as well as after their return to the community.

Stress levels for stroke caregivers and stroke survivors have been correlated positively throughout the first year after hospital discharge. Stress levels for both members of the caregiving dyad were at a moderate level and had decreased by the end of the first year, but stroke survivors experienced a greater decrease in stress than stroke caregivers. Predictors of lower levels of stroke caregiver stress during the first year after hospital discharge include being older, a greater number of people in the caregiver's support network, greater caregiving preparedness, use of a reframing coping style, and higher functioning of the stroke survivor. Predictors of higher levels of stroke caregiver stress during the first year after hospital discharge include being female, using a passive coping style, and having a lower self-rated health status at the time the stroke survivor is discharged from the hospital (Ostwald, Bernal, Cron, & Godwin, 2009).

Other studies suggest a complementary—if not reciprocal—relationship of caregiver distress and well-being to stroke survivor emotional adjustment and functioning (Grant et al., 2013; Perrin, Heesacker, Stidham, Rittman, & Gonzalez-Rothi, 2008). Although causal effects are difficult to disentangle, these studies indicate that stroke survivors have more emotional difficulties, physical impairments, and isolation as caregiver distress increases during the first year after discharge. Of the various factors that predicted stroke survivor adjustment significantly after return to the community, Klinedinst and colleagues (2009) found caregiver depression at baseline was the only clinical predictor that could be considered potentially modifiable.

Long-Term Adjustment

Stroke caregiving stress later during the stroke disease trajectory consists of a plateau in the survivor's functioning, caregiver and survivor health problems, finances, and dealing with the caregiver's emotions. Balancing work and caregiving is a stressor that is present in both the early and later stages of stroke caregiving; but, overall, the specific difficulties of stroke caregiving change over time and there is individual variation in needs as well (King & Semik, 2006). Stroke caregivers report greater burden and lower overall quality of life when compared with age- and sex-matched population norms during the first 2 years of caregiving (White et al., 2003). White et al. (2003) found caregivers experienced an average of four to five physical symptoms each month. The most frequently reported of these physical symptoms were feeling tired, headaches, stiff joints, and trouble falling asleep. Although other evidence indicates that burden may decrease during the first 3 years of caregiving, this work also found caregiver–care recipient dyads experienced steady and significant decreases in interpersonal and social relations (Visser-Meily et al., 2009). A recent study found a population-based sample of family caregivers had significantly poorer adjustment on several psychosocial dimensions at nine months post-stroke than a matched non-caregiving control group, but by three years these differences dissipated (Haley, Roth, Hovater, & Clay, 2015). This work illustrates the value of longitudinal studies of population-based samples in understanding the long-term adjustment of family caregivers.

Cultural influences on caregiver adjustment range from the subtle to the obvious throughout the literature. Across cultures and nations, financial issues loom prominently in the burden reported by caregivers (Lurbe-Puerto, Leandro, & Baumann, 2012; Mak, Mackenzie, & Lui, 2007). Deteriorations in personal health can vary by nationality (Lurbe-Puerto et al., 2012), and by corresponding disparities and differences in health care and support services. Caregiver needs vary over time among caregivers of different nationalities, consistent with findings from studies of American samples. Cultural values such as *familismo*, the value of placing family over the individual, may account for differences observed in time spent in caregiving, support received from other family members and a larger social network, and emotional reactions to care-recipient adjustment in comparisons of Puerto Rican caregivers with white and black caregivers (Hinojosa & Rittman, 2007; Perrin, Heesacker, Uthe, & Rittman, 2010). Collectively, the available literature indicates that individually tailored, culturally sensitive interventions and services for caregivers are warranted.

SYSTEMATIC REVIEWS AND META-ANALYSES
OF THE INTERVENTION RESEARCH

Several systematic reviews of the intervention literature concerning family caregivers of stroke survivors have appeared during the past 13 years, and several of these are listed in the evidence table (Table 3.1). In one of the more influential reviews (cited 123 times to date, according to Google Scholar), Visser-Meily and colleagues examined the effectiveness of different types of interventions for caregivers of stroke survivors: provision of specialist services, psychoeducation, counseling, and social support from peers (Visser-Meily, van Heugten, Post, Schepers, & Lindeman, 2005). Of the 22 studies reviewed, 10 reported positive results on one or more of the outcome measures used, including a significant reduction in depression, improvement of knowledge, improvement in satisfaction with care, improvement in family functioning, improvement in quality of life, better problem-solving skills, more social activities in daily life, more social support, and less burden. Four of the six psychoeducation studies had positive results, three of the four counseling studies had positive results, and the only study that concerned social support from peers study had no positive results. These researchers concluded that they could not recommend a specific type of intervention that is most beneficial for stroke caregivers. However, they suggested that future research base interventions on the needs of caregivers according to a caregiver needs assessment, as opposed to providing a "prepackaged" intervention. They also asserted that counseling interventions seem to be promising because they have been shown to be effective and because they focus on the needs of caregivers specifically, as opposed to focusing on the needs of both stroke survivors and stroke caregivers.

A substantive review by Liu and colleagues specifically examined interventions for caregivers that tried to improve their problem-solving skills across a variety of formats, including training, education, and support (Liu, Ross, & Thompson, 2005). Eleven studies met the criteria for review, six of which were randomized controlled trials (RCTs). Although the authors concluded the overall evidence supported the use of problem-solving approaches to treat caregiver depression, this literature was plagued by a lack of theoretical grounding, poor operational definitions of "problem solving," and lack of diversity in the samples. Moreover, all the studies were confined to the early "poststroke" phase of caregiving.

Only two of the reviews listed in Table 3.1 featured meta-analytic procedures. The meta-analysis by Lee, Soeken, and Picot (2007) was restricted to studies written in English that used the Short Form Health Study-36 (Ware & Sherbourne, 1992) to measure caregiver adjustment, resulting in only four studies for analysis. All four were RCTs; two were studies of education programs and two studied support programs. Although the effect sizes provided evidence for efficacy, the strict criteria for inclusion and the small number of studies limit the

Table 3.1. Intervention Studies for Family Caregivers of Stroke Patients

Author (Year)	Sample (Baseline)	Racial/Cultural Factors			Design	Interventions	Results	Evaluation
		Diversity of Study Sample	Cultural Diversity Training Received?	Comparisons of Racial/Cultural Factors				
					INTERVENTION STUDIES			
Bakas et al., 2009b	50 caregivers; phase 4	25% black, 73% white, 2% other	NR	NR	RCT	TASK	Increased optimism, and decreased task difficulty and threat appraisal were noted.	Caregiver needs met earlier in intervention group than in attention control group.
Bakas et al., 2009a	40 caregivers; phase 4	NR	NR	NR	Program evaluation	TASK	Content validity rated as 4.56 points on a scale of 1 to 5 points. Satisfaction with TASK rated as 4.41 points on a scale of 1 to 5 points.	Satisfaction with TASK (4.41 points) was significantly greater statistically than satisfaction with attention control (3.94 points).
Bjorkdahl et al., 2007	35 caregivers; phases 4 and 5	NR, but study took place in Sweden	NR	NR	RCT	Home setting intervention; day rehabilitation	No statistically significant differences in caregiver burden between the two interventions were noted.	There was a tendency for lower burden in stroke caregivers to be evidenced immediately after a 3-week home-setting intervention.
Grant et al, 2002	74 caregivers; phase 4	74% white, 26% black	NR	NR	RCT; three-group, repeated-measures experimental design	Social problem-solving telephone intervention	Improved problem-solving skills, greater caregiver preparedness, and decreased depression were noted.	Effectiveness may be the result of addressing unique caregiver concerns as opposed to using a standardized protocol.

Study	Sample	Race/Ethnicity		Design	Intervention	Results	Conclusion
Hartke & King, 2003	88 caregivers; phase 5	81% white, 15% black, 4% other	NR	RCT	Structured psychoeducational telephone support group intervention	There was a statistically significant reduction in stress, but no statistically significant changes in depression, burden, loneliness, or competence.	Intervention was effective in preventing accumulation of burden over time, but it was ineffective in reducing burden over time.
Kim et al., 2012	73 caregivers; phases 3 and 4	NR, but study was conducted in South Korea	NR	Repeated-measures quasi-experimental design	Hospital-based group intervention, home-based individual telecare intervention	There was a statistically significant decrease in caregiver burden in the home-based individual telecare intervention group.	Home-based individual telecare intervention was more effective in reducing caregiver burden than hospital-based group intervention.
King et al., 2007	30 caregivers; phases 3 and 4	83% white, 10% Hispanic, 7% black	NR	Single-group repeated-measures design	CPSI	A statistically significant improvement in depression, preparedness, and anxiety was noted; however, caregiver burden and taking care of one's own needs declined over time.	Effectiveness of intervention was attributed to it being tailored to each individual caregiver.
King et al., 2012	255 caregivers; phases 3, 4, and 5	64% white, 36% nonwhite	NR	RCT	CPSI	Statistically significant changes in depression, life change, and health were observed at 3 months, but faded by 6 months.	A second round of intervention was recommended because caregiver needs change over time.
Oupra et al., 2010	140 caregivers; phases 1–4	NR, but study conducted in Thailand	NR	Two-group nonrandomized experimental design	SELF	The SELF group had a better quality of life and lower levels of strain than the control group.	Providing education and support can reduce strain and improve quality of life.

(continued)

Table 3.1. CONTINUED

Author (Year)	Sample (Baseline)	Racial/Cultural Factors			Design	Interventions	Results	Evaluation
		Diversity of Study Sample	Cultural Diversity Training Received?	Comparisons of Racial/Cultural Factors				
Perrin et al., 2010	89 caregivers; phases 3 and 4	16.3% African American/ black, 1.6% Asian American, 16.4% non-Hispanic white/white, 62.3% Hispanic/ Latino Puerto Rican, 3.3% Hispanic/ Latino Mexican	Yes; primary tool of intervention is a guidebook with two different versions designed specifically for Mainland and Puerto Rican stroke caregivers	NR	Experimental design with random assignment of participants to either the treatment group or the control group	TAP, consisting of skill development, education, and supportive problem solving	At 3 months, the treatment group had lower depression scores than the control group when controlling for baseline differences. A decrease in strain in the treatment group and an increase in strain in the control group were observed.	TAP may be an effective intervention during the transition from hospital to home. Caregivers in the treatment group were highly satisfied with the intervention; caregiver satisfaction was associated with reduced depression and strain.
Pfeiffer et al., 2014	122 caregivers; phase 5	82% native German, 8% ethnic German repatriates from Eastern European states, 10% of various European migration backgrounds	NR	NR	RCT	Problem-solving intervention	Statistically significant improvements were noted in caregiver depression and competence at the 3-month and 12-month assessments, but not in caregiver problem-solving ability.	The effects of the intervention on caregiver outcomes were most pronounced during the first 3 months of intervention.
Schure et al., 2006	127 caregivers; phase 5	NR	NR	NR	Program evaluation	Group program intervention, home visit program intervention	Overall, stroke caregivers expressed a preference for the group program intervention.	Intervention type should be matched to the caregiver based on caregiver preference or screening procedures.

Shyu et al., 2010	158 caregivers; phases 4 and 5	NR, but study took place in Taiwan	NR	RCT	Telephone call and home visit intervention	Intervention did not improve stroke caregivers' quality of life.	The intervention focus on preparedness and balancing competing needs was ineffective.
Smith et al., 2012	32 caregivers; phase 4	NR	NR	RCT	Web-based psychoeducational intervention	Depression was significantly lower statistically for the intervention group than for the control group.	Intervention targeted at stroke caregivers specifically, as opposed to stroke caregivers and survivors, was effective.
Wilz & Barskova, 2007	124 caregivers; phases 4 and 5	NR	NR	Controlled, three-group, repeated-measures design	Cognitive–behavioral group therapy (using different evidence-based therapeutic techniques)	A decrease in depression and anxiety, and an improvement in physical and environmental quality of life in the intervention group were noted.	Multicomponent group interventions that are tailored to stroke caregivers can be effective.
SYSTEMATIC REVIEWS AND META-ANALYSES							
Brereton et al., 2007	8 stroke caregiver intervention studies (N = 1,294 caregivers); phases 3, 4, and 5	Only reported by three of the eight studies, but not reported in the systematic review	NR	Systematic review of RCTs	Noninformation-giving interventions (e.g., problem solving, support, training, counseling) designed specifically for stroke caregivers	All interventions had positive outcomes. Only training, problem solving, and support improved quality of life and well-being.	The quality of the included RCTs was low, thus it is not possible to draw conclusions on the effectiveness of the interventions because of the heterogeneity of the interventions and of the outcome measures.
Lee et al., 2007	4 stroke caregiver intervention studies (N = 718 caregivers); phases 3, 4, and 5	NR	NR	Meta-analysis of RCTs	Two education programs, two support programs	There was a mean weight effect size of 277. Overall, the interventions were effective in improving caregiver mental health (as measured by the Short Form Health Study-36).	This study was limited by specific outcome measures. Future meta-analyses should study additional outcome variables and outcome measures.

(continued)

Table 3.1. Continued

| Author (Year) | Sample (Baseline) | Racial/Cultural Factors | | | Design | Interventions | Results | Evaluation |
		Diversity of Study Sample	Cultural Diversity Training Received?	Comparisons of Racial/ Cultural Factors				
Legg et al., 2012	8 stroke caregiver intervention studies (N = 1,007 caregivers); phase(s) NR	NR	NR	NR	Systematic review and meta-analysis of RCTs	Three intervention types: support and information, vocational training, psychoeducation	Mean weight effect size was NR. Only the vocational training intervention showed a reduction in stroke caregiver stress and strain.	No intervention was effective in reducing depression or anxiety, or in improving health-related quality of life.
Lui et al., 2005	11 stroke caregiver studies, but only information pertaining to the six intervention studies is included here (N > 1,400 caregivers; one study did not report sample size); phases 3, 4, and 5	Only reported by two of the six studies: n = 30, with 60% of stroke caregivers black; n = 74, with 74% of stroke caregivers white and 26% black	NR	NR	Systematic review of RCTs	Problem-solving interventions	Improvements in depression, preparedness, vitality, and coping were observed. No improvements in physical health, stress, or burden were noted.	Teaching problem solving may be more effective via telephone than by home visits. There was no difference between individual home visits and group support programs.

| Visser-Meily et al., 2005 | 22 stroke caregiver intervention studies (N > 2,300 caregivers; not all studies reported sample size); phases 1–5 | NR | NR | NR | Systematic review of intervention studies (18 of the 22 studies were RCTs) | Four intervention types: provision of specialist services, psychoeducation, counseling, social support from peers | Ten of the 22 studies reported positive results on one or more outcome measures. | Interventions should be based on the results of stroke caregiver needs assessments. |

NOTE. CPSI, Caregiver Problem-Solving Intervention; NR, not reported; RCT, randomized controlled trial; SELF, Supportive Education Learning Program; TAP, Transition Assistance Program; TASK, Telephone Assessment and Skill-Building Kit.

[a]The five phases of caregiving after a stroke are (1) event/diagnosis, (2) stabilization during acute care, (3) preparation during acute care and in-patient rehabilitation, (4) implementation during the first few months after the patient returns home ("learning the ropes"), and (5) long-lasting adaptation in the home and community (Cameron & Gignac, 2008).

generalizability of the results. However, a recent Cochrane review of nonphar-macological interventions for stroke caregivers restricted to RCTs—and with no restrictions on date of publication or language of publication—resulted in only eight studies for analysis (Legg et al., 2012). There was no evidence that these interventions were effective in reducing caregiver depression, anxiety, or quality of life. Understandably, these researchers observed the need for more interven-tion research because the evidence to date is insufficient (Legg et al., 2012).

RANDOMIZED CONTROLLED TRIALS

In our review of the literature, two RCTs published earlier this century, and sub-sequently included in some of the literature reviews discussed previously, war-rant further attention in this chapter. In addition, several noteworthy RCTs have appeared in the current literature. All of these are listed in the Table 3.1. The two RCTs included in some of the published literature reviews that merit comment are the evaluations by Grant and colleagues (Grant, Elliott, Weaver, Bartolucci, & Giger, 2002) and Hartke and King (2003). Both studies relied on telephone contacts to interact with participants and both featured interventions that were informed by contemporary theories of coping and adjustment: the social problem-solving model (Grant et al., 2002) and the stress and coping model (Hartke & King, 2003). Both also had unique methodological features that stand out in contrast to other studies listed in Table 3.1. Grant and colleagues (2002) assigned participants to either a problem-solving "partnership" group (that pro-vided training in problem-solving skills) or to one of two comparison condi-tions: a "sham" intervention group and a control group. In addition, Grant and colleagues (2000) were among the first to analyze intraindividual trajectories of response to the intervention over time with hierarchical linear modeling, in a manner congruent with most theoretical models of therapeutic changes in coun-seling (Kahn & Schneider, 2013). The study by Hartke and King (2003) stands out because it is among the few in the literature with a majority of participants who were beyond their second year in the caregiver role.

The results of these telephone-based, theory-driven interventions were also interesting. Grant and colleagues (2002) found that caregivers in the problem-solving group reported a significant decline in depression, and sig-nificant increases in problem-solving abilities and caregiver preparedness compared with those in the comparison groups. No differences were found, however, in burden between the groups during the 12 weeks of participation postdischarge. In contrast, Hartke and King (2003) found no differences dur-ing 6 months between the telephone "group conference" support group and the control group, but those in the control condition experienced a significant increase in their sense of burden compared with the treatment group. Although the reasons for this pattern are unclear, these results provide evidence that home-based interventions may benefit "experienced" caregivers despite clini-cal lore that they live with chronic, intractable problems. Grant and colleagues

(2002) suspected their results may be attributable, in part, to the way in which the intervention was tailored to address the specific problems identified by each caregiver at each contact. Collectively, both studies demonstrate the potential of long-distance, home-based technologies in providing strategic, theory-driven interventions for stroke caregivers.

Similar to the study by Grant et al. (2002), many recent RCTs focus almost exclusively on family caregivers identified during rehabilitation and use some variation of telephone contacts to provide or enhance the intervention upon return to the community. For example, Bakas and colleagues developed the Telephone Assessment and Skill-Building Kit (TASK), an 8-week intervention program that assesses caregivers' unmet needs and then helps them obtain knowledge and skills after hospital discharge (Bakas et al., 2009b). The intervention was designed to meet caregivers' needs in four areas: finding information about stroke, managing the survivors' emotions and behaviors, providing personal care, and providing instrumental care. Caregivers in the TASK intervention group received tip sheets addressing needs and concerns, a stress management workbook, a brochure on family caregiving from the American Stroke Association, and eight weekly calls from a nurse who conducted assessments of needs and delivered individualized interventions. Caregivers in the TASK intervention group displayed statistically significant increases in optimism at 4 weeks, 8 weeks, and 12 weeks, and significant decreases in task difficulty at 4 weeks and in threat appraisals at 8 weeks and 12 weeks. These caregivers also had greater satisfaction with their experience in the intervention group than those assigned to the comparison group (Bakas et al., 2009a).

Other RCTs that featured telephone contacts after discharge include a study of an enhanced, home-based, postdischarge program that resulted in improved quality of care for stroke survivors at the 12-month follow-up, but no effects on quality of life (Shyu, Kuo, Chen, & Chen, 2010). Another study, building on positive results from an earlier, quasi-experimental pilot of a problem-solving intervention for caregivers (King, Hartke, & Denby, 2007), found caregivers receiving the intervention reported significant gains during the first 4 months of participation, but these were no longer present at the 6-month evaluation (King et al., 2012). The intervention included problem-solving and cognitive–behavioral therapy techniques individualized to each caregiver. The systematic nature of this research provides an excellent example of the kind of programmatic research that is needed to advance our understanding of interventions for stroke caregivers.

A novel application of a contemporary long-distance technology involved a Web-based psychosocial intervention guided by a stress process model to benefit caregivers and care recipients (Smith, Egbert, Dellman-Jenkins, Nanna, & Palmieri, 2012). The intervention consisted of five components: a professional guide, educational videos, online chat sessions, e-mail and message boards, and a resource room. In comparisons with those assigned to an education-only group, caregivers in the treatment group reported less depression postintervention and at the 1-month follow-up assessment. More caregivers and stroke survivors in the intervention group showed at least a 50% decrease in Center for Epidemiologic Studies–Depression (Radloff, 1977) scale scores postintervention and at the 1-month follow-up than caregivers and stroke survivors in the control group. In addition, more participants in the intervention group than in the control group dropped below the clinical cutoff score for depression postintervention and at the 1-month follow-up. This work demonstrates the potential of other long-distance technologies to assist family caregivers in the community.

A recent RCT conducted in Germany for family caregivers of stroke survivors illustrates how long-distance technology and cognitive–behavioral interventions are integrated with beneficial effects (Pfeiffer et al., 2014). This project differs from much of the work discussed previously because it focuses on the issues facing family members who have been caregivers for some time and who face the personal consequences of providing care, such as restrictions in social life, competing demands and roles in their lives, need for respite, increasing awareness of an uncertain future with regard to possible new adverse health events, and changes in their own health or ability to continue caregiving. To provide more information about this project, we have included two case studies that demonstrate how caregiver issues are assessed and how a problem-solving intervention (D'Zurilla & Nezu, 2006) based, in part, on Lazarus' relational model of stress (Lazarus & Folkman, 1984) is provided in the context of an ongoing, collaborative partnership with a provider.

The components of the problem-solving intervention in this project were (a) problem definition and facts using a card-sorting procedure for problem identification, (b) optimism and orientation, (c) goal setting, (d) generation of alternatives, (e) decision making, and (f) implementation and verification. The card-sorting task was developed to identify problems of each caregiver. The essential element of this approach was a set with 40 cards marked with possible challenging issues in stroke caregiving. The card-sorting task included the following steps: (a) sorting out applicable cards (e.g., "My sleep is disturbed"), (b) labeling additional blank cards with problems that were not covered by the set, (c) allocating the selected and labeled cards to a 5-point scale ranging from "not at all burdensome" to "very burdensome," and (d) grouping cards that belong to the same problem (optional step). This technique helped the caregiver, with minimal instruction by the therapist, to realize there are common problems in caregiving, to break down one's own situation into specific challenges and problems, to identify one's own resources and strategies of successful coping (cards that were allocated to the categories "not at all" or "little" burdensome), to think about how problems might overlap or share similar characteristics, and to select problems that need immediate attention.

The main intervention period in the experimental condition of this study included an initial in-home visit, five weekly (month 1), and four biweekly (months 2 and 3) telephone sessions. The following maintenance period (months 4–12) consisted of another in-home visit (month 4) and nine monthly telephone sessions, with the option of four additional telephone calls in case of crisis or severe symptomatology. The intervention was delivered by clinical psychologists.

Assessments were delivered at baseline, after 3 months, and after 12 months. Depressive symptoms were reassessed at 24 months and 36 months.

The following two case studies demonstrate the positive effect of the problem-solving approach on caregivers' depressive symptoms. Case study 1 (Mrs. V) is an example for an implementation according to the study protocol with regard to frequency and duration of contacts, as well as the numerous repetitions of the problem-solving steps accompanied by an improvement in social problem-solving abilities. Case study 2 (Mrs. W) is an example of a slow start of the intervention with short telephone contacts, low initial compliance, difficulties in implementing a selected solution, very few repetitions of the problem-solving steps, and no improvement of social problem-solving abilities during the 12 months of intervention, but one very effective solution implementation after 8 months.

Case Study 1: "Mrs. V"

Mrs. V, a 59-year-old retired pediatric nurse and former head of a daycare facility for children is the informal caregiver for her mother, who is 89 years old. In addition, Mrs. V has been caring for her mother-in-law, who has been living with Mrs. V and her husband for 10 years. Her mother has mild cognitive impairment as a result of a stroke that occurred 18 months before the caregiver intervention began. Mrs. V has four grown children. After her mother had the stroke, Mrs. V's husband wanted to place her in long-term care, but Mrs. V was very offended by this suggestion. The arrangement they agreed on was to have Mrs. V's mother live in their house 5 days a week and spend the other 2 days each week living in her own apartment in a house belonging to Mrs. V's cousin.

During the initial home visit of the interventionist, Mrs. V completed a card-sorting task to categorize caregiving aspects as either not burdensome at all or as very burdensome. Caregiving aspects that Mrs. V identified as not burdensome at all were housekeeping, lacking knowledge about disease and caring, being responsible for organization and finances, being responsible for caregiving, fear that something could happen to her mother (e.g., another stroke), and her mother's incontinence. Caregiving aspects that were burdensome or very burdensome for Mrs. V were change of life planning, conflicts and tensions, testy and aggressive interactions, feelings of guilt, divergences, her mother's negative attitude toward everything, difficulty communicating with her mother, and partnership problems that were written down on an additional blank card. Superior problem areas were sleep, interaction with her mother, partnership, and support.

A problem-solving telephone intervention was conducted for 12 months and consisted of 19 telephone calls, with a mean duration of 51 minutes, and two home visits. During these 12 months, several major events occurred in Mrs. V's life. Specifically, during the first month her third grandchild was born; in the third month, her mother experienced pulmonary inflammation. During the fourth month her mother-in-law passed away; during the seventh month, her son and daughter-in-law separated. During the twelfth and final month of the intervention, her daughter-in-law became severely ill and, as a result, Mrs. V had to help her son and daughter-in-law care for their two young children.

The goals of the intervention were to improve Mrs. V's interactions with both her mother and her husband, to organize various responsibilities (e.g., children, grandchildren, mother), to cope with the death of her mother-in-law and the divorce of her son, to alleviate her insomnia, to organize her own leisure time, and to enhance self-care. The problem-solving steps were applied to one to five different problems at each contact. During the intervention, a wide range of problem- and emotion-focused goals were covered, and numerous selected solutions were implemented (e.g., clear and nonjudgmental communication with her husband, self-awareness, giving voice to own needs, being kind to oneself, asking cousin for support, dealing with own impatience and aggressions, integrating moments of respite during the day).

At the baseline, 3-month, and 12-month assessments, Mrs. V was above the cutoff score for depression, but her depression decreased to below the cutoff at a 24-month assessment (Table 3.2). Her satisfaction with her own

Table 3.2. BASELINE AND OUTCOME MEASURES FOR THE CASE STUDIES

Individual Case	Baseline	3 Months	12 Months	24 Months
CASE STUDY 1: MRS. V				
Depressive symptoms (CES-D)	35	31	26	11
Physical complaints (GBB-24)	36	37	43	—
Satisfaction with own performance as caregiver (SCQ-subscale 2)	18	29	28	—
Social problem-solving abilities (SPSI-R(S))	63	69	81	—
CASE STUDY 2: MRS. W				
Depressive symptoms (CES-D)	21	18	12	16
Physical complaints (GBB-24)	33	25	20	—
Satisfaction with own performance as caregiver (SCQ-subscale 2)	39	44	44	—
Social problem-solving abilities (SPSI-R(S))	67	73	63	—

NOTE: CES-D, Center for Epidemiologic Studies–Depression scale (Radloff, 1977); GBB-24, Giessen Subjective Complaints List (Brähler, Hinz, & Scheer, 2008); SCQ, Sense of Competence Questionnaire Subscale 2 (Vernooij-Dassen, 1993); SPSI-R(S), Social Problem-Solving Inventory–Revised: Short Version (D'Zurilla, Nezu, & Maydeu-Olivares, 2002).

performance as a caregiver increased from the baseline to the 3-month assessment and had remained relatively stable by the 12-month assessment. Mrs. V's social problem-solving abilities increased from the baseline to the 3-month assessment and had increased again by 12 months. The intensity of her physical complaints increased from the baseline to the 3-month assessment and from the 3-month assessment to the 12-month assessment. Mrs. V was very satisfied with the total time of the intervention and with the telephone-based delivery of the intervention as well as the frequency and duration of the telephone calls, but she wished she had this kind of counseling earlier. Mrs. V perceived the intervention as very helpful (98 on an analogue scale from 0 to 100) and summarized her experience with the intervention after 12 months this way: "The talks helped me not to feel responsible for everything any longer and to let things slide from time to time … and not to feel bad about this like before … . But it was an abyss to realize that I am completely at a loss what to do during the achieved leisure time … that I have to relieve strain even in such moments … . Taken as a whole I can take things as they come much easier in the future … . I'm thankful about the received individual support."

Case Study 2: "Mrs. W"

Mrs. W is a 69-year-old retired office assistant. She is the informal caregiver for her husband who is 82 years old and has been living with various severe diseases for the past 20 years. He had a stroke 23 months before the start of the caregiver intervention and has frontal temporal symptoms, such as lack of impulse control and depression. Although Mrs. W has one child from a previous marriage and her husband has four children from a previous marriage, none of their children are providing them with any support. They also are not receiving support from any other family members or friends and have no money for additional support. They maintain a range of sporadic to no contact with their family members and have lost nearly all their previous social contacts. Mrs. W can only leave the house during her husband's afternoon nap. When talking about her life and her situation in her initial in-home face-to-face session, Mrs. W was very embittered and reported that the only relaxation she can actually experience is smoking.

Before the implementation of the caregiving intervention, Mrs. W completed the card-sorting task. Caregiving aspects that Mrs. W identified as little or not burdensome at all were inadequate recognition of her role as a caregiver, the inability to speak openly, her husband's wish to die, lack of common activities, her husband's incontinence, and the impossibility of having her intimacy and sexual needs met. Caregiving aspects that were burdensome or very burdensome for Mrs. W were being bothered by her husband's misery and suffering, being responsible for caregiving, testy and aggressive interactions, and the fact that she couldn't leave her husband alone. Superior problem areas include rumination, lack of time for her own interests, missing her husband as a partner, and being responsible for everything. Her major goal was to be free of any caregiving obligations for at least one afternoon per week. The selected possible solution was to contact one of the local volunteer services to arrange a first meeting.

A problem-solving telephone intervention was conducted for 12 months, consisting of 13 calls, with an average time per call of 15 minutes, and two home visits. The first three telephone contacts after the initial home visit were shorter than 10 minutes. With these brief calls we informed Mrs. W that we wanted to keep contact without putting any pressure on her and hoped to overcome her skepticism about the intervention. Her skepticism stemmed, in part, from her depressive attitudes and former negative experiences with the healthcare system. Even after establishing a more stable and confidential therapeutic partnership, Mrs. W was still not able to contact any volunteer service, but successfully organized an inpatient rehabilitation program for her husband after 4 months. However, instead of the wished-for relief, her husband lost a great amount of weight during rehabilitation and Mrs. W suffered burnout and exhaustion during this time. During the sixth month, Mrs. W experienced severe frustration, accompanied by suicidal ideation after her husband shouted at her relatives during the only family celebration in her home after many months. During this time the intervention goals were to find feasible solutions to deal with the aggressive behaviors of her husband (e.g., time out, cognitive strategies, contact a volunteer service to make some respite possible) and to agree on an emergency strategy in the case of repeated suicidal ideations. During the seventh month, she had severe hives. Finally, during the eighth month of the intervention, Mrs. W was able to contact a volunteer service despite the skepticism and refusal of her husband. The first volunteer who introduced herself was a couple years older than Mrs. W and was immediately declared to be unqualified by Mrs. W. The interventionist encouraged Mrs. W not to drop this solution at all, and practiced with her how to communicate her concerns openly to the volunteer service. Finally, Mrs. W organized two volunteers with weekly visits and experienced, as a consequence of this support, a relief of her burdensome situation. Despite his earlier skepticism, her husband looked forward to each volunteer visit and enjoyed the new contacts as well.

At the baseline and 3-month assessments, Mrs. W was above the cutoff score for depression, but her depression decreased to below the cutoff at the 12-month assessment (Table 3.2). Her satisfaction with her own performance as a caregiver increased from the baseline to the 3-month assessment and remained the same by the 12-month assessment. Mrs. W's social problem-solving abilities increased from the baseline to the 3-month assessment, but then declined by the 12-month assessment to below the baseline score. The intensity of her physical complaints decreased from the baseline to the 3-month assessment and from the 3-month assessment to the

12-month assessment. Mrs. W was very satisfied with the total time of the intervention and mostly satisfied with the telephone-based delivery of the intervention as well as the frequency and duration of the telephone calls. She perceived the intervention as very helpful (100 on an analogue scale from 0 to 100) and summarized her experience with the intervention after 12 months: "I liked the telephone calls. I felt well regarded and could talk about things nobody else is interested in … . Get on with it [this kind of intervention]. The talks helped me. Many thanks for your efforts."

ADDITIONAL INTERVENTION STUDIES

The more noteworthy quasi-experimental intervention studies also focused on caregivers during hospitalization and postdischarge, and used telephone contacts as part of the intervention. In one of these, a home-based individual telecare intervention, consisting of 14 phone calls over 3 months to provide emotional and social support and information specific to the family's needs, was examined (Kim et al., 2012). The home-based individual telecare intervention was more effective in reducing caregiver burden than a hospital-based group intervention. The significant decrease in caregiver burden in the home-based individual telecare intervention group was apparent 12 weeks after discharge.

A study conducted in Thailand examined the implementation and effectiveness of the Supportive Educative Learning Program (SELF) in reducing caregiver strain and improving caregiver quality of life, with stroke caregivers located in two different hospitals (Oupra, Griffiths, Pryor, & Mott, 2010). The SELF intervention consists of didactic education sessions, hands-on training for caregivers, a booklet describing stroke care, and three follow-up phone calls. Both the SELF intervention and the usual-care groups showed improvement in quality of life, but caregivers in the intervention group had better quality of life at the time of hospital discharge and 3 months after discharge. Both groups showed statistically significant declines in strain at the 3-month follow-up, but the caregivers in the control group reported greater levels of strain than the caregivers in the SELF intervention group at both discharge and at the 3-month follow-up.

COSTS

All the intervention studies discussed to this point were implemented in community and/or hospital settings. The types of interventions ranged from telephone calls to home visits, from hospital and rehabilitation settings to home settings, from individual to group interventions, from problem solving to supportive education, and from an in-person format to an online format. These studies demonstrate that community implementation of stroke caregiver interventions can be effective, but a potential barrier to continued community implementation is cost of the intervention per caregiver. For this reason, stroke caregiver intervention

cost templates have been developed. For example, after Bakas and colleagues created and implemented the TASK intervention for stroke caregivers (Bakas et al.,
2009b), they developed a cost template to determine the cost of the intervention
per caregiver (Bakas, Yong, Habermann, McLennon, & Weaver, 2011).

Bakas and colleagues (2011) developed the cost template by accounting for the
costs of organizing and implementing the intervention, and the costs of the caregivers' time. The cost of the intervention included training the nurses to deliver
the intervention, preparing for the intervention, delivering the intervention,
supervising the delivery of the intervention, and wrapping up the intervention.
The number of nurses and supervisors needed, as well as the number of hours
spent preparing for and delivering the intervention, were measured. Caregiver
time was measured as the amount of time it took to deliver the intervention
and was valued at $10.39 per hour, which is the mean wage for home-care aides.
Because TASK is a telephone-based intervention, there were no travel costs, but
costs were incurred when mailing printed materials to caregivers, which cost $43
per caregiver. The personnel cost was estimated to be $20/hour for nurses and
$22/hour for supervisors. The two nurses who delivered the intervention spent
18 hours being trained by the supervisors, and for each intervention delivery the
nurses spent 15 minutes preparing and 15 minutes wrapping up. For the caregivers who participated in the TASK intervention, they received, on average, 3.95
hours of intervention across eight phone calls. After intervention delivery, the
nurses met with supervisors for 1.5 hours of evaluation after each phone call, creating a sum of 12 hours of evaluation per caregiver. Supervisors also held weekly
meetings throughout the course of a year, totaling 26 hours. The mean cost per
caregiver was calculated to be $421, which the researchers evaluated as low cost
(Bakas et al., 2011).

Some of the costs of the intervention are fixed. For example, regardless of the
number of caregivers receiving the intervention, the cost of training and supervision is fixed. Supervisory costs might be reduced with video or computer training
resources. The researchers also suggest that costs can be reduced by streamlining the weekly meetings and by communicating the necessary information only.
As stated earlier, the mean cost of $421 per caregiver is considered low cost;
moreover, the cost also should be evaluated in terms of the effectiveness of the
intervention (Bakas et al., 2011). The TASK intervention was shown to be effective in increasing stroke caregiver optimism and in decreasing stroke caregiver
task difficulty and threat appraisal. Furthermore, stroke caregiver needs were
met more quickly in the TASK intervention group than in the attention control
group (Bakas et al., 2009b). Based on the effectiveness of the TASK intervention,
the costs of delivering the intervention may be balanced by the lower subsequent
costs as a result of the positive outcomes of the intervention. Ultimately, cost
templates are important in developing and evaluating intervention programs
(Bakas et al., 2011). The development of cost templates for other interventions
can highlight their cost-effectiveness as well as denote areas in which cost reduction is possible.

CONCLUSION

Stroke is one of most frequent and debilitating health conditions in modern society, and its deleterious effects on family functioning and family members are well documented. Therefore, the paucity of caregiver research in general and of high-quality research specifically is surprising. Although there are several interesting themes and trends in the literature, we understand why the Cochrane review adroitly observes that a critique of this work "highlights the opportunities for improvements" in the area (Legg et al., 2012; p. e31). There are several key themes apparent in the literature at this point. We understand that caregivers value information and want emotional support (Schure et al., 2006). When effects are found in response to interventions, they involve reductions in distress, negative moods, and depressive symptoms, but lack promotion of positive attributes (e.g., caregiver competence, life satisfaction). Long-distance technologies appear to be quite suitable for providing home-based interventions (and caregivers seem to appreciate them [Pfeiffer et al., 2014]). And the research to date has attended almost exclusively to interventions for caregivers in the transition from hospital to home.

There are interesting trends embedded in the literature as well that have not yet become as well developed as the aforementioned key themes. Information-only programs appear insufficient to help caregivers; some degree of counseling and "tailoring" of the intervention is required to address caregivers' emotional needs and unique problems. Interventions that attend to the specific problems reported by caregivers appear to be promising, and there is emerging evidence as caregivers benefit from an intervention, changes may also be observed in the care recipient. Yet, the lack of ethnic and racial diversity in the research poses a serious threat to its generalizability, and this must be remedied in future work. In addition, benefits of interventions provided in the weeks postdischarge may not persist throughout the remainder of the inaugural year of caregiving. Perhaps the trajectory of the caregiver career does, in fact, pose new problems and challenges over time that require ongoing support and training as needed.

In a comprehensive, integration of the cross-sectional, longitudinal, and qualitative studies of stroke caregiver adjustment, Gaugler (2010) observed that this research relied heavily on samples recruited from clinical settings. Studies of caregivers recruited from the community might reveal different patterns of adjustment. Indeed, a nationwide study of a matched sample of stroke caregivers ($N = 3,503$) and noncaregivers using an empirical, propensity score matching procedure found noncaregivers had significantly higher mortality rates over an average of 6 years (Roth et al., 2013). Although the study lacks information about the actual degree of assistance provided, and lacks detail about the psychological and physical health of the caregivers during the 6-year time frame, the findings illustrate dramatically the need to consider the possible benefits of the "caregiving career." The authors speculated that the positive psychological benefits of caregiving might facilitate personal health over time. A recent systematic review of benefits reported by stroke caregivers concluded that individual differences may account, in part, for positive experiences such as increased self-esteem, feeling appreciated, and improved relationships (Mackenzie & Greenwood, 2012). Some of these benefits may be apparent within a year of assuming the caregiver role (Haley et al., 2009). Yet, the degree to which these experiences are amenable to psychosocial interventions is essentially unknown.

The mechanisms underpinning positive adjustment among caregivers are unclear, but it is reasonable, theoretically, to assume that these would operate in a manner anticipated by popular stress and coping process models in which cognitive appraisals influence coping behaviors (which can include positive reappraisals and spiritual beliefs) and subsequent emotional experiences (Folkman, 2008). However, cognitive appraisal activity does not assume such a primary role in other compelling models of positive adjustment. For example, the broaden-and-build model of resilience maintains that experiences of positive affect facilitate increased flexibility, personal well-being, and an ability to integrate new information over time in times of stress (Fredrickson, 2013). Indeed, in a current student of family members during the initial year of caregiving for a relative with a traumatically acquired disability, resilient caregivers were distinguished significantly from distressed caregivers by their elevated experiences of positive mood throughout the year (Elliott, Berry, Richards, & Shewchuk, 2014). Resilient caregivers were not significantly different from other caregivers on measures of personal gain, positive comparisons, or caregiver competence. Furthermore, there is evidence that resilience among family caregivers may be an extension of a resilient personality, consistent with Block's (1993) ego resilience and control model that accounts, in part, for the lower levels of distress they experience in comparison with other caregivers (Elliott et al., 2014). Understanding the theoretical mechanisms that promote positive adjustment among caregivers is necessary for strategic, informed interventions that facilitate personal growth and meaning.

Historically, family caregivers are expected to operate as extensions of the healthcare system, performing complex medical and therapeutic tasks, and ensuring care recipient adherence to prescribed regimens (Shewchuk & Elliott, 2000). This is certainly true of family caregivers of stroke survivors. However, these caregivers do not receive adequate training, preparation, or ongoing support from the healthcare system. Although stroke caregivers often receive information and instruction during inpatient hospitalization or rehabilitation, it is illogical and unreasonable to assume this prepares them adequately for the challenges and problems that will evolve and appear over time. The complex and evolving issues faced by stroke caregivers cannot be addressed in brief, educationally based training during the inpatient rehabilitation program or in brief, infrequent outpatient visits arranged with the survivor's care providers, who are concerned primarily with the medical care and therapeutic needs of the survivor.

Viewing caregiver needs from the lens of a chronic care model requires the development of interventions that prepare stroke caregivers to address the challenges they face and to "help them become more active and expert in their own self-management and to operate competently as formal extensions of health care systems" (Shewchuk & Elliott, 2000, p. 561). This kind of "partnership" recognizes the active and essential role of the individual caregiver in health care; respects their needs for ongoing training, support, and assistance; and is responsive to problems often encountered by caregivers in general, and to those experienced specifically by the individual caregiver. Elliott and Parker (2012) recently argued that the success of these partnerships requires ongoing assessments of the needs, health, and capacity of the caregiver, and of the problems experienced by the dyad at any point in time, and sensitivity to changes to their status, challenges, and needs. For these reasons, many favor cognitive–behavioral interventions that address emotional issues and provide training in instrumental skills for coping with specific and unique problems. These interventions can be conducted by low-cost (i.e., nondoctoral-level) providers, they can address the specific issues identified and prioritized by the caregiver, and they can be delivered effectively to the home via long-distance technologies.

REFERENCES

Bakas, T., Farran, C. J., Austin, J. K., Given, B. A., Johnson, E. A., & Williams, L. S. (2009a). Content validity and satisfaction with a stroke caregiver intervention program. *Journal of Nursing Scholarship, 41*, 368–375.

Bakas, T., Farran, C. J., Austin, J. K., Given, B. A., Johnson, E. A., & Williams, L. S. (2009b). Stroke caregiver outcomes from the Telephone Assessment and Skill-Building Kit (TASK). *Topics in Stroke Rehabilitation, 16*, 105–121.

Bakas, T., Yong, L., Habermann, B., McLennon, S. M., & Weaver, M. T. (2011). Developing a cost template for a nurse-led stroke caregiver intervention program. *Clinical Nurse Specialist, 25*, 41–46.

Berg, A., Palomaki, H., Lonnqvist, J., Lehtihalmes, M., & Kaste, M. (2005). Depression among caregivers of stroke survivors. *Stroke, 36*, 639–643.

Bjorkdahl, A., Nilsson, A. L., & Sunnerhagen, K. S. (2007). Can rehabilitation in the home setting reduce the burden of care for the next-of-kin of stroke victims? *Journal of Rehabilitation Medicine, 39*, 27–32.

Block, J. (1993). Studying personality the long way. In D. C. Funder, R. D. Parke, C. Tomlinson-Keasey, & K. Widaman (Eds.), *Studying lives through time* (pp. 9–41). Washington, DC: American Psychological Association.

Brähler, E., Hinz, A., & Scheer, J. W. (2008). *Gießener Beschwerdebogen (GBB-24) [Giessener Symptom List (GBB-24)]* (3rd ed.). Bern, Switzerland: Huber.

Brereton, L., Carroll, C., & Barnston, S. (2007). Interventions for adult family carers of people who have had a stroke: A systematic review. *Clinical Rehabilitation, 21*, 867–884.

Cameron, J. I., & Gignac, M. A. (2008). "Timing it right": A conceptual framework for addressing the support needs of family caregivers to stroke survivors from the hospital to the home. *Patient Education and Counseling, 70*, 305–314.

D'Zurilla, T. J., & Nezu, A. (2006). *Problem-solving therapy: A positive approach to clinical intervention* (3rd ed.). New York: Springer.

D'Zurilla, T. J., Nezu, A. M., & Maydeu-Olivares, A. (2002). *Social Problem-Solving Inventory–Revised (SPSI-R)*. North Tonawanda, NY: Multi-Health Systems.

Elliott, T. R., Berry, J. W., Richards, J. S., & Shewchuk, R. M. (2014). Resilience in the initial year of caregiving for a family member with a traumatic spinal cord injury. *Journal of Consulting and Clinical Psychology, 82*, 1072–1086.

Elliott, T. R., & Parker, M. W. (2012). Family caregivers and health care providers: Developing partnerships for a continuum of care and support. In R. C. Talley & J. E. Crews (Eds.), *Multiple dimensions of caregiving and disability* (pp. 135–152). New York: Springer.

Elliott, T. R., Warren, R. H., Blucker, R., Berry, J. W., Chang, J., & Warren, A. M. (2013b). Resilience among family caregivers of children with severe neurodisabilities requiring chronic respiratory management. *Developmental Medicine and Child Neurology, 55*(3 Suppl), 58.

Folkman, S. (2008). The case for positive emotions in the stress process. *Anxiety, Stress and Coping, 21*, 3–14.

Fredrickson, B. L. (2013). Positive emotions broaden and build. *Advances in Experimental Social Psychology, 47*, 1–53.

Gaugler, J. E. (2010). The longitudinal ramifications of stroke caregiving: A systematic review. *Rehabilitation Psychology, 55*, 108–125.

Grant, J. S., Bartolucci, A., Elliott, T., & Giger, J. N. (2000). Sociodemographic, physical, and psychosocial characteristics of depressed and non-depressed family caregivers of stroke survivors. *Brain Injury, 14*, 1089–1100.

Grant, J. S., Clay, O. J., Keltner, N. L., Haley, W. E. Wadley, V. G., Perkins, M. M., et al. (2013). Does caregiver well-being predict stroke survivor depressive symptoms? A mediation analysis. *Topics in Stroke Rehabilitation, 20*, 44–51.

Grant, J. S., Elliott, T. R., Weaver, M., Bartolucci, A. A., & Giger, J. N. (2002). Telephone intervention with family caregivers of stroke survivors after rehabilitation. *Stroke, 33*, 2060–2065.

Grant, J., Elliott, T., Weaver, M., Glandon, G., & Giger, J. (2006a). Social problem-solving abilities, social support, and adjustment of family caregivers of stroke survivors. *Archives of Physical Medicine and Rehabilitation, 87*, 343–350.

Grant, J. S., Glandon, G. L., Elliott, T. R., Giger, J. N., & Weaver, M. (2004a). Caregiving problems and feelings experienced by family caregivers of stroke survivors the first month after discharge. *International Journal of Rehabilitation Research, 27*, 105–111.

Grant, J. S., Glandon, G. L., Elliott, T. R., Giger, J. N., & Weaver, M. (2006b). Problems and associated feelings experienced by family caregivers of stroke survivors the second and third month postdischarge. *Topics in Stroke Rehabilitation, 13*, 66–74.

Grant, J., Weaver, M., Elliott, T., Bartolucci, A., & Giger, J. (2004b). Family caregivers of stroke survivors: Characteristics of caregivers at-risk for depression. *Rehabilitation Psychology, 49*, 172–179.

Hackett, M. L., Yapa, C., Parag, V., & Anderson, C. S. (2005). Frequency of depression after stroke: A systematic review of observational studies. *Stroke, 36*, 1330–1340.

Hafsteinsdóttir, T. B., Vergunst, M., Lindeman, E., & Schuurmans, M. (2011). Educational needs of patients with a stroke and their caregivers: A systematic review of the literature. *Patient Education and Counseling, 85*, 14–25.

Haley, W. E., Allen, J. Y., Grant, J. S., Clay, O. J., Perkins, M., & Roth, D. L. (2009). Problems and benefits reported by stroke family caregivers: Results from a prospective epidemiological study. *Stroke, 40*, 2129–2133.

Haley, W. E., Roth, D. L., Hovater, M., & Clay, O. J. (2015). Long-term impact of stroke on family caregiver well-being. *Neurology, 84*, 1323–1329.

Hartke, R. J., & King, R. B. (2003). Telephone group intervention for older stroke caregivers. *Topics in Stroke Rehabilitation, 9*, 65–81.

Hinojosa, M. S., & Rittman, M. R. (2007). Stroke caregiver information needs: Comparison of Mainland and Puerto Rican caregivers. *Journal of Rehabilitation Research and Development, 44*, 649–658.

Hoffmann, T., McKenna, K., Worrall, L., & Read, S. J. (2004). Evaluating current practice in the provision of written information to stroke patients and their carers. *International Journal of Therapeutic Rehabilitation, 11*, 303–307.

Kahn, J. H., & Schneider, W. J. (2013). It's the destination and the journey: Using multilevel modeling to assess patterns of change in psychotherapy. *Journal of Clinical Psychology, 69*, 543–570.

Kim, S. S., Kim, E. J., Cheon, J. Y., Chung, S. K., Moon, S., & Moon, K. H. (2012). The effectiveness of home-based individual tele-care intervention for stroke caregivers in South Korea. *International Nursing Review, 59*, 369–375.

Kim, J. W., & Moon, S. S. (2007). Needs of family caregivers caring for stroke patients: Based on the rehabilitation treatment phase and the treatment setting. *Social Work in Health Care, 45*, 81–97.

King, R. B., Ainsworth, C. R., Ronen, M., & Hartke, R. J. (2010). Stroke caregivers: Pressing problems reported during the first months of caregiving. *Journal of Neuroscience Nursing, 42*, 302–311.

King, R. B., Hartke, R. J., & Denby, F. (2007). Problem-solving early intervention: A pilot study of stroke caregivers. *Rehabilitation Nursing, 32*, 68–76.

King, R. B., Hartke, R. J., Houle, T., Lee, J., Herring, G., Alexander-Peterson, B. S., et al. (2012). A problem-solving early intervention for stroke caregivers: One year follow-up. *Rehabilitation Nursing, 37*, 231–242.

King, R. B., & Semik, P. E. (2006). Stroke caregiving: Difficult times, resource use, and needs during the first 2 years. *Journal of Gerontological Nursing, 32*, 37–44.

Klinedinst, N. J., Gebhardt, M. C., Aycock, D. M., Nichols-Larsen, D. S., Uswatte, G., Wolf, S. L, et al. (2009). Caregiver characteristics predict stroke survivor quality of life at 4 months and 1 year. *Research in Nursing & Health, 32*, 592–605.

Ko, J. Y., Aycock, D. M., & Clark, P. C. (2007). A comparison of working versus nonworking family caregivers of stroke survivors. *Journal of Neuroscience Nursing, 39*, 217–225.

Lai, S. M., Studenski, S., Duncan, P. W., & Perera, S. (2002). Persisting consequences of stroke measured by the Stroke Impact Scale. *Stroke, 33*, 1840–1844.

Lazarus, R. S., & Folkman, S. (1984). *Stress, appraisal, and coping.* New York: Springer.

Lee, J., Soeken, K., & Picot, S. J. (2007). A meta-analysis of interventions for informal stroke caregivers. *Western Journal of Nursing Research, 29*, 344–356.

Legg, L. A., Quinn, T. J., Mahmood, F., Weir, C. J., Tierney, J., Stott, D. J., et al. (2012). Nonpharmacological interventions for caregivers of stroke survivors. *Stroke, 43*, e30–e31.

Lui, M. H., Ross, F. M., & Thompson, D. R. (2005). Supporting family caregivers in stroke care: A review of the evidence for problem solving. *Stroke*, *36*, 2514–2522.

Lurbe-Puerto, K., Leandro, M., & Baumann, M. (2012). Experiences of caregiving, satisfaction of life, and social repercussions among family caregivers, two years post-stroke. *Social Work in Health Care*, *51*, 725–742.

MacIsaac, L., Harrison, M. B., Buchanan, D., & Hopman, W. M. (2011). Supportive care needs after an acute stroke: A descriptive enquiry of caregivers' perspective. *Journal of Neuroscience Nursing*, *43*, 132–140.

Mackenzie, A., & Greenwood, N. (2012). Positive experiences of caregiving in stroke: A systematic review. *Disability & Rehabilitation*, *34*, 1413–1422.

Mak, A. K. M., Mackenzie, A., & Lui, M. H. L. (2007). Changing needs of Chinese family caregivers of stroke survivors. *Journal of Clinical Nursing*, *16*, 971–979.

Ostwald, S. K., Bernal, M. P., Cron, S. G., & Godwin, K. M. (2009). Stress experienced by stroke survivors and spousal caregivers during the first year after discharge from inpatient rehabilitation. *Topics in Stroke Rehabilitation*, *16*, 93–104.

Oupra, R., Griffiths, R., Pryor, J., & Mott, S. (2010). Effectiveness of Supportive Educative Learning programme on the level of strain experienced by caregivers of stroke patients in Thailand. *Health and Social Care in the Community*, *18*, 10–20.

Perrin, P. B., Heesacker, M., Stidham, B. S., Rittman, M. R., & Gonzalez-Rothi, L. J. (2008). Structural equation modeling of the relationship between caregiver psychosocial variables and functioning of individuals with stroke. *Rehabilitation Psychology*, *53*, 54–62.

Perrin, P. B., Heesacker, M., Uthe, C. E., & Rittman, M. R. (2010). Caregiver mental health and racial/ethnic disparities in stroke: Implications for culturally sensitive interventions. *Rehabilitation Psychology*, *55*, 372–382.

Perrin, P. B., Johnston, A., Vogel, B., Heesacker, M., Vega-Trujillo, M., Anderson, J., et al. (2010). A culturally sensitive Transition Assistance Program for stroke caregivers: Examining caregiver mental health and stroke rehabilitation. *Journal of Rehabilitation Research and Development*, *47*, 605–616.

Pfeiffer, K., Beische, D., Hautzinger, M., Berry, J. W., Wengert, J., Hoffrichter, R., Becker, C., van Schayck, R., & Elliott, T. (2014). Telephone-based problem-solving intervention for family caregivers of stroke survivors: A randomized controlled trial. *Journal of Consulting and Clinical Psychology*, *82*, 628–643.

Radloff, L. S. (1977). The CES-D Scale: A self-report depression scale for research in the general population. *Applied Psychological Measurement*, *1*, 385–401.

Rosamond, W., Flegal, K., Friday, G., Furie, K., Go, A., Greenlund, K., et al. (2007). Heart disease and stroke statistics—2007 update: A report for the American Heart Association statistics committee and the stroke statistics committee. *Circulation*, *115*, e69–e171.

Roth, D. L., Haley, W. E., Hovater, M., Perkins, M., Wadley, V. G., & Judd, S. (2013). Family caregiving and all-cause mortality: Findings from a population-based propensity-matched analysis. *American Journal of Epidemiology*, *178*, 1571–1578.

Schure, L. M., van den Heuvel, E. T., Stewart, R. E., Sanderman, R., de Witte, L. P., & Meyboom-de Jong, B. (2006). Beyond stroke: Description and evaluation of an effective intervention to support family caregivers of stroke patients. *Patient Education and Counseling*, *62*, 46–55.

Shewchuk, R., & Elliott, T. (2000). Family caregiving in chronic disease and disability: Implications for rehabilitation psychology. In R. G. Frank & T. Elliott (Eds.), *Handbook of rehabilitation psychology* (pp. 553–563). Washington, DC: American Psychological Association Press.

Shyu, Y. L., Kuo, L., Chen, M., & Chen, S. (2010). A clinical trial of an individualised intervention programme for family caregivers of older stroke victims in Taiwan. *Journal of Clinical Nursing, 19*, 1675–1685.

Smith, G. C., Egbert, N., Dellman-Jenkins, M., Nanna, K., & Palmieri, P. A. (2012). Reducing depression in stroke survivors and their informal caregivers: A randomized clinical trial of a Web-based intervention. *Rehabilitation Psychology, 57*, 196–206.

Smith, L. N., Lawrence, M., Kerr, S. M., Langhorne, P., & Lees, K. R. (2004). Informal carers' experience of caring for stroke survivors. *Journal of Advanced Nursing, 46*, 235–244.

Vernooij-Dassen, M. J. F. J. (1993). *Dementie en thuiszorg: Een onderzoek naar determinenten van het competentiegevoel van centrale verzorgers en het effect van professionele interventie* [Dementia and Home Care: Determinants of the Sense of Competence of Primary Caregivers and the Effect of Professionally Guided Caregiver Support]. Lisse, The Netherlands: Swets & Zeitlinger.

Visser-Meily, A., Post, M., van de Port, I., Maas, C., Forstberg-Wärleby, G., & Lindeman, E. (2009). Psychosocial functioning of spouses of patients with stroke from initial inpatient rehabilitation to 3 years poststroke: Course and relations with coping strategies. *Stroke, 40*, 1399–1404.

Visser-Meily, A., van Heugten, C., Post, M., Schepers, V., & Lindeman, E. (2005). Intervention studies for caregivers of stroke survivors: A critical review. *Patient Education and Counseling, 56*, 257–267.

Ware, J. E., & Sherbourne, C. D. (1992). The MOS 36-item short-form health survey (SF-36): Conceptual framework and item selection. *Medical Care, 30*, 473–483.

White, C. L., Mayo, N., Hanley, J. A., & Wood-Dauphinee, S. (2003). Evolution of the caregiving experience in the initial 2 years following stroke. *Research in Nursing & Health, 26*, 177–189.

Wilz, G., & Barskova, T. (2007). Evaluation of a cognitive behavioral group intervention program for spouses of stroke patients. *Behaviour Research and Therapy, 45*, 2508–2517.

4

Caregiving for Patients with Cancer

BARBARA A. GIVEN AND CHARLES W. GIVEN ■

As a result of the development of more aggressive treatment protocols and targeted drugs, individuals with cancer are living longer with the disease. Although these developments are positive, family caregivers are now expected to provide immediate and long-term care to family members with cancer, often without the ongoing support of the formal healthcare system. These caregivers participate actively in helping the patient achieve treatment goals and manage side effects, while coping with their own emotional responses to the patient's diagnosis. Family members provide a combination of physical, practical, and emotional care and support to their loved ones with cancer.

Complicating the provision of care, cancer and cancer-related treatments might alter family functioning, occupational and social roles, and communication patterns. Changes occur at multiple time points across the cancer care trajectory, through the diagnosis, treatment, and survivorship phases. The advanced stage of cancer and end-of-life care is especially difficult for caregivers (Northouse, Templin, & Mood, 2001, Northouse, Katapodi, Song, Zhang, & Mood, 2010).

Although more than half the care needed by cancer patients is provided by family members, these caregivers assume this role with no assessment or preparation by the formal care system with regard to whether they have adequate knowledge, resources, or skills to assume this role. Clearly, interventions are needed to address family caregivers' needs (Kane, 2011, McCorkle, Siefert, Dowd, Robinson, & Pickett, 2007; Silveira et al., 2011).

The purpose of this chapter is to provide a description of existing intervention studies that assist family caregivers while providing care to older patients undergoing cancer treatment. To frame the context of these interventions, we first describe the characteristics of the caregiver's role in cancer care. The effects of the intervention on caregiver outcomes are summarized, and we include recommendations for future research.

THE CAREGIVING ROLE

Caregivers of cancer patients become involved in a wide array of tasks and care activities that include learning new psychoeducational skills, supervision, and clinical judgments. Care demands include interpreting and managing symptoms, monitoring nutrition, and providing emotional, spiritual, and social support. In addition, for varying periods during treatment, caregivers may have to assume new roles related to housekeeping, transportation, and financial management. Changes during the cancer trajectory may include providing care such as direct physical care, assistance in activities of daily living, the administration of complex medication regimens, assistance with decision making, and the provision of comfort to the patient.

Caregivers are actively involved in navigating the healthcare system and gaining access to needed community services. The responsibility of negotiating and communicating with healthcare professionals continues as effects of treatment and the disease occur. Each form of caregiver involvement demands different skills and knowledge, organizational capacities, and social and psychological strengths (Schumacher, Stewart, Archbold, Dodd, & Dibble, 2000).

Caregivers' distress can increase as their responsibilities multiply (Andrews, 2001; Given et al., 2004; Kurtz, Kurtz, Given, & Given, 2004; Morita, Chihara & Kashiwagi, 2002). Even if patient symptoms and functional abilities improve, caregivers report they continue to provide assistance and center their lives on cancer care (Northouse et al., 2001). Family members adjust their schedules and relinquish valued personal activities to provide care (Given et al., 2004; Kurtz et al., 2004). Family and work responsibilities, role strain, and role overload may cause difficulty as demands on the caregiver change (increase or decrease) over time.

Caregivers have a variety of responses to the care they provide that depends on the nature of care demands, their complexity, and the duration of the care they provide (Stenberg, Ruland, & Miaskowski, 2010). Changing demands create uncertainty that makes planning and establishing routines very difficult, which in turn raises caregivers' levels of distress. Negative sequelae of taking on the caregiving role include increases in anxiety, depression, and burden, as well as a negative impact on physical health. This is especially challenging when the caregiver is an older adult with his or her own chronic diseases. In the remainder of this section we discuss areas of family member's lives most affected by the caregiving role.

Emotional Well-being

Caregivers describe being on an emotional roller coaster during cancer care that may be as short as a few months or may last for years. As a result, in part, of the trajectory of cancer treatment and symptoms, families may undergo the stresses related to diagnosis and initial treatment, reduction in cancer symptoms resulting in less provision of hands-on care (albeit ongoing stress related to monitoring the health and well-being of the relative with cancer), the emotional upheaval related to recurrence, and end-of-life cancer care. These emotional reactions to the demands for cancer care are often called *burden* and result when perceived demands outweigh personal resources for meeting these demands (Sherwood et al., 2004).

Burden is multidimensional and evolves from the imbalance between the social, psychological, and economic consequences that permeate a care situation and caregivers' coping strategies to meet demands. Caregivers who are unable to use strategies to cope effectively with care demands may experience burden, which if sustained may lead to depression (Kozachik et al., 2001, Sherwood, Given, Given, & von Eye, 2005; Sherwood et al., 2006, Sherwood et al., 2007). Disruption of usual daily activities, competing demands, and increasing physical care demands and decreased patient functional capacity have all been shown to result in caregiver burden (Pinquart & Sörenson, 2004). Patients' poor coping also poses concern to caregivers. Hagedoorn and colleagues (Hagedoorn, Sanderman, Bolks, Tuinstra, & Coyne, 2008), Hodges and colleagues (Hodges, Humphris, & Macfarlane, 2005), and Northouse and colleagues (Northouse et al., 2010) examined the relationship between reports of stress and the emotional distress reported by patients and caregivers.

Caregiver *depression* is considered to be a secondary or long-term mood disturbance that may follow continued burden and my develop as a result of providing care over a sustained period (Braun, Mikulincer, Rydall, Walsh, & Rodin, 2007; Fortinsky, Kercher, & Burant, 2002; Harris, Godfrey, Partridge, & Knight, 2001). Caregiver depression may be manifested by feelings of loneliness, sadness, isolation, irritability, and fearfulness, and being easily bothered (Cameron, Franche, Cheung, & Stewart, 2002; Carter, 2003; Grunfeld et al., 2004; Pavalko & Woodbury, 2000; Sherwood et al., 2005; Sherwood et al., 2012; Stephens, Townsend, Martire, & Druley, 2001).

The cancer trajectory poses challenges for patients and their caregivers. Initially, there is the suspicion of cancer. Uncertainty is the hallmark emotion during this phase. Patients and family caregivers replay imagined scenarios and seek reasons to explain their dilemma, all of which challenge the emotions and strain relationships between the patient and their closest relations and friends. When the diagnosis is confirmed, patients and families are focused on the extent of the disease and the treatment options offered. During this time, caregivers and their patients seek information about treatment effectiveness. Knowledge acquisition and sorting through large numbers of research reports that they are poorly equipped to interpret sets into motion different demands (Given & Sherwood, 2006; Grunfeld et al., 2004).

When treatment begins caregivers face problems related to carrying on their own work roles while ensuring appointments are kept and regimens are followed. Family members begin to undertake more traditional caregiving roles; they may assume added responsibilities at home, assist in symptom management, and navigate insurance claims and the financial implications of cancer treatment. After treatment is completed, caregivers have to continue to support patients while encouraging them to resume their normal work and family roles.

This latter phase is especially challenging; there are no regular appointments so families can query the oncologist, and as a result they may feel isolated. Each untoward event is met with hypervigilence. Last, caregivers are concerned about the frequency and appropriateness of follow-up care. It is the diversity of the challenges, the multiple periods of uncertainty, along with the disruption of family life, work, and the threat of financial disaster that can lead initially to burden and later to more serious and sustained emotional responses, then to depression (Grunfeld et al, 2004; Sherwood et al. 2007; Sherwood et al., 2012; Stenberg et al., 2010). These periods of change can serve as triggers for formal risk appraisal.

Physical Well-being

Given the shifting demands throughout treatment and into posttreatment survivorship, a number of negative physical consequences may result from providing care to a patient with cancer (Given & Given 1992; Given, Given, Azzouz, Stommel, & Kozachik, 2000; Given et al., 2006; Kurtz et al., 2004). Caregivers are at risk for fatigue and sleep disturbances, increased risk for infection, loss of physical strength, loss of appetite, lower immune functioning, altered response to influenza shots, slower wound healing, and higher blood pressure. Caregivers describe being physically exhausted and having fatigue (Stenberg et al., 2010). Exacerbations of chronic disease and altered lipid profiles have been described, but extensive work has not been conducted in this area (Bevans & Sternberg, 2012; Carter, 2002; Kiecolt-Glaser et al., 2003; Northouse, Williams, Given, & McCorkle, 2012; Vitaliano, Zhang, & Scanlan, 2003;, Kim, Carver, Cannady, & Shaffer, 2013). Bevans and Sternberg (2012) suggest that the physical health effects of distress are mediated in part by immune and autonomic regulation. Long-term studies are not available on the impact of these physiological changes, nor are there data on the effect of concomitant chronic diseases for the older cancer caregiver.

Social Well-being

Social functioning and impaired social well-being encompass financial difficulties, work problems, role strain, problems managing their environment, and negative sexual and marital relationships (Manne, Babb, Pinover, Horwitz, & Ebbert, 2004; McCorkle et al., 2007; Scott, Halford, & Ward 2004). Caregivers may have information about social support services, yet knowing when and how to use them remains a challenge (Brodaty, Thomson, Thompson, & Fine, 2005; Collins, Stommel, King, & Given, 1991). Cancer caregivers report they do not use many assistive services; however, service utilization would increase if they were offered services tailored to their needs.

To be valuable, social support must be offered according to the type and amount needed by caregivers. This calls for a appraising risk and tailoring interventions to caregivers needs. For example, early during the disease, family and friends come to the caregiver's assistance; over time, however, this support wanes and caregivers describe loneliness.

Feelings of isolation may also occur as spouse caregivers become fixed or enmeshed in family care, and social and marital interactions becomes difficult (Manne et al., 2004). Finding social support strategies appropriate to specific caregiver needs is complex—some may need information regarding treatment, finances, or other demands; others require social support or emotional support. Anticipating each in advance is beyond translational mechanics for the healthcare system. Recognizing that the health system does not meet caregiver needs and that this affects patient care is only now emerging.

Family Relationships

Gender has been shown to be related differentially to caregiver distress. Overall, caregiving is reported to be more stressful for women (wives and daughters) than for men (husbands and sons) (Given & Sherwood, 2006; Given et al., 2006). Age has also been related to caregiver distress, with younger caregivers being more distressed, which may be the result of competing demands of multiple family and work roles (Given et al., 2004). Low personal and household incomes, loss of income, substantial out-of-pocket costs, and overall limited financial resources can place caregivers at risk for negative outcomes. Intervention researchers should consider these sociodemographic factors as they plan their studies (Hayman et al., 2001; Stephens et al., 2001).

Premorbid family discord may be aggravated by the demands for caregiving and may affect the care process, decision making, and roles of caregivers in response to the challenges of cancer care (Northouse et al., 2001; Northouse, Kershaw, Mood, & Schafenacker, 2005). Adult children are often caregivers for the older patient. Adult children and other nonspousal caregivers may experience more lifestyle adjustment and exhibit lower levels of well-being than spouses (Coristine, Crooks, Grunfeld, Stonebridge, & Christie, 2003). Adult children are forced into negotiating these life-style adjustments as they deal with competing demands, which may open familial conflicts that result in negative emotional reactions as care begins. These factors and family dynamics that precede the onset of cancer contribute to and are exacerbated by caregiving.

Family role expectations, relationships, and responsibilities change when a loved one has cancer and is aging. Communication between the dyad is an important component of examining family relationships among cancer patients and their family caregivers (Manne et al., 2004). The time spent communicating with the patient about care, emotions, and decisions can be challenging (Blanchard, Toseland, & McCallion, 1996; Budin et al., 2008; Northouse et al., 2005; Northouse et al., 2007).

Positive Responses to Providing Care

Although the difficulties and negative emotional and physical reactions to care are widely reported, less research has been devoted to the circumstances that produce positive reaction among family members caring for a patient. Providing care may engender satisfaction and meaning (Pinquart & Sörenson, 2004). Positive consequences that derive from caregiving may include a personal sense of a tough job well done, as well as personal rewards, self-esteem, support, and satisfaction, each of which may act as a buffer to the negative effects of caregiving (Kurtz et al., 2004; Pinquart & Sörenson, 2004).

Caregivers report feelings of increased closeness as both the relative with cancer and the family caregivers experience cancer together (Kim, Schulz, & Carver, 2007). These positive responses to care may lead to a sense of optimism that accrues from the care situation and the experiences, meaning, and purpose that family members derive from providing care. (Gaugler et al., 2005; Gitlin, Corcoran, Winter, Boyce, & Hauck, 2001; Moody & McMillan, 2003; Northouse et al., 2005). Focus on positive responses should be considered, but few are examined in caregivers of cancer patients.

INTERVENTIONS FOR CANCER CAREGIVERS

Interventions directed at improving various aspects of family caregivers' lives as they care for cancer patients are summarized in the evidence-based table (Table 4.1). There are a limited number of studies that used rigorous designs and methods; moreover, the sample sizes are small and results are modest. Follow-up data beyond 3 months are rare. Most interventions designed to improve caregivers' quality of life (QOL) are derived from cognitive–behavioral theory (Holland & Greenberg, 2006). This broad-based framework seeks to enhance personal control over situations by using cognitive-behavioral techniques to alter emotions, and behavioral and social problems, and to alleviate anxiety and depression.

Among the interventions included in this chapter there was very little focus on racial, ethnic, or cultural diversity. Those studies that mentioned diversity in their samples are noted in Table 4.1. Beyond this, no analyses or subanalyses were undertaken comparing outcomes between different racial/ethnic groups.

In this section we discuss the most frequently cited studies from meta-analyses and systematic and integrated reviews (Griffin et al., 2013; Harding, List, Epiphaniou & Jones, 2012; Hartmann, Bazner, Wild, Eisler & Herzog, 2010; Northouse et al., 2010; Waldron, Janke, Bechtel, Ramirez & Cohen, 2012). Some of the interventions are directed toward improving caregivers' involvement in patient care (symptoms, management, and direct physical care) and some are directed toward the needs of family caregivers themselves, with most focusing on emotional reactions. Among the studies reviewed, the majority of the interventions were delivered jointly (Campbell et al., 2007) to patients and caregivers (50%–63%) and less often to caregivers only (37%); however, some interventions

Table 4.1. Intervention Studies for Family Caregivers of Cancer Patients

Author (Year)	Design/ Sampling	Subject Characteristics	Methods/Interventions	Data/Measures	Findings/Outcomes	Limitations
Badger et al., 2007	RCT, three arms	N = 96 77% spouse Breast stages I–III 74% male caregivers Median caregiver age, 52 years (range, 44–65 years) 87% white, 11% Hispanic, 2% other	Role transitions Delivered separately to patient and caregiver Six weeks Psychiatric registered nurse Interpersonal Counseling/Education Intervention type: dyadic Caregiver: problem solving, health self-care, emotional self-care; managing depression, anxiety, and social support **Arm I:** n = 38 Therapeutic counseling, Psychoeducational Telephone caregiver only Three calls **Arm II:** n = 23 Skills training Telephone and caregiver only Exercise-related telephone calls Three calls Caregiver self-care and health self-care, emotional self-care; low-impact self-managed exercise-related calls **Arm III:** n = 35 Attention control group Caregiver receiving biweekly phone calls during the 6 weeks No counseling or encouragement to exercise; everything referred back to the primary physician	Outcome measures Depression CES-D, Anxiety SF12, Index of Clinical Stress, CES-D Positive and negative affect schedule of PANAS	Patients and partners in Arm I couples intervention (cancer education and communication skills training) and Arm II (couples exercise protocol) experienced decreased anxiety relative to control subjects over 10 weeks. Symptoms of depression also improved in the two intervention groups. (There was a strong correlation of emotional distress between women and their partners.) Improved quality of life was noted.	Various stages Limited follow-up Only 10 weeks Patients condition not considered 12% attrition Small study

Citation	Design	Sample	Intervention	Outcome measures	Results	Limitations
Blanchard et al., 1996[a] and Toseland et al., 1995[a]	RCT Oncology social worker Caregiver counseling sessions in counselor's office.	N = 86 100% spouse Heterogeneous group of cancer Stage not known 52% male caregivers Median caregiver age, 52 years (age range not available) 97% white, 3% other No mention of comparison by race or culture	Caregivers apply problem-solving strategies to manage patient care needs and to communicate with the patient. Self-care: coping skills, problem solving, health self-care, emotional self-care, self-efficacy and esteem, social support Skills training Psychoeducational counseling Problem solving/coping 6 weeks Face-to-face and caregiver only Four to six 1-hour individuals contacts	Outcome measures CES-D Barret Burden Scale State trait anxiety Marital relationship	Significant decrease in depressive symptom in patients but no effects for caregivers. Anxiety assessed for caregivers only was found to be significantly greater for caregivers than for a community sample. Caregivers reported significantly better scores on marital consensus and social functioning.	Small study Short follow-up Attrition, 23% Stage of cancer not known Brief interaction Various diagnosis 97% white
Budin et al., 2008	RCT No mention of training of interveners	N = 249 54% spouse, 12% children, 34% other Breast stages 0–3, 58% male caregivers, Median caregiver age, 52 years (range, 30–89 years) 70% white, 13% black, 7% Hispanic, 10% other No comparison of racial or ethical differences No mention of culture	Four-arm intervention trial Arm I: n = 59 Psychoeducational Counseling Stress and coping, crisis intervention Nurses 32 weeks Patient–partner dyads Disease management only Face-to-face, caregiver only Arm II: n = 66 Education Psychoeducational with videos, disease management Four 1-hour caregiver with telephone and caregiver only Arm III: n = 58 trained nurses Psychoeducational plus therapeutic counseling (skill development and training) Four 1-hour telephone counseling sessions to patient and partner delivered by nurse	Outcome measures Psychological well-being PALC (Profile of adaptation to Life) Side effect: distress BCTRI (Breast Cancer Treatment Response Index) Physical adjustment Side effects severity PALC Physical Health SRHS: self-rated overall health Social and emotional adjustment, PAIS (Psychosocial adjustment to illness)	There was no impact on psychological well-being or overall health of the caregivers. Partners in Arm IV reported significantly fewer physical symptoms than partners in Arm III. The disease management group had poorer adjustment over time. Caregiver scores improved significantly over time in physical symptoms and social adjustment in the vocational and social environments.	32% attrition Breast only Few blacks

(continued)

Table 4.1. Continued

Author (Year)	Design/ Sampling	Subject Characteristics	Methods/Interventions	Data/Measures	Findings/Outcomes	Limitations
			Arm IV: $n = 58$ Psychoeducation and telephone counseling, disease management. Four-phase specific psychoeducation videos for both patient and partner (viewed separately).			
Campbell et al., 2007	All caregivers African American (AA) AA interventionists Used some cultural sensitivity strategies	$N = 30$ 100% spouse Prostate, early stage 100% female caregivers Median caregiver age, 59 years (range, 50–71 years) 100% black	Used AA medical psychologists as interventionists Coping skills training Telephone based, caregiver and patient (joint) Six-week intervention Dyads **Arm I:** $n = 12$ Coping skills training Six 1-hour joint telephone sessions (speakerphones provided for joint sessions) Marital/family care relationship, communication, teamwork; effects of cancer on marital relationship and communication skills; planning of mutually pleasant activities Self-care: coping skills, problem solving, self-efficacy and esteem; progressive muscle relaxation, activity-rest cycles, and cognitive restructuring; communication skills **Arm II:** $n = 18$ Usual-care condition received the routine care provided through the medical outpatient program; neither patient or caregiver received training in coping skills	Outcome measures Caregiver Strain Index POMS QOL Vigor SF36 Self-efficacy Symptom Control Index (SESCI)	In coping skills group, partners had less caregiver strain, less depression, less fatigue, and more vigor and more self-efficacy. Couples reported benefits of communication. Cultural sensitivity was important.	25% attrition Small study

Study	Design	Sample	Intervention	Outcome measures	Results	Racial/ethnic considerations
Given, et al, 2006[b] and Kurtz et al., 2005[b]	RCT Nurse interveners and interviewers had training on cultural and racial sensitivity	N = 237 65% spouse, 35% others Heterogeneous diagnosis: 33% early stage, 67% advanced stage 54% female caregiver Median caregiver age, 55 years (range, 42–69 years) 92% white, 5% black, 3% other No comparison of race or ethnicity	Cognitive–behavioral Skills training, symptom management 20 weeks (10 contact interventions) Nurses with oncology experience Communication as a device to help caregiver assist in patient care (symptom management) and other care tasks Caregiver problem solving, self-care, emotional self-care, self-efficacy and esteem, depression, burden Face-to-face and caregiver and patient (joint) plus telephone for caregiver only **Arm I:** n = 118 Three joint sessions at clinic alternating with two individual telephone calls to caregivers only to focus on problem solving, symptom management for patients, emotional support, role coping, self-care, communication, reframing **Arm II:** n = 119 Receive usual care	Outcome measures CES-D, depression Caregiver reaction (burden) Reaction to providing assistance Number of caregiver tasks Symptom assistance Self-efficacy SF36 (physical and social functioning)	Males had a more negative reaction to tasks. Patients of female caregivers had lower levels of symptom severity than control subjects and thus needed less caregiver assistance over time. Mastery was indicated. Younger caregivers were more depressed. Ten-week and 20 week outcomes indicated that the intervention was effective in decreasing caregiver reactions to symptom assistance and was effective in improving social functioning. Caregivers had less depressive- related symptoms and more self-efficacy of care.	31% caregiver attrition Few minorities No culturally sensitive considerations Both early and late stages
Jepson et al., 1999	Psycho-educational 4 weeks skills training	N = 161 88% spouse Heterogeneous Newly diagnosed 35% stages 3–4 68% female caregivers Median caregiver age, 62 years (24.2% were 70 years of age or older) 85% white, 15% other No comparison of race or ethnicity	Oncology nurse specialist Face-to-face, telephone, and caregiver and patient (joint) Caregiver activities: include problem solving, health, emotional self-care, accessing resources; assess patient; use resources; care for own health problems, Monitoring and symptom management. **Arm I:** n = 90 Three 1.5-hour joint home visits alternating with six telephone calls (45 minutes each); skills to care and coordinate care **Arm II:** n = 71 Usual care	Outcome measures Caregiver burden CES-D, depression Caregiver self-esteem	Psychosocial status in treatment group improved by 3 months and was the same at 6 months. No improvement in self-esteem or burden For Caregivers with their own physical problems, the psychosocial status of those in treatment group declined at the first 3 month period but improved after 3 months	No racial/ ethnic analysis, mixed-disease group and mixed stage of disease Mostly female

(continued)

Table 4.1. CONTINUED

Author (Year)	Design/ Sampling	Subject Characteristics	Methods/Interventions	Data/Measures	Findings/Outcomes	Limitations
Kozachik et al., 2001	RCT No special training on culture	$N = 120$ 100% spouse Heterogeneous diagnosis: 48% stages I and-II, 52% stage III and IV, and newly diagnosed 51% female caregivers Median caregiver age, 52 years, (range, 39–64 years) 5% AA, 3% other No comparison of race in analysis	Symptom management Psychoeducational Skills training Face-to-face, caregiver and patient (joint) for in person and telephone, caregiver only Masters' registered nurses certified in oncology Caregiver burden: communication, emotional support, decisions; problem solving, health self-care, emotional self-care, self-efficacy, and accessing resources **Arm I:** $n = 61$ Nine contacts Five 1-hour joint meetings alternating biweekly with four individual caregiver telephone calls; symptom monitoring/management, emotional support, coordination, information for preparation for care **Arm II:** $n = 59$ Attentional control group 5 hour joint Alternating every other week	Outcome measure Caregiver depression (CES-D)	In intervention group, lagged improvement (Time 2) in caregiver depression Depressed caregivers require more intensive intervention	Very limited diversity Multiple-disease diagnosis, all disease stages All spouses

| Manne et al., 2004 | Psycho-education and coping skills | N = 68

100% spouse

Prostate, 80% early stage I and −II, 18% stages III and IV

100% female caregivers

Median caregiver age, 60 years (range, 51–69 years)

84% white, 13% AA, 3% other | 6 week intervention

Coping skills training

Group, caregiver only

Doctor, masters-level social worker, psychologist, and nutritionist

Arm I:
Six 1-hour weekly caregiver group sessions held in clinical setting, 6 consecutive weeks were used. They focused on coping, communication, skills training, and stress management

Arm II:
Usual care | Outcome measures

General psychological distress (MHI)

Impact of Events Scale (IES)

Coping (COPE)

Posttraumatic growth

Cancer-specific marital interaction | Caregivers receiving intervention reported more positive aspects of caregiving and more adaptive coping. General distress declined over time. IES declined but was not significant.

Participants receiving the intervention perceived that they had made positive contributions to their lives, gains in reappraisal coping and reduced denial coping

Small differences occurred in coping.

There was more personal growth in intervention groups. | 12% attrition

All spouse caregivers |

(*continued*)

Table 4.1. CONTINUED

Author (Year)	Design/ Sampling	Subject Characteristics	Methods/Interventions	Data/Measures	Findings/Outcomes	Limitations
McCorkle et al., 1998	Compares 2 home care-based interventions	*N* = 91 100% spouse Lung cancer Terminal stage Majority female caregivers Median caregiver age, 58 years (age range unclear) Cultural/ethic information not available	**Home care:** Masters-level nurses with expertise in terminal care **Arm I:** 1–24 weeks Psychoeducational Skills training Face-to-face, telephone, caregiver and patient (joint), and printed materials Ten 70-minute weekly home visits (on average) plus weekly follow-up telephone calls Specialized home care Emphasis on physical and psychosocial assessment, symptom management, coordination of healthcare resources, communication, problem solving, emotional and social support, access and use of resources, receiving emotional and bereavement support **Arm II:** 6 weeks Face-to-face and caregiver and patient (joint) Multidisciplinary team (not cancer-specific) standard medicine Reimbursed home care, communication Accessing resources **Arm III:** Usual care	Outcome measures Brief Symptom Inventory with nine dimensions of psychological distress Use of resources	Home-visit caregivers had less depression at 6 weeks, and at 6 months had less hostility paranoid ideation. No difference was noted at 25 months. The bereavement course among survivors was influenced positively. In caring for patients, the home nurses were able to reduce the overall level of psychological distress among spouses. Psychological distress was lower in the intervention group. The same difference was noted with regard to hostility and psychoticism in Arm 1.	43% attrition Race/ethnicity of sample not described

McCorkle et al., 2007	RCT	N = 126	100% spouse	Psychoeducational, coaching, skills training	Outcome measures	Outcomes were measured at 1, 3, and 6 months. A SNIP delivered by APNs may assist patients and their spouses with developing realistic perceptions of their sexual function and may increase their ability to interact with each other. The intervention had no group effect on depressive symptoms; however, depressive symptoms improved significantly in both patients and spouses over time. There was a positive effect on sexual function.	Need longitudinal follow-up 15% attrition Small number of non-white subjects
	16 contacts over 8 weeks	Prostate, early stage	100% female caregiver	**Arm I:** *n* = 62 SNIP	CES-D, depression		
	No mention of cultural component or special training	Median caregiver age, 56 years (range 39–63; 8% older than 65)	85% white, 15% other	Face-to-face, telephone, caregiver and patient (joint), printed materials, counseling	Cancer Rehabilitation Evaluation System (CARES)		
				APNs	Sexual function		
				Eight 1.5-hour joint weekly home visits alternating with eight weekly telephone calls (45 minutes each)	Marital interaction (relationships)		
				16 contacts (eight in home, eight-telephone)			
				Monitoring and managing symptoms			
				Use of community resources			
				Marital communication			
				Examine sexual functioning issues resulting from side effects of surgery			
				Coping skills, problem solving, emotional support, social support, accessing resources			
				Arm II: *n* = 64			
				Usual care			

(continued)

Table 4.1. CONTINUED

Author (Year)	Design/ Sampling	Subject Characteristics	Methods/Interventions	Data/Measures	Findings/Outcomes	Limitations
McMillan et al., 2006	Coping and skills training No information on special cultural training	N = 329 Unknown patient–caregiver relationship Mixed advanced stage, hospice patients 85% female caregivers Median caregiver age, 74 years (range, 44–76 years)	1 and 2 weeks, and 16- and 30-day assessments Family COPE model Registered nurses and home healthcare aides (not employed at hospice site) **Arm I:** n = 109 Control group, received hospice usual care and participated in data collection **Arm II:** n = 109 Therapeutic counseling Face-to-face and caregiver only Standard hospice care plus three 1-hour caregiver sessions to provide individual emotional support. Discussing relationship with patient health self-care; discussing caregiver's fears and feelings **Arm III:** n = 111 Coping, skills training Face-to-face and caregiver only Hospice care plus problem solving method by the intervention nurse to assist with assessing and managing patient symptoms Three 1-hour caregiver sessions to teach problem-solving methods (COPE) relationship, teamwork; involve patient in care planning; work as a team (coping skills, problem solving, emotional self-care, self-efficacy and esteem, accessing resources)	Outcome measures Coping, caregiver QOL index (CQOL-C) Caregiver task burden (Caregiver Demands Scale) Caregiver mastery Memorial Symptom Assessment Scale (MSAS) Burden of cancer symptoms	At the 30-day follow-up, the coping skills intervention led to significantly greater improvement in caregiver QOL and caregiving task burden. None of the groups showed significant change in overall caregiving mastery, or mastery specific to caregiving tasks or to problem-focused or emotional-focused coping.	69% caregiver attrition Race/ethnicity of sample not described Mixed diagnosis Female caregivers over-sampled

Source	Design	Sample	Intervention	Outcome measures (3–6 mo)	Results	Notes
Northouse et al., 2005	RCT/dyads No mention of special cultural training of interveners	N = 182 62% spouse, 16% children, 22% other Breast, advanced stage 69% male caregivers Median caregiver age, 54 years (range, 22–86 years) 77% white, 19% AA, 4% other	Psychoeducational stress, coping Skills training Family relationships, communication, family functioning, coping skills, emotional self-care, social support, management uncertainty, use of community/social resources Home visits for 13 weeks then telephone calls during the next 13 weeks Stress and coping Face-to-face, telephone, caregiver and patient (joint), and printed materials using FOCUS (Family involvement, Optimistic attitude, Coping effectiveness, Uncertainty reduction, and Symptom management), a family level intervention. Family/couples intervention for informal caregivers to provide emotional support, manage uncertainty, and promote optimism Masters-level registered nurses **Arm I:** n = 94 Usual care and 13-week home visits (initial phase), two 30-minute joint telephone calls (booster phase) **Arm II:** n = 88 Usual care	QOL Physical distress, SF36, coping, FACT-G Caregiver appraisal	Outcomes indicated a significantly less negative appraisal of caregiving. The experimental family intervention showed a significant decrease in the negative appraisal of caregiving from baseline to 3 months. This change was not evident at 6 months. No difference on QOL was noted.	26% attrition No cultural/ethnic comparison

(continued)

Table 4.1. CONTINUED

Author (Year)	Design/ Sampling	Subject Characteristics	Methods/Interventions	Data/Measures	Findings/Outcomes	Limitations
Northouse et al., 2007	RCT/dyadic 13 weeks No mention of special training of interveners	N = 263 100% spouse Prostate, 65% localized, 21% advanced, 14% recurrent 99% female caregivers Median caregiver age, 59 years (range, 42–90 years) 84% white, 14% AA, 2% other	Face-to-face, telephone, caregiver and patient (joint) videos and audiotapes, and printed materials Follow-up at 4, 8, and 12 months Marital/family: communication, hope, mutual support, maintenance of optimism and management of uncertainty were components of the intervention. Trained masters-level registered nurses Coping skills, emotional self-care, self-efficacy and esteem, access of resources, effective coping with stress, maintenance of social support system, and use of available resources effectively **Arm I:** n = 129 Three 90-minute monthly joint home visits alternating with two joint telephone calls (30 minutes each) for 13 weeks **Arm II:** n = 134 Usual care, standard clinic care	Outcome measures QOL, medical outcomes Appraisal of caregiver Mishel Uncertainty Scale, Beck Hopelessness Scale, and Lewis Self Efficacy of Coping Scale FACT-G	Treatment led to improved communication, less uncertainty in caregivers, and improved QOL. Negative appraisals of caregiving, hopelessness, and symptom distress in caregivers were noted. Some sustained at 8 months and 12 months, communication and self-efficacy sustained.	17% attrition No cultural/ethnic comparison Mixed stage of disease

| Scott et al., 2004 | RCT, couple coping Cognitive–behavioral therapy/ stress–coping therapy No mention of special training of interventionists | N = 94 100% spouse Breast and gynecological, stages I–III 100% male caregivers Median caregiver age, 53 years and as old as 63 years 98% white | 7 weeks plus a 6-month follow-up session Social–cognitive processing model of emotional adjustment to cancer **Arm I:** Face-to-face, telephone, caregiver and patient (joint), skills, printed materials, and medical information Five brief (maximum, 15-minute duration) telephone calls, no advice Female psychologists as interveners Caregivers received no intervention in this arm; focus on patient only and diagnosis **Arm II:** Patient coping skills training Psychoeducational Face-to-face, telephone, home psychological reactions, problem solving, supportive (patient only) Four 2-hour patient (individual) home visits plus two patient telephone calls (30 minutes each) **Arm III:** Couples (patient and caregiver) focus on teaching of supportive communication skills and coping (CanCope). CanCope is a couples focused communication – coping skills intervention. Five 2-hour sessions and two 30-minute phone calls, face-to-face with couple Educational materials, coping skills, supportive counseling, partner support, sexual counseling, supportive, mental communication | Outcome measures Couples communication Ways of coping Psychosocial Adjustment to Illness (PAIS) Impact of events Sexual self-functioning Brief Index of Sexual Function | Couples-family intervention led to significant improvement in caregiver communication, reduced psychological distress, better coping effort, and sexual adjustment. The intervention increased the partners' perceptions of the couples' supportive communication. | 20% attrition No cultural/ethnic comparison White caregivers over-sampled All spouse Disease stages 1–3 |

(continued)

Table 4.1. CONTINUED

Author (Year)	Design/ Sampling	Subject Characteristics	Methods/Interventions	Data/Measures	Findings/Outcomes	Limitations
Walsh et al., 2007	RCT No special training mentioned	N = 271 64% spouse Heterogeneous Advanced stage 79% female caregivers Median caregiver age, 56 years (range, 43–69 years) 86% white, 14% other	Follow-up at 4, 9, and 12 weeks **Arm I:** n = 137 Six 50-minute weekly caregiver home visits over 6 weeks Care provided by a team of clinical nurse specialists, with medical support; nurse and social worker as interveners The intervention found in health self-care, emotional self-care, social support, access of resources; respite, survivor benefits, finances, and maintenance of social networks **Arm II:** n = 134 Usual care	Outcome measures General health questionnaire Patient Health Questionnaire PHQ-28 Caregiver strain (Robinson) Caregiver QOL (Weizer)	Caregivers receiving the intervention reported a qualitative benefit but the study results did not show a significant reduction in psychological symptoms for caregivers. There was no significant impact of treatment on distress, although one third reduced QOL strain, bereavement outcomes, satisfaction with care after patient death. Caregivers reported intervention was helpful.	Rigor of interval Switched methods 55% attrition "Race/ethnicity of sample adequately described" Heterogeneous cancers

NOTE: AA, African American; APN, advance practice nurse; CARES, Cancer Rehabilitation Evaluation System; CES-D, Center for Epidemiological Studies–Depression scale; COPE, Creativity, Optimism, Planning, Expert Information; FACT-G, Functional Assessment of Cancer Therapy—General; IES, impact of events scale; MHI, Mental Health Inventory; MSAS, Memorial Symptom Assessment Scale; PAIS, psychosocial adjustment to illness; PALC, profile of adaptation to life; PANAS, Positive and Negative Affect Schedule; PHQ28, Patient Health Questionnaire-28; POMS, Profile of Mood States; QOL, quality of life; RCT, randomized controlled trial; SESCI, Self Efficacy Symptom Control; SF36, Short Forum-36; SNIP, Standardized Nursing Intervention Protocol; SRHS, Self Rated Overall Health.

[a]Same studies, but different reports. Thus, we combined them to get a full view

[b]Same study, reported in two different ways.

appeared to be sequenced (e.g., provided to the patient first, followed by provision to the caregiver [Badger, Segrin, Dorros, Meek, & Lopez, 2007; Northouse et al., 2010; Waldron et al., 2012]). A combination of face-to-face and telephone sessions were used (Given et al., 2006; Kozachik et al., 2001; McCorkle et al., 2007). Caregiver intervention trials were delivered by nurses, social workers, and psychologists (Campbell et al., 2007; Manne et al., 2004; Northouse et al., 2010; Scott et al., 2004).

Three types of interventions were identified:

1. *Therapeutic counseling* (17%), which focused primarily on strengthening patient–caregiver relationships; managing conflict, and marital and family relationships; and dealing with loss (Northouse et al., 2007, Northouse et al., 2010).
2. *Psychoeducational* (57%), which provided primarily evidence-based information about disease, treatment, management of patients' symptoms, physical aspects of patient care, and some attention to emotional and family aspects of care.
3. *Skills training* (26%), which addressed primarily the development of caregivers' coping, acquisition of skills, communication, problem-solving skills, and social support facilitation (Campbell et al., 2007; McMillan et al., 2006; Regan et al., 2012; Waldron et al., 2012; Walsh et al., 2007).

Psychoeducation and skills training strategies are often combined in intervention studies, and are discussed in a combined section later in the chapter.

Therapeutic Counseling

Northouse and colleagues (2010) found that intervention characteristics that had a positive impact on coping outcomes included face-to-face protocols as well as group interventions with at least 7 hours over five or more sessions. Greater number of hours and more sessions resulted in better outcomes. Longer interventions (e.g., >7 hours) versus shorter interventions were more likely to improve coping outcomes in cancer caregivers (Hartmann et al., 2010; Northouse et al., 2010).

Depression in caregivers has not had a consistent response to the interventions studies (Given et al., 2006). The Center for Epidemiological Studies–Depression (CES-D) scale seems to be the most common measure for depression. In general, the interventions did have a positive effect that was small but significant for caregiver burden and strain from demands. There were small but significant outcomes assessed at 3 months—not longer (Given et al., 2006, McMillan et al., 2006). In addition to depression, distress was assessed primarily by measures of worry, anxiety, and coping (Badger et al., 2007; Blanchard et al., 1996; Campbell et al., 2007; Jepson, McCorkle, Adler, Nuamah & Lusk, 1999; McCorkle, Robinson,

Nuamah, Lev, & Benoliel, 1998; McCorkle et al., 2007; Northouse et al., 2005; Northouse et al., 2007; Scott et al., 2004; Toseland, Blanchard, & McCallion, 1995; Walsh et al., 2007).

Improved well-being and coping has been shown to result in moderate to significant improvement during the first 3 months after the onset of the intervention (Northouse et al., 2005; Northouse et al., 2007; Northouse et al., 2010). Only a few investigators have looked beyond 3 months, but for those who did, effects were still significant at 6 months and beyond. (Blanchard et al., 1996; McMillan et al., 2006; Northouse et al., 2005; Northouse et al., 2007; Toseland et al., 1995).

Therapeutic interventions that focus on marital satisfaction, family support, or communication had small but significant positive effects (Blanchard et al., 1996; McCorkle et al., 2007; Northouse et al., 2005; Northouse et al., 2007; Toseland et al., 1995). Studies focusing on relationships between patients and caregivers as an outcome showed improvement in anxiety, depression, or distress in the patient and/or caregiver (Badger et al., 2007; McMillan et al., 2006; Northouse et al., 2005; Northouse et al., 2007; Scott et al., 2004), but Walsh and colleagues (2007) did not find these improved outcomes.

Social functioning relates to the caregiver interaction with family and friends. The effects of interventions that focus on enhancing social functioning are often not significant, yet this is an area of family-stated need (Badger et al., 2007; Campbell et al., 2007; McMillan et al., 2006). Goldstein and colleagues suggest that social networks and social interaction are essential to alleviate and prevent caregiver burden (Goldstein et al., 2004). Despite the increased likelihood of caregivers with lower levels of social support suffering caregiver distress, there are a limited number of interventions aimed solely at increasing and improving social support (Budin et al., 2008, Northouse et al., 2007, Walsh et al., 2007).

Case Study 1: "Sociodemographic and Diagnostic Information"

Steve is a 71-year-old semiretired high school history teacher who has just begun to care for his 66-year-old wife, Jennifer, who was diagnosed with recurrent breast cancer 2 months earlier. She is HIV negative and has received one cycle of paclitaxel administered at 3 weeks on and 1 week off, repeat every 4 weeks. Follow-up appointments monitor the levels. Communications with specialty pharmacies are also required.

Steve enjoys his role as a history teacher. He recalls that Jennifer's initial treatment was very difficult for her, both emotionally and physically, because of the number and severity of the symptoms and side effects she experienced.

The Presenting Problem

In this setting, nurses provide general guidance to patients and caregivers after a medical plan is in place. In other settings, other interdisciplinary team members may be involved to help the dyads understand the plan of care. Steve and Jennifer are quite frightened and depressed by the recurrence of the cancer and the coming months of treatment. They indicate they are having trouble talking about it. Both the suddenness of this news and its gravity led Steve to consult their nurse to discuss his fears and the impact this new treatment phase will have on their lives. The nurse listens to Steve's concerns. She tells both Steve and Jennifer about a telephone program they have for patients and caregivers that helps them cope with care responsibilities and also fosters good communication.

The nurse notes that Jennifer appears somewhat withdrawn and sad, but also anxious. Jennifer admits she is beginning to feel some fatigue, achiness, and depression. She indicates she is very frightened and needs Steve to help around the house and help manage appointments. Jennifer indicates that Steve is also depressed and anxious, that they are having trouble coping, and that he is sullen and uncommunicative.

Specifics of the Intervention

The nurse assesses Jennifer's symptoms and asks her to rate each symptom according to its severity and its interference with her daily activities. The nurse then explains to Jennifer and Steve the importance of their working together and helping one another to manage her symptoms, but also to communicate about this phase of treatment.

The nurse introduces them to materials, including a 6-week phone intervention for couples designed to help patients and family members cope with their anxieties. The nurse reviews several of the strategies for pain, fatigue, and insomnia, and discusses when to call the oncologist or nurse and what to report. Jennifer is encouraged to organize her day so she can accomplish her most important activities when she is least fatigued. She is encouraged to take short walks and that Steve accompany her on these walks. The nurse recommends they take advantage of the Better Family Communication telephone program the cancer center offers. The nurse makes sure they have the cancer center call numbers, and encourages them to talk and to communicate their needs to one another and to spend time anticipating how they can support one another.

At a subsequent visit, to address the conflict around Steve's teaching and providing care for Jennifer, the nurse begins by assessing how much they have communicated. They have discussed the conflict but have not reconciled their differences. The nurse asks Jennifer to define her priority needs for Steve. The needs are relatively few and manageable (help with dinner preparation, laundry, grocery shopping, and medication management); Steve should be able to fit these tasks into his current schedule, and he has already begun doing many of them. Soon it becomes clear that Jennifer is worried about being alone with her symptoms. After some further discussion, the nurse suggests Jennifer move her appointments for infusion to Friday afternoons so that Steve can accompany her and be available during the weekend. The strategies proposed are accepted by Steve and Jennifer, and will be reviewed at the next visit.

Last, the nurse queries Jennifer about her feelings. Jennifer begins to tear up and to acknowledge that she is depressed sometimes and frightened at other times. The nurse reminds her of the center's telephone-based program on communication. The nurse encourages Jennifer to discuss her feelings with Steve when they arise and to talk with each other. If the telephone-based program does not help, the nurse suggests that Jennifer raise these problems at her next visit so a consulting referral can be made if needed. The nurse acknowledges that this is a difficult and stressful period.

Evaluation of the Strategies

The nurse schedules two follow-up visits. At the first follow-up visit, both Steve and Jennifer report the symptom strategies are helping Jennifer to manage and continue with her current dosage of chemotherapy. Moving the infusion visits to Fridays was viewed as very helpful and supportive. Steve indicates, and Jennifer agrees, that her depression is worsening. The nurse suggests a referral to a social worker.

Psychoeducational Skills Training Interventions

In general, caregiver interventions designed to improve caregivers' knowledge had greater effects on patient or caregiver outcomes than those designed to decrease caregivers' depression or emotional health (Sörensen, Pinquart, & Duberstein, 2002). Waldron and colleagues (2012) showed that interventions targeting problem-solving and communication skills improved burden related to care and improved caregiver QOL. The consensus from these meta-analyses and systematic reviews indicates that when the patient–caregiver dyad is treated as the unit of care, important synergies are achieved that contribute to the well-being of both patients and caregivers (Harding et al., 2012; Hartmann et al., 2010; Hodges et al., 2005; Northouse et al., 2010; Sörenson et al., 2002; Waldron et al., 2012).

Studies targeting QOL vary in the measures included, and range from the Caregiver Quality of Life Index-Cancer, the Functional Assessment Cancedr Therapy—General (FACT-G) Scale, and the Short Form (SF)36 Health Survey. Anxiety, depression, general mood, and burden measures varied (Badger et al., 2007; Blanchard et al., 1996' Budin et al., 2008; Toseland et al., 1995). The Profile of Mood States subscales, the CES-D scale and the Caregiver Strain Index have been used in some QOL studies, with the focus on the physical and emotional functioning component of the QOL (Campbell et al., 2007; Given et al., 2004).

Outcomes show improvement in overall QOL (McMillan et al., 2006) but not in all factors of QOL. (Carter, 2003; Northouse et al., 2005). Problem-solving and communication skills interventions related to patient care and role changes had the most effect on patients' overall QOL (Northouse et al., 2007; Waldron et al., 2012; Walsh et al., 2007).

Although many studies give information to the caregivers, there are few that look at or address caregiver information needs and, when addressed, only immediate needs are examined, with no reports to determine whether those needs were met. There is some focus on the preparation for care, and a few studies focus on caregiving mastery (Sherwood et al., 2005) or tasks of care for which skills could be taught and their uptake evaluated (Kurtz, Kurtz, Given, & Given, 2005; McMillan et al., 2006).

Psychoeducational studies that focus on self-efficacy help caregivers gain confidence and achieve a greater level of mastery. Small but significant responses during the first 3 months have been documented, with a few reporting changes slightly beyond 3 months (Campbell et al., 2007; Given et al., 2006; Kurtz et al., 2005; McMillan et al., 2006; Northouse et al., 2005; Northouse et al., 2007).

The effect on outcomes of the caregivers include physical function—activity, leisure, or overall daily functioning—and other dimensions of QOL. Interventions did have a small but positive effect on caregivers' physical function, even beyond 3 months of follow-up (Blanchard et al., 1996; Given et al., 2006; Kurtz et al., 2004; Northouse et al., 2005; Northouse et al., 2007; Toseland et al., 1995). Skill building with communication skills may facilitate the coordination of care to help caregivers gather information needed for patient care or to communicate with healthcare providers.

Couples intervention for improving communication (Badger et al., 2007) among partners may be used to develop skills to enhance coping ability (Campbell et al., 2007; Kozachik et al., 2001; Kurtz et al., 2005; Northouse et al., 2005; Northouse et al., 2007). Baik and Adams (2011) have indicated that couples-based interventions can improve dyadic coping and dyadic adjustment, and facilitate emotional support (Hopkinson, Brown, Okamoto, & Addington-Hall, 2012). After a systematic review there is little evidence of an advantage of a simultaneous patient–family caregiver pair intervention compared with either the patient or caregiver alone to improve the outcomes for either partner (Baik & Adams, 2011).

Few of the interventions have focused on helping caregivers to acquire skills to perform care tasks, find access to resources, or manage their own health status. No studies focused on assessing the quality of care provided by family members related to patient safety, or overall patient outcomes.

Case Study 2: "Sociodemographic and Diagnostic Information"

Brenda is a 41-year-old, divorced white female who is the division head for a major software engineering firm. Brenda has a PhD in computer design, she was divorced more than 10 years ago, and she has no children and few friends. Brenda's mother is 68 and has been diagnosed with stage III breast cancer after a routine breast examination and mammogram. She is on her second cycle of paclitaxel delivered for 3 weeks with 1 week off.

The Presenting Problems

Brenda is very concerned about her mother, who lives a considerable distance away. Brenda's father died some years back and her mother has a close social group. Her mother is beginning to experience severe limiting fatigue, nausea, loss of appetite, and insomnia. All these symptoms have forced her to withdraw from her daily activities with her friends because she does not feel "up to it" and because the treatments are having an impact on her cognitive functioning, which makes her depressed and compounds the difficulty of dealing with her cancer.

Specifics of the Interventions

Faced with attempting to care for her mother at a distance, Brenda begins with an extended conversation with her mother regarding how the symptoms she is experiencing are affecting her. Brenda's mother reveals that she simply cannot maintain her home the way she would like and she is reluctant to ask her friends in because the house is "not up to her standards." Brenda learns there are several days after her treatment when her mother spends most of the day in bed. Before her mother's third cycle of treatment, Brenda seeks a telephone appointment with a nurse practitioner. The nurse practitioner is unaware of how severely the treatments are affecting Brenda's mother. She has the oncologist prescribe supporting medications to stimulate appetite, manage the nausea, and to promote sleep for those nights when insomnia occurs. In addition, the nurse practitioner suggests Brenda participate in the telephone Caregiver Intervention sessions available at the cancer center. This is a 6-week intervention to help Brenda (the long-distance caregiver) cope, solve problems, obtain support, and communicate with her mother during the cancer experience.

Brenda has another extended phone conversation with her mother and urges her mother to accept help. Reluctantly, her mother agrees. Brenda hangs up, exhausted, but glad she is able to convince her mother of the value of accepting help. Brenda contacts a couple of her mother's close friends. She tells each about her concerns and her mother's growing sense of loneliness. While problem solving, Brenda's barriers included a reluctance on the part of her mother to accept help, side effects from treatment, and lack of the availability of friends.

Brenda discovers the cancer center website has a symptom management toolkit (Given, Given, & Majeske, 2012) with strategies to manage symptoms. Brenda purchases a tablet for her mother and sets it up with Internet access. To help her mother further, Brenda installs icons to several Internet applications—one to report symptom severity to the cancer center provider and another to access on the center's symptom management toolkit. Brenda adds websites of resources from the list that the nurse practitioner gave her, including Web-based support groups. Brenda and her mother agree to set up regular communication.

Evaluation of the Strategies

Caregiving at a distance is becoming more the norm. Brenda and her mother were happy with the support they received from the cancer center nurses. The oncologist was quick to prescribe supportive care drugs. The nurse used the symptom management toolkit for both the patient and caregiver. The symptom management strategies that she and Brenda worked on together through the telephone intervention and the websites enabled her mother to manage her symptoms. She is no longer spending days in bed after each cycle of treatment. For Brenda, she has an approach to helping her mother.

CONCLUSION

It is noteworthy that none of the intervention studies discussed appear to have been disseminated to clinical settings. Caregivers of cancer patients are distressed and want help. Interventions for family caregivers of cancer patients have been limited by unimpressive outcomes. Recommendations for best practices are needed to foster more standardized care across the care continuum for caregivers of patients with cancer. A key to advancing this work would be to take strategies that are supportive and introduce mobile and e-health technology to assist dyads. We need to identify and target those dyads that are at higher risk/need, and are willing and can be served by this technology (National Alliance for Caregiving, 2011). There needs to be more studies that focus on older caregivers.

In the studies outlined, the use of technology, the Internet, mobile health, and social media is limited, and the reasons for this are unclear. Current evidence (National Alliance for Caregiving, 2011) clearly suggests that caregivers are interested in using technology to gain information targeted to their needs at the points when they deliver care to their family members (Silveira et al., 2011). Outcomes from tailored technology-driven interventions should focus on caregiver burden or depression, coping strategies, or changes in patient health states. Additional research is needed to determine whether technology-driven interventions produce similar or better results.

Caregiver intervention trials must include outcomes of interest to payers. Caregiving has remained outside the mainstream components of supportive care largely because there is little evidence to support how caregiving improves treatment or survival outcomes, or its impact on rehospitalizations, emergency department use, and unscheduled visits to oncologists or primary care providers. Until caregiving interventions demonstrate how they make unique contributions to these outcomes, it is not likely that support for caregiving research will gain additional allies and enter the larger debate regarding quality, cost-effective cancer care.

We have more than a decade of research reporting successful interventions, and recently a number of systematic reviews and meta-analyses have emerged to evaluate the potential benefits of cancer caregiver interventions. However, few of these interventions have been introduced to or implemented in practice settings. As a result of constraints of the healthcare system and financing, there are few caregiver programs. Interventions to increase support for family caregivers have lagged far behind those provided for patients, despite research that shows that spouses of cancer patients have significantly little support given the care demands (Northouse et al., 2010).

Lau and colleagues found that caregivers' negative emotional states, cognitive and physical impairment, and low literacy were serious impediments to being effective caregivers to cancer patients (Lau et al., 2010). Thus, dealing with the emotional responses of the caregivers should be considered as important interventions for the quality care for cancer patients. Well-prepared caregivers are needed to ensure high-quality cancer care to the patient (Northouse et al., 2012). Perhaps dealing with physical, emotional, and social health of caregivers is the first step; now it is time to move the research and care forward.

Many of the existing interventions are underpowered and have high attrition rates, which is expected from stressed caregivers. It is not clear that the interventions described here best meet the multifaceted set of caregiver needs. Do the interventions contribute to the overall quality of patient care? Are we focusing on caregivers with the greatest needs or just those who are willing to participate in research studies? We know little about patient needs from the described intervention studies, thus we have little ability to compare the effect on caregivers. Unfortunately, most of the intervention studies did not consider potential confounding or risk variables, such as prior family relationships, cultural variation, caregiver health status, stage of disease, hours of care, or competing caregiver role demands. Last, few studies provide any data on patient outcomes.

To understand the variation in family caregiving, we need more research focused on racial, literacy, and cultural issues. Few studies provide any comparison or separate analysis by race or culture. We need to have studies that examine caregiver problems and responsibilities throughout the cancer care trajectory. Are those caregivers who do well at the end of interventions, often 3 months, able to cope with changes from early to late disease psychologically as well as physically?

We need more studies on older patients and their caregivers, and those on younger patients (<40 years) and their caregivers. The mean age of these studies is in the 50s whereas most cancer patients with solid tumors are almost a decade older. Do men and women experience differential improvement? Do male and female caregivers who have different needs experience different problems related to caring? Are interventions gender neutral or must interventions be targeted differently for men than for women?

There has been very little research on patient outcomes as a result of the hours of family care. Moreover, little work has been done to identify specific caregiver needs, offer tailored interventions designed to address these needs, and document their uptake, use by caregivers, and what specific responses from patients occur. Understanding uptake and patient response is important for caregivers and can produce a greater sense of efficacy/mastery and willingness to continue in the caregiving role. Might explicit recognition of the value of such interventions, if delivered formally to patients, forestall caregiver anxiety and depression?

Research questions should address whether caregiver distress affects caregiver decision making, judgment, and ability to provide quality patient care. Few studies described the nature of care tasks of the caregiver. Therefore, it is not known whether caregivers were managing symptoms effectively, providing emotional support, providing direct care, monitoring patient status, or performing a combination of these tasks. Also, it is not clear how needed care tasks vary by diagnosis, treatment modality, and stage of disease. Improving caregiver preparedness and providing adequate formal support on care tasks may lead to fewer patient hospital and emergency readmissions, and fewer interruptions in cancer treatment cycles. Along with this quality and safety focus is the need to examine cost of care and use of resources.

REFERENCES

Andrews, S. (2001). Caregiver burden and symptom distress in people with cancer receiving hospice care. *Oncology Nursing Forum, 28*(9), 1469–1474.

Badger, T., Segrin, C., Dorros, S. M., Meek, P., & Lopez, A.M. (2007). Depression and anxiety in women with breast cancer and their partners. *Nursing Research, 56*(1), 44–53.

Baik, O. M., & Adams, K. B. (2011). Improving the well-being of couples facing cancer: A review of couples-based psychosocial interventions. *Journal of Marital and Family Therapy, 37*(2), 250–266.

Bevans, M., & Sternberg, E. M. (2012). Caregiving burden, stress, and health effects among family caregivers of adult cancer patients. *Journal of the American Medical Association, 307*(4), 398–403.

Blanchard, C., Toseland, R., & McCallion, P. (1996). The effects of a problem solving intervention with spouses of cancer patients. *Journal of Psychosocial Oncology, 14*(4), 1–21.

Braun, M., Mikulincer, M., Rydall, A., Walsh, A., & Rodin, G. (2007). Hidden morbidity in cancer: spouse caregivers. *Journal of Clinical Oncology, 25*, 4829–4834.

Brodaty, H., Thomson, C., Thompson, C., & Fine, M. (2005). Why caregivers of people with dementia and memory loss don't use services. *International Journal of Geriatric Psychiatry, 20*(6), 537–546.

Budin, W. C., Hoskins, C. N., Haber, J., Sherman, D. W., Maislin, G., Cater, J. R., et al. (2008). Breast cancer: Education, counseling, and adjustment among patients and partners: A randomized clinical trial. *Nursing Research, 57*(3), 199–213.

Cameron, J., Franche, R., Cheung, A., & Stewart, D. (2002). Lifestyle interference and emotional distress in family caregivers of advanced cancer patients. *Cancer, 94*(2), 521–527.

Campbell, L. C., Keefe, F. J., Scipio, C., McKee, D. C., Edwards, C. L., Herman, S. H., et al. (2007). Facilitating research participation and improving quality of life for African American prostate cancer survivors and their intimate partners: A pilot study of telephone-based coping skills training. *Cancer, 109*(2 Suppl), 414–424.

Carter, P. A. (2002). Caregivers' descriptions of sleep changes and depressive symptoms. *Oncology Nursing Forum, 29*(9), 1277–1283.

Carter, P. A. (2003). Family caregivers' sleep loss and depression over time. *Cancer Nursing, 26,* 253–259.

Collins, C., Stommel, M., King, S., & Given, C. W. (1991). Assessment of the attitudes of family caregivers toward community services. *Gerontologist, 31*(6), 756–761.

Coristine, M., Crooks, D., Grunfeld, E., Stonebridge, C., & Christie, A. (2003). Caregiving for women with advanced breast cancer. *Psycho-Oncology, 12,* 709–719.

Fortinsky, R., Kercher, K., & Burant, C. (2002). Measurement and correlates of family caregiver self-efficacy for managing dementia. *Aging and Mental Health, 6*(2), 153–160.

Gaugler, J. E., Hanna, N., Linder, J., Given, C. W., Tolbert, V., Kataria, R. et al. (2005). Cancer caregiving and subjective stress: A multi-site, multi-dimensional analysis. *Psycho-Oncology, 14*(9), 771–785.

Gitlin, L., Corcoran, M., Winter, L., Boyce, A., & Hauck, W. (2001). A randomized controlled trial of a home environmental intervention: Effect on efficacy and upset in caregivers and on daily function of persons with dementia. *Gerontologist, 41*(1), 4–14.

Given, B., & Given, C. W. (1992). Patient and family caregiver reaction to new and recurrent breast cancer. *Journal of the American Medical Women's Association, 47*(5), 201–212.

Given, C. W., Given, B., Azzouz, F., Stommel, M., & Kozachik, S. (2000). Comparison of changes in physical functioning of elderly patients with new diagnoses of cancer. *Medical Care, 38*(5), 482–493.

Given, B. A., Given, C. W., & Majeske, C. (2012). *Symptom management toolkit.* East Lansing, MI: Michigan State University.

Given, B., Given, C. W., Sikorskii, A., Jeon, S., Sherwood, P., & Rahbar, M. (2006). The impact of providing symptom management assistance on caregiver reaction: Results of a randomized trial. *Journal of Pain and Symptom Management, 32*(5), 433–443.

Given, B., & Sherwood, P. (2006). Family care for the older person with cancer. *Seminars in Oncology Nursing, 22*(1), 43–50.

Given, B., Wyatt, G., Given, C. W., Sherwood, P., Gift, A., DeVoss, D., et al. (2004). Burden and depression among caregivers of patients with cancer at the end of life. *Oncology Nursing Forum, 31*(6), 1105–1117.

Goldstein, N., Concato, J., Fried, T., Kasl, S., Johnson-Hurzeler, R., & Bradley, E. (2004). Factors associated with caregiver burden among caregivers of terminally ill patients with cancer. *Journal of Palliative Care, 20*(1), 38–43.

Griffin, J. M., Meis, L., Greer, N., Jensen, A., MacDonald, R., Rutks, I., et al. (2013). *Effectiveness of family and caregiver interventions on patient outcomes among adults with cancer or memory-related disorders: A systematic review.* VA-ESP Project #09-009. Washington, DC: Department of Veterans Affairs.

Grunfeld, E., Coyle, D., Whelan, T., Clinch, J., Reyno, L., Earle, C., et al. (2004). Family caregiver burden: Results of a longitudinal study of breast cancer patients and their principal caregivers. *Canadian Medical Association Journal, 170*(12), 1795–1801.

Hagedoorn, M., Sanderman, R., Bolks, H. N., Tuinstra, J., & Coyne, J. C. (2008). Distress in couples coping with cancer: A meta-analysis and critical review of role and gender effects. *Psychological Bulletin, 134*(1), 1–30.

Harding, R., List, S., Epiphaniou, E., & Jones, H. (2012). How can informal caregivers in cancer and palliative care be supported? An updated systematic literature review of interventions and their effectiveness. *Palliative Medicine, 26*(1), 7–22.

Harris, J., Godfrey, H., Partridge, F., & Knight, R. (2001). Caregiver depression following traumatic brain injury: A consequence of adverse effects on family members? *Brain Injury, 15*(3), 223–238.

Hartmann, M., Bäzner, E., Wild, B., Eisler, I., & Herzog, W. (2010). Effects of interventions involving the family in the treatment of adult patients with chronic physical diseases: A meta-analysis. *Psychotherapy and Psychosomatics, 79*, 136–148.

Hayman, J., Langa, K., Kabeto, M., Katz, S., DeMonner, S., Chernew, M., et al. (2001). Estimating the cost of informal caregiving for elderly patients with cancer. *Journal of Clinical Oncology, 19*(13), 3219–3225.

Hodges, L. J., Humphris, G. M., & Macfarlane, G. (2005). A meta-analytic investigation of the relationship between the psychological distress of cancer patients and their carers. *Social Science and Medicine, 60*(1), 1–12.

Holland, J., & Greenberg, D. (Eds.). (2006). *Quick reference for oncology clinicians.* Charlottesville, VA: IPOS Press.

Hopkinson, J. B., Brown, J. C., Okamoto, I., & Addington-Hall, J. M. (2012). The Effectiveness of patient–family carer (couple) intervention for the management of symptoms and other health-related problems in people affected by cancer: A systematic literature search and narrative review. *Journal of Pain and Symptom Management, 43*(1), 111–142.

Jepson, C., McCorkle, R., Adler, D., Nuamah, I., & Lusk, E. (1999). Effects of home care on caregivers' psychosocial status. *Image: The Journal of Nursing Scholarship, 31*(2), 115–120.

Kane, R. L. (2011). *The good caregiver: A one-of-a-kind compassionate resource for anyone caring for an aging loved one.* New York: Penguin Group.

Kiecolt-Glaser, J. K., Preacher, K. J., MacCallum, R. C., Atkinson, C., Malarkey, W. B., & Glaser, R. (2003). Chronic stress and age-related increases in the proinflammatory cytokine IL-6. *Proceedings of the National Academy of Sciences of the United States of America, 100*(15), 9090–9095.

Kim, Y., Carver, C. S., Cannady, R. S., & Shaffer, K. M. (2013). Self-reported medical morbidity among informal caregivers of chronic illness: The case of cancer. *Quality of Life Research. 22*(6), 1265–1272.

Kim, Y., Schulz, R., & Carver, C. S. (2007). Benefit finding in the cancer caregiving experience. *Psychosomatic Medicine, 69*(3), 283–291.

Kozachik, S., Given, C., Given, B., Pierce, S., Azzouz, F., Rawl, S., et al. (2001). Improving depressive symptoms among caregivers of patients with cancer: Results of a randomized clinical trial. *Oncology Nursing Forum, 28*(7), 1149–1157.

Kurtz, M., Kurtz, J., Given, C. W., & Given, B. (2004). Depression and physical health among family caregivers of geriatric patients with cancer: A longitudinal view. *Medical Science Monitor,* 10(8), CR447–CR456.

Kurtz, M., Kurtz, J., Given, C. W., & Given, B. (2005). A randomized, controlled trial of a patient/caregiver symptom control intervention: Effects on depressive symptomatology of caregivers of cancer patients. *Journal of Pain and Symptom Management,* 30(2), 112–122.

Lau, D. T., Berman, R., Halpern, L., Pickard, A. S., Schrauf, R., & Witt, W. (2010). Exploring factors that influence informal caregiving in medication management for home hospice patients. *Journal of Palliative Medicine,* 13(9), 1085–1090.

Manne, S., Babb, J., Pinover, W., Horwitz, E., & Ebbert, J. (2004). Psychoeducational group intervention for wives of men with prostate cancer. *Psycho-Oncology,* 13(1), 37–46.

McCorkle, R., Robinson, L., Nuamah, I., Lev, E., & Benoliel, J. Q. (1998). The effects of home nursing care for patients during terminal illness on the bereaved's psychological distress. *Nursing Research,* 47(1), 2–10.

McCorkle R., Siefert M. L., Dowd M. F., Robinson J. P., & Pickett M. (2007). Effects of advanced practice nursing on patient and spouse depressive symptoms, sexual function, and marital interaction after radical prostatectomy. *Urologic Nursing,* 27(1), 65–77; discussion 78–80.

McMillan, S. C., Small, B. J., Weitzner, M., Schonwetter, R., Tittle, M., Moody, L., et al. (2006). Impact of coping skills intervention with family caregivers of hospice patients with cancer: A randomized clinical trial. *Cancer,* 106(1), 214–222.

Moody, L. E., & McMillan, S. (2003). Dyspnea and quality of life indicators in hospice patients and their caregivers. *Health and Quality of Life Outcomes,* 1(1), 9.

Morita, T., Chihara, S., & Kashiwagi, T. (2002). Family satisfaction with inpatient palliative care in Japan. *Palliative Medicine,* 16(3), 185–193.

National Alliance for Caregiving. (2011). *e-Connected family caregiver: Bringing caregiving into the 21 Century.* Washington, DC: Author.

Northouse, L. L., Katapodi, M. C., Song L., Zhang, L., & Mood, D. W. (2010). Interventions with caregivers of cancer patients: Meta-analysis of randomized trials. *CA: A Cancer Journal for Clinicians,* 60, 317–339.

Northouse, L., Kershaw, T., Mood, D., & Schafenacker, A. (2005). Effects of a family intervention on the quality of life of women with recurrent breast cancer and their family caregivers. *Psycho-Oncology,* 14(6), 478–491.

Northouse, L., Mood, D. W., Schafenacker, A., Montie, J. E., Sandler, H. M., Forman, J. D., et al. (2007). Randomized clinical trial of a family intervention for prostate cancer patients and their spouses. *Cancer,* 110(12), 2809–2818.

Northouse, L., Templin, T., & Mood, D. (2001). Couples' adjustment to breast disease during the first year following diagnosis. *Journal of Behavioral Medicine,* 24(2), 115–136.

Northouse, L., Williams, A., Given, B., & McCorkle, R. (2012). Psychosocial care for family caregivers of patients with cancer. *Journal of Clinical Oncology,* 30, 1227–1234.

Pavalko, E. K., & Woodbury, S. (2000). Social roles as process: Caregiving careers and women's health. *Journal of Health and Social Behavior,* 41(1), 91–105.

Pinquart, M., & Sörensen, S. (2004). Associations of caregiver stressors and uplifts with subjective well-being and depressive mood: A meta-analytic comparison. *Aging and Mental Health,* 8(5), 438–449.

Regan, T., Lambert, S., Girgis, A., Kelly, B., Kayser, K., & Turner, J. (2012). Do couple-based interventions make a difference for couples affected by cancer? A systematic review. *BMC Cancer, 12*, 279.

Schumacher, K., Stewart, B., Archbold, P., Dodd, M., & Dibble, S. (2000). Family caregiving skill: Development of the concept. *Research in Nursing and Health, 23*(3), 191–203.

Scott, J. L., Halford, W. K., & Ward, B. G. (2004). United we stand? The effects of a couple-coping intervention on adjustment to early stage breast or gynecological cancer. *Journal of Consulting and Clinical Psychology, 72*(6), 1122–1135.

Sherwood, P., Given, B., Given, C. W., Schiffman, R., Murman, D., & Lovely, M. (2004). Caregivers of persons with a brain tumor: A conceptual model. *Nursing Inquiry, 11*(1), 43–53.

Sherwood, P., Given, B., Given, C. W., Schiffman, R., Murman, D., Lovely, M., et al. (2006). Predictors of distress in caregivers of persons with a primary malignant brain tumor. *Research in Nursing and Health, 29*(2), 105–120.

Sherwood, P., Given, B., Given, C. W., Schiffman, R., Murman, D., von Eye, A., et al. (2007). The influence of caregiver mastery on depressive symptoms. *Journal of Nursing Scholarship, 39*(3), 249–255.

Sherwood, P., Given, B., Given, C. W., Sikorskii, A., You, M., & Prince, J. (2012). The impact of a problem-solving intervention on increasing caregiver assistance and improving caregiver health. *Supportive Care in Cancer, 20*(9), 1937–1947.

Sherwood, P. R., Given, C. W., Given, B. A., & von Eye, A. (2005). Caregiver burden and depression: Analysis of common caregiver outcomes. *Journal of Aging and Health, 17*(2), 125–147.

Silveira, M. J., Given, C. W., Cease, K. B., Sikorskii, A., Given, B., Northouse, L. L., et al. (2011). Cancer carepartners: Improving patients' symptom management by engaging informal caregivers. *BMC Palliative Care, 10*, 21.

Sörensen, S., Pinquart, M., & Duberstein, P. (2002). How effective are interventions with caregivers? An updated meta-analysis. *Gerontologist, 42*, 356–372.

Stenberg, U., Ruland, C., & Miaskowski, C. (2010). Review of the literature on the effects of caring for a patient with cancer. *Psycho-Oncology, 19*(10), 1013–1025.

Stephens, M., Townsend, A., Martire, L., & Druley, J. (2001). Balancing parent care with other roles: Interrole conflict of adult daughter caregivers. *Journal of Gerontology, Series B, Psychological Sciences and Social Sciences, 56*(1), 24–34.

Toseland, R., Blanchard, C., & McCallion, P. (1995). A problem solving intervention for caregivers of cancer patients. *Social Science in Medicine, 40*(4), 517–528.

Vitaliano, P., Zhang, J., & Scanlan, J. (2003). Is caregiving hazardous to one's physical health? A meta-analysis. *Psychological Bulletin, 129*(6), 946–972.

Waldron, E., Janke, E. A., Bechtel, C., Ramirez, M., & Cohen, A. (2012). A systematic review of psychosocial interventions to improve cancer caregiver quality of life. *Psycho-Oncology, 22*(6), 1200–1207.

Walsh, K., Jones, L., Tookman, A., Mason, C., McLoughlin, J., Blizard, R., et al. (2007). Reducing emotional distress in people caring for patients receiving specialist palliative care: Randomised trial. *British Journal of Psychiatry, 190*, 142–147.

5

HIV/AIDS Caregiving

HELEN M. LAND AND BROOKLYN LEVINE ■

Family caregiving for a loved one with HIV/AIDS was born in a context of disease stigma and a broad meaning of family. Because HIV is a transmittable virus, the populations that contract it are affected by geopolitical forces influencing service provision for both caregiver and care recipient. Crucial to understanding the caregiving context is the recognition that the caregiver may also be carrying the virus and thus may have compromised health issues while providing care for another. This chapter addresses the highly diverse characteristics and needs of HIV/AIDS caregivers. Here, we provide the historical background of HIV/AIDS caregiving set within the context in which AIDS is recognized. We then review the multiple roles of the caregiver and the challenges, which are unique to this experience. We follow with a review of research on AIDS caregiving and provide implications for treatment for each subgroup. We then discuss intervention studies aimed at stemming the burden of AIDS caregiving.

BACKGROUND

Since the early 1980s, when an unknown, perplexing, virulent, and terminal virus appeared in gay men in New York and California, HIV caregivers have assumed roles of support giver, nurse, psychotherapist, spiritual provider, breadwinner, housekeeper, and advocate. Often carrying the virus themselves, the majority of caregivers were partners and friends of young gay men requiring care (Pearlin, Mullan, Aneshensel, Wardlaw, & Harrington, 1994). Mothers, sisters, and other family members who were less visible to the public eye also enacted caregiving during the relatively short and steep decline of the care recipient. Because AIDS was first manifested in gay men who had contracted the virus through unprotected anal sex and through illicit intravenous drug use, people living with HIV/AIDS have been heavily stigmatized, as have their caregivers. At the dawn of this new disease in the United States,

AIDS caregivers, many of whom were not related to the patient, faced striking challenges as they were denied access to hospital rooms, doctor visits, and other support services required for ongoing HIV care. Despite the circumstances, these caregivers stood as a protective bulwark giving direct and indirect support, and advocating for access to dental care, nurse visits, health insurance, job security, and medical clinical trials for those with this fatal disease. Providing hope, humor, distraction, and information, HIV caregivers traveled an emotional rollercoaster across days and weeks, administering medication, diapering and bathing the care recipient, changing soiled sheets, cooling raging fevers, keeping house, and feeding their loved ones (Land, Hudson, & Stiefel 2003). Many caregivers confronted anger, sadness, fear, and anticipatory grieving as the focus of their care changed from long-range planning to day-to-day realities of declining health and disease manifestation (Le Blanc & Wight, 2000). Providing activities of daily living (ADLs) with little preparation, and managing cognitive problems and dementia in the care recipient, many of these young men experienced role overload with too much to do and too little time to do it, and role strain and loss, altering their roles from partner to caregiver (Land et al. 2003; Pearlin et al., 1994). Frequently, in emerging adulthood themselves, the caregiver for a terminally ill loved one was often developmentally premature and unprepared to take on the unexpected caregiving duties required. Many who were seropositive themselves evidenced poorer outcomes than their seronegative counterparts, including significantly more depression and burden (Centers for Disease Control & Prevention, 2006).

Moreover, because countless caregivers were at an earlier stage of disease manifestation, they saw into their future what they were likely to endure themselves: extreme fatigue, vomiting, previously unknown opportunistic infections, wasting syndrome, purple blotches covering the body (Kaposi's sarcoma), nausea, vomiting, and, ultimately, death. The illness was named the *20th-century plague*. Stigma's wide reach resulted in gay caregivers being discouraged from attendance at funerals and memorial services of their loved one. And unlike other caregivers, they received little compensation for caregiving—no days off work, no death benefits, and, frequently, no inheritance. The funerals, memorial services, and burials mounted, and cause of death was often relabeled as cancer, leukemia, or other wasting syndrome. Over time, multiple losses left a kind of posttraumatic stress reaction in the bereaved and in their communities. Yet, fortitude remained. They mourned their losses, formed support groups for other caregivers, organized AIDS service organizations (ASOs) out of their living rooms, and lobbied for funding for AIDS research. In fact, the *Names Project* was born as caregivers sewed quilt patches together so in the days ahead others would remember their loved ones. Many times, these caregivers garnered their strength and went on to provide care for another friend or family member with AIDS, until they themselves needed care.

Throughout the course of a decade, stigma continued for AIDS caregivers and care recipients, but the face of AIDS began to change. HIV spread from larger white gay enclaves in New York and California across the country to the Midwest and South, and from large cities to smaller towns and rural areas where service provision was scant. In addition, women and men of color residing in poverty-ridden, urban communities and neighborhoods held the AIDS spotlight (Wyatt, Carmona, Loeb, & Williams, 2005). Previously a bulwark in black communities, black churches said little of the viral killer dwelling in their midst. Reports document that, by the 1990s, AIDS was the leading cause of death for young to middle-age black women (Centers for Disease Control & Prevention, 2006). Often infected through intravenous (IV) drug use or heterosexual contact with an IV drug user, these young mothers were likely refused treatment because they were labeled poor candidates as a result of polydrug use (Wingood, 2003). Children orphaned by AIDS commanded the attention of child welfare agencies as aging black mothers and grandparents became primary caregivers for their infected daughters and grandchildren (Land, 2010).

Concomitantly, as medications improved quality and length of life, AIDS caregiving moved from hospital to home. Again, new groups of AIDS caregivers emerged with needs that differed from those previously known. AIDS spread to Latino communities and border towns as Latin women infected through heterosexual contact became caregivers for their HIV-infected partners and their seropositive children born with the virus. The Roman Catholic Church's ban on condoms (as artificial birth control) saw the spread of HIV in Latinas, whose serostatus converted to being positive. Many were monolingual Spanish speaking from rural areas in the Caribbean, Mexico, and Central America. Often, these female caregivers had little education, scarce income, and few connections to power escalators needed to advocate for their sick loved ones. Because stigma in HIV is powerful in Latino communities, even family members residing in the same household as the care recipient were often unaware of the AIDS diagnosis. Soon entire households became HIV infected in Latin communities. Because this group was largely represented by undocumented residents, their knowledge of complex services systems and willingness to access care have been limited. Disempowerment remained a powerful force for this caregiver group. Few providers served caregivers who were Spanish speaking and had distinct cultural values from those who were U.S. born. Often, caregivers came from rural communities where medical provision is lacking. Thus, caregivers were and are an extremely varied group. Although all caregivers are subject to the stress process of HIV/AIDS caregiving, the needs of caregivers vary because not everyone goes through the same stress process. Background variables such as length of time caregiving, education, income, age, migration experience, gender, and culture all affect the dynamics of stress proliferation.

Today, ASOs continue to be challenged to provide care as the demands of new groups of HIV infected become identified. For example, one relatively new subgroup at risk are adolescents and emerging young adults living on the streets of urban America who are drawn to the entertainment industry and soon turn to subsistence sex work and drug use. New information technologies, including *sexting,* set this group apart from others. Often, these individuals are without medical insurance or stable care providers who will meet their needs (Land, 2010).

CAREGIVER STRESS HEALTH MODEL

How does academic literature address vulnerabilities of AIDS caregivers and their care recipients? Similar to other groups of caregivers, the stress of HIV/AIDS caregiving is a process comprised of interrelated conditions, including (a) the sociodemographic background characteristics of the caregiver that may render vulnerable statuses; (b) primary stressors that are inherent in the daily acts of caregiving, and financial and psychological burdens stemming from the health and psychological needs of the care recipient; and (c) secondary stressors that evolve out of caregiving, including diminishment of control or mastery over life, worries about one's health, developmental life transitions, and job–caregiving conflict. Thus, stress may proliferate as caregiver burden grows (Pearlin, 2010). Often, the outcomes are depression or other mental health concerns and threats to physical health. Psychological mediators, such as high self-esteem, and positive coping methods along with life conditions, such as strong social support, may explain why not all caregivers negotiating difficult circumstances go through the same stress process. Response differences may arise because caregivers are exposed to different constellations of stress and strain (Pearlin et al., 2009; Knight & Sayegh, 2010). In fact, stressors and mental health differences may reduce the capacity to harness personal resources that buffer the stress process (Land & Hudson, 2004). Stress proliferation may occur as a result of life and role transitions, the bunching of stressors particularly around exit events (involving loss), and available coping resources such as accessing social support (Pearlin et al., 2009; Knight, 2009). Differences in the cycle of caregiving and in the stress proliferation process may explain why some people fare better as AIDS caregivers. Studies of the stress process in HIV/AIDS groups demonstrate that white family caregivers, black women, Latinas, and gay male partners and friends differ substantially with respect to the stress process and its outcomes (Land & Hudson, 2004). Thus, care plans for caregivers must vary accordingly.

In the western world and globally, HIV caregivers continue to provide care to their sick or dying loved ones. In addition, in many communities HIV continues to hold profound stigma, which provokes a cascade of stress proliferation in caregiving for someone with AIDS. The advent of combination treatment of highly active antiviral therapy (HAART) became known as the resurrection drug for those who had access to medication and were able to follow strict regimens needed for effective treatment. Throughout the course of two decades, HIV in industrial countries has become more and more a chronic and sometimes fatal disease of the poor and people of color.

THE TYPE OF CAREGIVING RELATIONSHIP
AND EMOTIONAL WELL-BEING

Because HIV caregiving often plays out with both caregiver and care recipient being infected, recent research investigations have focused on the type and quality of the caregiving relationship and its effect on the emotional well-being of the caregiving dyad.

Gay Men

HAART has reduced viral load substantially, and has given new and extended life for those who take it. Although newer forms of combination therapies continue to evolve, their long-term use has deficits. For those gay men who were infected during the 1990s and have taken HAART, accelerated aging is a very real problem. Thus, for some, caregiving continues to be needed, and HIV caregivers who are infected are also subject to these adverse side effects. The negative side effects of HAART affect both care recipient and caregiver, with the role of caregiving being ever more difficult. Side effects can be particularly troubling depending on which combination of therapies is used. Resulting physical problems include arrhythmia and breathing problems; liver damage; bone death; mineral loss and osteoporosis; diarrhea; elevated blood sugar levels (hyperglycemia); excessive acidity of the blood, which is detrimental to cells; disfiguring fat deposits (lipodystrophy); nausea; and skin eruptions (Engel, 2008). Thus, for some, informal caregivers continue to be needed. This group is often represented by partners and friends providing care. Gay male caregivers who are seropositive consistently report more stressors than their female counterparts (Land et al., 2003). Reported in the literature over time is role overload—that is, feeling overwhelmed and overloaded in the caregiver role. Perhaps this is because men are less likely to be socialized to perform caregiving. Enduring stressors such as managing problematic behavior and cognitive impairment in the care recipient often result in more severe depressive episodes for gay male caregivers, especially those who are seropositive (Wight, 2000). Vulnerability to depression increases as ecological background risk factors increase. Younger age, lower educational level, lower income, and unemployment render greater probabilities of experiencing depression in gay male caregivers. For older gay caregivers, internalized homophobia, perceptions of HIV alienation, stigma, and conflict in the social network are associated with higher rates of depression. In fact, both discrimination and poor relationship quality are associated with greater depression in both care recipient and caregiver. Furthermore, when one partner experiences the role transition to caregiver, the bunching of developmentally unexpected life transitions interacting with the stress proliferation process renders a recipe for poorer mental health outcome (Land & Hudson, 2004). Moreover, findings suggest that relationship quality moderates the impact of discrimination as a risk factor for gay and bisexual adults (Fredriksen-Goldsen, Kim, Muraco, & Mincer, 2009). Last, experiencing exit events, particularly multiple-loss and HIV bereavements, culminates in a powerful equation for depression for older gay caregivers (Fredriksen-Goldsen, 2007; Fredriksen-Goldsen, Muraco, Mincer, & Kim, 2009). Conditions that buffer the relationship between stress and depression include higher self-esteem, dispositional optimism, and feelings of mastery over life.

Heterosexual Male Caregivers of HIV-Infected Children

Heterosexual male caregivers are a little known and understudied group. As mothers die as a result of HIV, fathers, uncles, and grandfathers have taken on the caregiving of these children when grandmothers and other female relatives are not present. The majority (about 75%) are birth and adoptive fathers; approximately 10% are providing care for more than one child with HIV(Land, 2010). About half have other children in the home for whom they provide care. A large percentage of these caregivers are black men (58%) and Latinos (23%) who provide care for children between the ages of 5 years and 12 years (Land, 2010). Roughly one quarter of the members of this population are estimated to be HIV infected themselves. These male caregivers of color experience problems that are absent from other caregiver groups. Most prominent is the stigma associated with the prototype of the absent father (McAdoo, 1993). Its influence affects the mentalities of medical and other service providers negatively. Too frequently, formal service providers hold the erroneous belief that male caregivers lack role models to set limits with children or that they are limited in caring for or communicating with a sick child. These are caregivers whose custodial rights have been challenged, thus adding additional stress to an already difficult situation. For others, placement of children has been discussed without adequate assessment of family life. Interrogation by school and medical providers is common and may be experienced as shaming and emotionally exhausting in this group.

Caring for HIV-infected children is not a simple task for heterosexual male caregivers who have little experience being a single parent or primary caregiver. Although some are children who have been orphaned by HIV, others continue to see their mothers who are debilitated by HIV and in a state of decline. Orphaned children often grow up with significant emotional, developmental, and physical limitations; hence, parenting these children poses a significant challenge (Land, 2010). Moreover, most of these caregivers live alone and have little instrumental and emotional support from relatives or friends. Within this context, both child and parent may be actively grieving the loss of the female relationship presence and thus may feel quite depleted. In addition, men and children may grieve quite differently; thus, the adult must be able to provide variable emotional responses to bereaved children while experiencing his own grief.

Those men with jobs outside the home face particular challenges. With potentially conflicting roles of breadwinner and caregiver, stress proliferation likely mounts. Reduced employment results, predictably, in anxiety about meeting financial concerns during economically depressed times. Under such circumstances it is little wonder that these male primary caregivers are hesitant to approach social services for assistance or are resistant to services when needed. These conditions often result in a cycle of growing need and little support (Land, 2010).

Within this context, service providers must take the time to build a strong working alliance and be cognizant of said caregiver issues. Comprehensive care plans should include an assessment of the developmental needs of all children living in the household as well as the idiosyncratic needs of each child. In addition, providers should determine the family dynamics in the home, the coping style of the adult caregiver, and an alcohol and drug history. In addition, it may be helpful to include an assessment of available supports to the family system and how the male caregiver runs the household. Thus, working within the system, the provider completes a comprehensive assessment of needs and coaches from a stance of trust. As one man said, "Children can be very demanding and repetitive in their needs for care. I love my children but I have to say that at times they drive *me crazy*. This is about children, and AIDS, and being the parents of these kids" (Strug, Rabb, & Nanton, 2002, p. 310).

White Women

In many communities, female caregivers constitute the backbone of family caregiving (Land & Hudson, 2004). In addition to providing care for HIV-infected children, partners, or friends, they often assume a non-HIV-related caregiving role for other family members, such as aging parents. This group of HIV female caregivers is largely composed of ethnic and racial minorities of color, particularly women of African and Latin heritage.

Stressors experienced and the needs of white women are quite distinct from those of their sisters of color. The majority of white female AIDS caregivers are better educated, have medical insurance, are HIV negative, and are caring for a partner or adult offspring with HIV (Centers for Disease Control & Prevention, 2006). Thus, background factors are less likely to render vulnerabilities. Moreover, this group of HIV caregivers has fewer non-HIV-related chronic illnesses than any other group of HIV caregivers. However, compared with their white male counterparts, they have lower education, lower income, and more years of providing care. Major stressors that affect and reflect elevated depression include feelings of role captivity in caregiving, poor quality in the caregiver–care recipient relationship, and loss of self-identity to the caregiving role. In fact, those women caring for partners often experience worse role functioning and poorer dyadic well-being, as manifested by diminished affect involvement, poorer medication adherence, and less ability to manage aberrant behaviors of the care recipient. These factors, along with greater depression in the care recipient, predict greater burden and depression in the caregiver (Miller, Bishop, Herman, & Stein, 2007).

Conversely, the presence of greater self-esteem and better relationship quality tends to lower the toxic effect of the feelings of discrimination and depression resulting from the stress proliferation process (Fredriksen-Golden et al., 2009). As with other research of white females, findings indicate that this group of HIV caregivers is more likely to seek services than any other HIV/AIDS caregiving group, perhaps indicating their heightened knowledge of available resources and strong potential for accessing help. However, compared with female cancer caregivers, white female HIV caregivers evidence lower functioning and greater restriction in socializing. Moreover, although they report less family support, they report greater rewards from caregiving (Stetz & Brown, 2004). As one woman put it, "That's what friends do" (Muraco & Fredriksen-Goldsen, 2011, p. 1073). Service plans may include support groups for caregivers, individual counseling, and couples counseling, as well as in-home services to stem feelings of captivity and loss of self to the caregiving role.

Black Women

Because the late 20th and early 21st centuries ushered in both increased drug use and increased incarceration of drug offenders, co-occurrence accompanied rapidly rising rates of HIV (Knowlton, 2003). Current prevalence of black men who have sex with men is quite high, yet the stigma associated with HIV is higher. Moreover, until recently, the black church took a small role in providing resources or support for those with HIV and their caregivers (Knowlton, 2003). Thus, the culmination of these contextual background factors increases both the psychological and physical burden in these female caregivers.

Black female caregivers often travel a difficult road. For generations, these women have been a strong resource of caregiving support, both formally and informally. Black female caregivers are a diverse group. They are young women providing care for HIV-infected children and male partners, and older women caring for daughters with HIV and providing care for their orphaned grandchildren. In addition, a sizeable minority of women with nonkin ties are providing care for another woman or man with HIV. These are caregivers who are disproportionately HIV infected, and often have a history of drug and alcohol use. Concomitantly, they experience great stigma within their communities. Background factors include poor general health and low educational attainment and the majority live below the poverty line (Knowlton, 2003). Of note, many who are injection drug users have a history of being sexually or physically abused and became homeless at a young age to escape abuse (Wyatt et al., 2005). Moreover, investigations suggest that, although caregivers report their ability to provide care is reduced because of financial deprivation, their care recipients report that burdens to caregiving are largely a result of health status (Knowlton, 2003).

Black female caregivers typically report less burden than their white counterparts, yet such is not the case with this group of HIV/AIDS caregivers (Redgrave,

Swartz, & Romanoski, 2003). Moreover, although informal caregiving is culturally normative in this group, HIV caregivers continue to cite HIV-related stigma as being associated directly with depressive symptoms. Despite strong stigma, disclosure of caregiving status is associated with fewer symptoms. In fact, significant decreases in depressive symptoms relate inversely to the number of disclosures, thus demonstrating the buffering effect of serostatus disclosure in this group (Mitchell & Knowlton, 2009). In addition, the presence of a strong female social network is associated with less role overload (Mitchell & Knowlton, 2012). More important, financial resources are much needed to support both the HIV caregiver and the support network. As one woman stated of providing care to another with HIV, "I feel I have lost my identity to what I was, ... I just always give ... my son, my grandson, my husband, my aunt who is sick, it's a constant" (Knowlton, 2003, p. 1308). Implications for practice are great and focus on both needed structural supports, such as financial and medical help, as well as emotional support. Same-sex support groups and telephone support have been found to be effective with this group of HIV/AIDS caregivers (Herbert, Weinstein, Martire & Schulz, 2006). Results suggest that religion and spirituality may also provide some support for these caregivers (Herbert et al., 2006). The tradition of caregiving is long and strong in this group; thus, services should be gender sensitive and focus on the needs of the black female experience. Programs must be designed to be relevant to these women who have cared for others across generations.

Latinas

With the rise in immigration to the United States during the past 30 years, the face of HIV/AIDS was evidenced in both Caribbean immigrants residing in large east coast cities, and Central and South Americans moving north to California's urban settings. These female caregivers constitute the great majority of HIV/AIDS caregivers in Latino communities (Oliveros, 2008). Often, women from the great variety of Latino subcultures share cultural values such as close-knit extended families (*familismo*), yet many continue to keep the AIDS diagnosis of husbands, children, and themselves silenced because the intensity of stigma prevails. Unfortunately, resulting loneliness occurs; thus, the buffering effects of familism are absent for many (Land & Hudson, 2002). Particularly for the newly emigrated, caregiving is allocated to women because of strong cultural role expectations. In fact, female caregivers in the Latin community dedicate an enormous portion of their life to family caregiving not only for their nuclear family, but also for sick relatives, the orphaned, and elderly parents and grandparents, in addition to HIV/AIDS caregiving.

For a variety of reasons, caregiving may be quite stressful for this group of caregivers, and especially for those who are poorer and newer to the United States. Frequently these are women coping with the stress of acculturation and accompanying isolation. Many have completed through the eighth grade of education only, because this is where compulsory education ends in Latin America. Moreover, a sizeable majority come from rural villages; thus, adjusting to complex urban environments with multilevel bureaucratic systems of care is foreign. The complexities of HIV treatment for both adults and children may involve multiple services to promote disease management. Moreover, to meet the needs of children or adults with HIV, the caregiver must first comprehend the nature of the illness, facilitate required services, and become involved in multilevel service systems instituting care plans. Research indicates that, often, Latinas are reluctant to seek outside help and early care for the illness (Land & Hudson, 2002). For those who are undocumented, fear of being deported delays treatment even further. In fact, there are few bilingual services that understand their cultural values, including the need for personalism with medical staff, the value of familism, and the acceptance of life's suffering (Magana, 2007). Most female caregivers who have emigrated from Central America reside in poverty where few resources exist, and the family may view them as unnecessary, insensitive to family needs, and intrusive, or these caregivers may be unaware of their existence altogether. Studies reveal that about half of all HIV family caregivers are seropositive themselves, with the HIV transmission route acquired by heterosexual contact with a partner who has had unsafe sex with another man or an injection drug user, or through unclean injecting equipment. Being seropositive while providing care to partners and children can leave the caregiver depleted and vulnerable to a variety of other chronic illnesses. It is common for Latina HIV/AIDS caregivers to put the needs of others ahead of themselves as a result of the cultural value of *sympatia* coupled with the value of *marianismo*—that is, being long suffering and strong in imitations of the Virgin Mary (Neff, Amodei, Valescu & Pomeroy, 2003).

Studies of Latina caregivers reveal that the stress process differs from that of other caregiving groups. For example, these caregivers report greater frequency of non-HIV-related chronic illnesses, including heart disease, hypertension, asthma, and diabetes. One study documents that a full 89% experienced one or more chronic illnesses (Land & Hudson, 2004). Thus, background factors of poverty, low levels of education, monolingualism, lack of documented status, acculturative stress, lack of health insurance, chronic illnesses, little to no knowledge of HIV, and the existence of few Spanish-speaking treatment centers leave the caregiver quite vulnerable to the stress process. In addition, major life events such as being forced to move the place of residence occur in greater frequency in this group of HIV caregivers. Of interest, despite multiple and heavy caregiving roles, stress resulting from providing assistance in ADLs was notably absent for this group as opposed to their male counterparts (Land & Hudson, 2004). As one woman put it when asked if she wanted respite care, "Why? It's my job." In one investigation, nearly all caregivers had refrained from disclosure to other family members that they were caring for someone with HIV/AIDS (Land, 2004). Thus, social constriction is common and social support is reduced.

Furthermore, compared with other cohorts, Latina HIV caregivers are more likely to experience anxiety over medication adherence. Study results suggest these caregivers may be more aware of lack of medication adherence, and hence become more anxious (Beals, Wight, Aneshensel, Murphy, & Miller-Martinez, 2006). Findings suggest that poorer health, exit events, managing cognitive difficulties in the care recipient, role captivity and isolation, and poor self-esteem predict poorer mental well-being, such as anxiety and depression (Land & Hudson, 2002).

Adequately addressing service to this group may be challenging because of low service use. *Promotoras* (health promoters) may be used to promote health services, educate about the disease transmission and day-to-day caregiving, and provide social support from within the microculture (Land, 2010). Also, prevention efforts have been noted that aim at disease prevention through abstinence and correct condom use in men (Herbst et al., 2007). Moreover, although familism is not a stress buffer, use of other cultural values has been noted to affect social support and specific coping strategies (Land, 2010).

Grandparents and Older Caregivers of HIV-Infected Children

The importance of grandparents was stable in black and Latino communities before the onset of the HIV pandemic. With the advent of HIV, grandparents have played a central role in raising grandchildren, especially those orphaned by HIV from the 1980s to the turn of the century. As these children age out of care and emerge into adulthood, often they continue to reside at home, and younger children with ill parents require more intensive parenting. Ultimately, aging grandparents may be stretched to the maximum in providing caregiving to adult offspring with HIV manifesting as a chronic condition as well as in providing direct parenting of grandchildren. The substantial needs of children and grandchild affected by HIV as well as the needs of the aging grandparent must be taken into account.

Often, the proliferation of the stress process involves the emotional and behavioral issues of grandchildren. For children, seeing a parent cope with a debilitating illness may be quite anxiety provoking and stressful. For those who lost a parent to HIV, bereavement may be difficult to manage for the aging grandparent. Children orphaned by HIV provide a challenging set of circumstances. For many, grandchildren have had to move several times as a result of financial instability, and thus must adjust to new schools, new primary attachment figures, new teachers, and a new set of friends. Some may be struggling with illness themselves. Multiple disruptions in life stability for these children culminate in many behavioral problems. Externalizing behaviors have been noted in the literature and may include acting out, stealing, lying, and causing disruptions in school. When schools complain, the grandparent must become involved with another system of care that requires further energy to monitor. Likewise, internalizing behaviors such as social withdrawal, mutism, overeating, nightmares, and night wandering may be perplexing and difficult to manage by an aging grandparent. Moreover, grandchildren may exhibit considerable anger toward their parents for being sick and dying, for past neglect, or for being victimized at school (Linsk & Mason, 2004). In such events, counseling may be needed. As one grandmother said, "You need to spend a lot of time with these children to help them understand that they are loved and have worth, and whatever happened to them is not their fault" (Linsk & Mason, 2004, p. 11). Other children may exhibit problems that are situated in living life in the 21st century, rather than being connected directly to HIV, including sexual acting-out, drug involvement, school failure, and early pregnancy. Still others have experienced emotional and physical abuse at home or at school. Many of the issues play out within a scenario of an aging grandparent who may be working and exhibiting work life–caregiver role conflict as secondary stressors to primary care issues. Should the grandparent experience illness and require care, the family systems may teeter on dissolution.

Complex care plans are challenging for AIDS service providers and must be multiply determined for this group of HIV caregivers and their care recipients. Both structural and emotional supports are often needed for the psychological and physical needs of these caregivers, the majority of whom are women. Structural supports may include food banks, and available financial support services may be needed for low-income groups. As with other female caregivers, grandmothers are likely to put the needs of their children and grandchildren ahead of their own; thus, the worker should make an extra effort to inquire about specific mental health issues such as anxiety, depression, eating and sleeping patterns, and somatic problems. Likewise, physical well-being should be screened and the grandparent referred to treatment when necessary. Because the needs are many within this family system, the worker would be wise to investigate after-school programs for children and telephone support for both parents (if living) and grandparents. Specific stress reduction exercises may also be taught through a psychoeducational approach. Thus, an approach that encompasses both sensitivity and knowledge of the many stressors of this group provides the best treatment.

CAREGIVER INTERVENTIONS

Much of the literature to date on HIV/AIDS caregiving has included cross-sectional studies that have identified caregiver stress and coping on emotional and physical well-being. We found that caregiver stress differs remarkably by caregiver socioeconomic group, cultural values, structural inequalities, access to emotional and care support, and level of stigma (Land & Hudson, 2004). The face of AIDS caregiving is ever changing, with new populations being identified as vulnerable. Thus, service provider care plans must take into account the complex set of interacting variables in the HIV/AIDS caregiving experience. A wide array of difficulties with which HIV/AIDS caregivers must cope include financial hardships, housing problems, interpersonal struggles, stigma, and legal issues.

The greater the vulnerability of the caregiver, the greater the need for a comprehensive care plan.

Far fewer intervention studies have been conducted with HIV/AIDS caregivers. In part, this situation exists because of the great diversity of caregiver groups and the associated diversity of need. Moreover, because infected groups often survive under the radar of identification, intervention studies often design treatment protocols for known groups of caregivers only. New groups (such as Orthodox religious groups and retirement communities where sexually transmitted diseases may be present but not identified) often go unrecognized for years, and thus intervention studies are delayed in documenting effective treatment. In addition, some vulnerable groups are migratory, such as those working in global sex trafficking. HIV/AIDS is a moving target and has increasingly become a global disease. Hence, investigators are called on to keep up with the curve of the disease rather than work behind it—a daunting task.

In this section we discuss intervention studies on HIV/AIDS caregiving. These studies are summarized in an evidence table (Table 5.1). In accordance with findings from cross-sectional studies of the stress health model, existing intervention research has centered on lowering depression and anxiety levels in caregivers (Boon et al., 2009; Herman et al., 2006; Li, Ji, Liang, Ding, Tian, & Xiao, 2011; Pakenham, Dadds, & Lennon, 2002; Pomeroy, Rubin, & Walker, 1995; Pomeroy, Walker, McNeil, & Franklin, 1996), increasing sense of social support (Esu-Willams et al., 2006; Hansell et al.,1998; Kmita, Baranska, & Niemiec, 2002; Li et al., 2011), decreasing feelings of isolation (Stewart et al., 2002), and lessening the burden of caregiving (Boon et al., 2009; Herman et al., 2006). Stigma associated with HIV/AIDS can be the catalyst to feelings of isolation and a lack of social support, thereby fueling a greater sense of burden related to care and higher rates of depression. Most of the interventions developed and examined have been integral in normalizing the experience of the caregiver, opening the space for communication, and increasing knowledge regarding both the disease as well as the transmission of the disease. Whether using face-to-face interactions or phone calls, interventions designed to help HIV/AIDS caregivers do show positive effects on the target symptoms.

Although the existing studies present promising results intervening at both the caregiver and patient–caregiver levels to yield the greatest outcomes, the availability of manuals to replicate interventions is rare. Pakenham and colleagues (2002) examined the effect of an intervention that targeted both the patient and the caregiver in one group, solely the caregiver in the second group, and a waitlist control group for the third group. Using psychoeducation and cognitive–behavioral therapy, the findings suggest that the greatest outcome for both the caregiver and the patient existed when the intervention targeted the dyad simultaneously. Psychoeducational interventions resulted in caregivers and people living with AIDS feeling better emotional functioning (Kmita et al., 2002; Mukherjee, 2010; Smith Fawzi, Eustache, Oswald, Surkan, Louis, Scanlan, et al., 2010), more positive attitude toward and knowledge about

Table 5.1. Intervention Studies for Family Caregivers of Patients with HIV/AIDS

Author (Year)	Sample (Baseline)	Racial/Cultural Factors			Design	Interventions	Results	Evaluation
		Diversity of Study Sample	Cultural Diversity Training Received?	Comparisons of Racial/ Cultural Factors				
INTERVENTION STUDIES								
Boon et al., 2009	209 caregivers	NR, but study took place in South Africa	NR	NR	Quasi-experimental	Health education intervention	No change in depression scores or burden scores were noted. Caregivers were better able to provide nursing care and had a more positive attitude toward and knowledge about people living with HIV/AIDS.	Greater control over nursing care activities, ability to relax, and coping skills were perceived.
Esu-Williams, 2013	Round 1, 365 youths; round 2, 496 youths	NR, but study took place in rural Zambia	NR	NR	Semistructured interviews	Training curriculum for youth to provide care and support for people living with AIDS	Caregiving increased among males (47%– 82%) and females (41%– 78%).	Findings suggest that young people respond well to responsibilities that require them to challenge gender norms.
Hansell et al., 1998	70 primary caregivers of children with HIV/AIDS	73% black, 13% white, 13% Hispanic	NR	NR	Experimental randomized controlled trial	Social support boosting interventions compared with no treatment control	Seronegative caregivers had increased levels of social support after intervention. The level of stress remained flat.	Stress and coping for the caregiver were not buffered by increased levels of social support. Stress was constant and separate from social support.

(continued)

Table 5.1. CONTINUED

Author (Year)	Sample (Baseline)	Racial/Cultural Factors			Design	Interventions	Results	Evaluation
		Diversity of Study Sample	Cultural Diversity Training Received?	Comparisons of Racial/Cultural Factors				
Kmita, 2002	30 HIV-positive children	NR, but study took place in Warsaw, Poland	NR	NR	Exploratory, descriptive study	Psychosocial intervention	Better emotional functioning of parent and child, more people in the family's social network, less silence about those who died, and more differentiated and flexible coping were observed.	Interventions in the medical and nonmedical contexts were most effective when children and caregivers were involved. Psychosocial interventions should be done in collaboration with different service providers.
Pakenham et al., 2002	36 caregivers and their care recipients with HIV	Recipients: 86% white Australian, 10% European, 1 New Zealander; caregivers: 93% white Australian, 1 Aboriginal Australian, 1 New Zealander	NR	NR	Quasi-experimental	Psychoeducation and cognitive–behavioral therapy	Best results were noted when both the caregiver and the patient were targeted simultaneously.	It is possible that treating the dyad adds up to more change.
Pomeroy et al., 1996	33 family members of people with AIDS	70% white 30% other	NR	NR	Quasi-experimental	Psychoeducational and task-oriented group intervention	Decreased stress, perceived stigma, depression, and anxiety were noted.	People with AIDS are blamed for their condition, so—by association—family members are also stigmatized. The opportunity to discuss their secret may have contributed to the success of the group intervention.

TELEPHONE INTERVENTIONS

	Sample			Design	Intervention	Findings	Themes/Notes
Herman et al., 2006	265 HIV patients, 176 caregivers.	NR, but study took place in Sweden	NR	Quasi-experimental	Telephone intervention calls	A higher T-cell count was associated with call adherence; cocaine use was associated with reduced call adherence for both patients and caregivers.	Telephone themes that emerged included problems with mood, relationships, finances, housing, and work. Interventions were initiated in response to these themes. Participant satisfaction was high.
Meier, 1996	9 mothers of gay men with AIDS	2 black, 7 white	NR	Pilot study, posttest participant questionnaires	Telephone support group	The study helped provide education about AIDS-related changes, validated the caregivers' commitment to care giving, and helped them to reconcile the extreme uncertainty of the future death of their sons.	Participants reported that not meeting face-to-face made it easier to express their feelings, and they appreciated the convenience of participating from home.
Stewart et al., 2001	3 people with HIV and hemophilia (all male, living in rural areas), 4 family caregivers of people with AIDS	NR, but study took place in Quebec, Canada	NR	Interviews	Telephone support group	The intervention enhanced their perceived support and lessened their isolation and loneliness. Caregivers reported increased confidence in personal knowledge and skills.	Participants believed they benefited from sharing information and that the support groups decreased their feelings of isolation and loneliness.

NOTE: NR, not reported.

people living with AIDS (Boon et al., 2009), and a decrease in stress, perceived stigma, depression, and anxiety (Pomeroy, Green, et al., 2002; Pomeroy et al., 2006). These findings support the cross-sectional literature, which has identified the importance of the caregiver dyad in designing efficacious interventions (Land & Hudson, 2004). However, in the absence of a formal manual to guide the intervention protocol, replicating the intervention will be difficult if not impossible.

Preliminary results from qualitative investigations using telephone interventions for HIV/AIDS caregivers and patients present positive outcomes and potentially diminish the financial and time demands required of other interventions (Herman et al., 2006). Findings in this study note that participants perceived that support made a difference in lessening feelings of isolation and loneliness while enhancing confidence, knowledge, and skills in caregiving. Similar conclusions were drawn from a telephone study conducted by Stewart and colleagues (2001), in which they found that participants experienced an increase in their sense of support and confidence in knowledge and skills, and a decrease in feelings of isolation and loneliness. Telephone support groups can be helpful for the caregivers because they are convenient to participant in from home, and the anonymity of participation counters the stigma many caregivers experience (Meier, Galinksy, & Rounds, 1995). Although such findings will not be useful in developing countries where caregiver telephones are less available, findings such as these point to the importance of boosting caregivers' sense of connection and confidence, as literature has long noted the importance of the subjective reality of the caregiving experience (Pearlin, Aneshensel, & Leblanc, 1997).

However, the lack of a quantitative measure of treatment fidelity is a limitation of these findings (Herman et al., 2006). In addition, the use of measures to target the observed behaviors is lacking in the existing intervention literature in this area. Boon and colleagues (2009) note that in training older caregivers to provide care for their children and grandchildren living with HIV/AIDS, authors measured the perceived ability to undertake care-relevant behavior only, and no measures of actual behavior were used. Thus, replicating such findings with reliable and valid measures of child behavior are an important aspect of establishing the ability to generalize findings.

With respect to cultural norms, research addressing the variable of gender roles in relation to caregiver issues is lacking. Yet, in one study conducted in Zambia (Esu-Williams et al., 2006), caregiving increased among males from 47% to 82% and among females from 41% to 78% after involvement in a training curriculum for youth to provide care and support to people living with HIV/AIDS. Researchers investigated gender roles associated with caregiving and found that females were more likely to carry out household tasks whereas males were more comfortable with public service tasks. Both groups responded well to challenging gender norms when caring for people living with HIV/AIDS. Although preliminary in nature, remarkable findings such as these point to the necessity of increasing a sense of efficacy in caregiving among youth. In fact, it may be that youth are far more flexible to care needs even when they challenge socialized gender norms. Yet, despite positive findings, this intervention study examined youth caregivers only, and thus results may not be generalizable to adults and older adults, or to other cultural groups.

Perhaps because of the nature of the work, the existing research in the area of intervention development of caregivers of those living with HIV/AIDS often lacks qualities necessary for generalizability. For example, most of the studies have a small sample size (Kmita et al., 2013; Li et al., 2011; Pakenham et al, 2002; Stewart et al., 2001), selection for participation uses nonprobability sampling methods (Esu-Williams et al., 2013; Kmita et al., 2013; Pakenham et al., 2002), and, most important, those administering the intervention are often not blind to the participants' group status and are, therefore, vulnerable to steering the interviews in a direction that could have caused bias in the emergent themes (Pakenham et al., 2002; Stewart et al., 2001). Again, these limitations may be a result, in part, of the fact that individuals affected by HIV/AIDS (both the patients and caregivers) often exist under the radar of identification because of stigma, thereby making it difficult to conduct large-scale randomized controlled trials.

In addition, too often there is limited, if any, information on whether those responsible for the actual intervention were trained appropriately in values of the culture under study. Although HIV/AIDS caregivers represent highly diverse cultures as a result of the spread of the virus from group to group, few if any investigations describe cultural awareness training and are, therefore, limited. Moreover, to our knowledge, there have been no attempts to translate interventions on the ground in communities affected by HIV/AIDS; thus, the facility or complexity of community outcomes cannot be measured. Therefore, future intervention research should support the use of manualized interventions, and larger sample sizes will yield greater potential for generalizability.

CONCLUSION

Because each group of HIV/AIDS caregivers presents a distinct set of cultural and gender circumstances, it is imperative for those who design programs to be knowledgeable about the wide range of populations infected by HIV. The storied lives of HIV/AIDS caregivers are at once similar and different. They are united in their steadfast support of a loved one with HIV/AIDS, sense of isolation, and likelihood of stigma. Most are strapped by financial insecurity. Often, the degree of social support received is spotty at best, and many carry substantial burdens of caregiving for others in their household in addition to the recipient of AIDS caregiving. Some live in neighborhood ravaged by drugs and are themselves drug addicted. Most have been strong resources for HIV/AIDS care provision whether the care recipient is a family member or a friend. Many have lost someone to the disease, whether that person is a partner, child, or grandchild. In developing countries, some caregivers are children and adolescents pressed into an adult role out of necessity. There are many uncertainties in the lives of these caregivers, yet findings from both cross-sectional and intervention studies point to caregivers who are bound together by their commitment and devotion to a loved one for whom they provide care. They are often bending but resilient figures in the global scene of HIV/AIDS caregiving.

Case Study 1: "Caring for My friend"

My friend, Rose, was about 45 when I started taking care of her, and I was 57. It all began one evening when she was rushed to the emergency room at MLK hospital one night as she was vomiting. Turns out she had a lot of infections due to the AIDS. She had been carrying it for years and just didn't know it. No one knew it and most people still don't know it because all you have to do in this neighborhood is even mention the word *AIDS* and people go running like they've seen a ghost—and, in a sense, you are a ghost when you have it because you're there like you always were but people act like you're not. Anyway, she had these infections that kept occurring, stomach problems, growths that had to come off, pneumonia, etc. After a week, Rose had to be released from the hospital because everything is outpatient now, even when it shouldn't be because she was mighty sick. That's when her family just dropped off the face of the Earth. Her kids don't want to see her now that she has no money—even less now than she had before, which was not very much. So she called me to ask for a ride back to her apartment and I could see she was in no condition to take care of herself. Her apartment is right across the hall from me and we've known each other for years. And let me tell you, in this neighborhood, if you're a single black woman, you got to stick together because no one else is going to be there for you. So Rose could barely climb the stairs to her apartment and I thought, "How in the world is she going to take care of herself?" and I saw she couldn't so, I made up my mind that I would just step in until she was stabilized. Folks told me not to do it, right? Like I could catch it just being in her presence. And these are the same folks who are in church on Sunday all decked out in their finest. Whatever happened to "Love your neighbor?" Now that's what they call stigma—just prejudice and stigma. So apparently, Rose got the AIDS from her boyfriend, who, by the way, hasn't been seen in quite a while. I knew he was a user but that's another story. So I do what I can for her because she's my friend and would do the same for me. She needs food, I get the food. She needs laundry done, it's not too much what she has.

And I remind her of all those pills she takes and I bring her down for her medi-van to take her to the doctor and help her back up the steps. I've become a regular nurse don't you know! Mostly, she needs a little support, a pep talk so to speak, because she can get depressed. Like she'll say, "What kind of a life is this? Why am I living?" And I remind her that the greatest fear is fear itself and you just got to take one day at a time and not go beyond that. They're discovering new things every day for AIDS. So she's had a heck of a time with it, but I can remember years back when everyone who got it was basically a dead man walking. She's weak and her system just picks up all kinds of things you didn't even know was out there to get. So when my kids ask if I'm tired—sure I'm tired. Who isn't tired by my age? My mamma always said, "If you have to ask if you're tired, you ain't doing enough yet." Or they'll say to look after myself first, or isn't it depressing taking care of her—like when is life all gumdrops and lollipops? If it wasn't Rose it'd be a grandchild or something. The important thing is I'm not too tired to do it. And we'll cross that bridge when we come it.

Case Study 2: "Spirituality"

My name is Carmen. I am willing to tell you my story, but please change my name and my son's name because my husband and other family members don't understand why I am taking care of my son when I should be looking after my grandchildren by now. Actually, I do take care of grandchildren, and my own mother who is in her 90s. I was born in El Salvador, but came North so my children could have a better life. I am 76 years old and my son, Jesus, is 56. He was one of the lucky ones who made it out alive, when many around his age died from AIDS. For many years I waited for Jesus to get married—and he tried, but it didn't last. I raised him to be a good Catholic, but what can you do but pray? Everything happens by God's grace and who are we to question God? Jesus says that God made everyone, so that must mean he made him gay as well. I don't know about that. Some people think that AIDS is a punishment because homosexuality is a sin, but I don't believe that either. Maybe I did something wrong. And then I think: his father isn't a strong man. Jesus is a good person, but he was careless in his youth. Too much high living, alcohol, and who knows what else? Now both he and his partner, Alex, are really sick. Alex doesn't talk to his family back in Indiana as they threw him out years ago—$50 and a bus ticket to Los Angeles. All he has is Jesus, and me I guess. I go over to their place, just a little way from my house, so I can cook for them, clean up their apartment, and get the laundry. Jesus tries to protect me, but I can always tell when he's having a bad day. He always says it could be worse, but as a mother, sometimes I don't know how. At times I pray to the blessed mother that God would call him home so he won't have to suffer every day. He has so many problems, and the ones that he doesn't have Alex does have! His liver isn't good and he has sugar. Alex has problems like an old man: arthritis, cholesterol, and always with the stomach and nausea. Sometimes I think the cure is as bad as the disease. At least they have the county hospital and they're on relief, but I have to give them a little money so they can get through the month. Someday I'm going to have to stop cleaning houses and the church because I'm not what I used to be. Then what will happen to them? No one else in the family really knows what's going on, and their own lives are busy enough without worrying about Jesus. Every time we have a family party people ask, Where is Jesus? I always make up a story, but some see through it. Last time my sister pulled me aside and told me to be strong and say a novena. I pray for strength every day, and for a better cure to this disease. Life is a struggle, so we must accept what God offers us and not ask why.

REFERENCES

Beals, K. P., Wight, R. G., Aneshensel, C. S., Murphy, D., & Miller-Martinez, D. (2006). The role of family caregivers in HIV medication adherence. *AIDS Care, 18*(6), 589–596.

Boon, H., Ruiter, R. A. C., James, S., Van Den Borne, B., Williams, E., & Reddy, P. (2009). The impact of a community-based pilot health education intervention for older people as caregivers of orphaned and sick children as a result of HIV and AIDS in South Africa. *Journal of Cross Cultural Gerontology, 24*, 373–389.

Centers for Disease Control and Prevention. (2006). *CDC HIV/AIDS fact sheet: HIV/ AIDS among women.* Atlanta, GA: CDC, National Center for HIV, STD and TB Prevention, Division of HIV/AIDS.

Engel, M.(2008, February 5). With HIV, growing older faster. *Los Angeles Times*, 14–15.

Esu-Williams, E., Schenk, K. D., Geibel, S., Motsepe, J., Zulu, A., Bweupe, P., et al. (2006). We are no longer called club members but caregivers: Involving youth in HIV and AIDS caregiving in rural Zambia. *AIDS Care: Psychological and Social-Medical Aspects of AIDS/HIV, 18*(8), 888–894.

Fredriksen-Goldsen, K. I. (2007). HIV/AIDS caregiving predictors of well-being and distress. *Journal of Gay and Lesbian Social Services, 18*(34), 53–73.

Fredriksen-Goldsen, K. I., Kim, H.- J., Muraco, A., Mincer, S. (2009) Chronically ill midlife and older lesbians, gay men, and bisexuals and their informal caregivers: The impact of the social context. *Journal of Sexuality Research and Social Policy*, 1–53.

Hansell, P. S., Hughes, C. B., Caliandro, G., Russo, P., Budin, W. C., Harman, B., et al. (1998). The effect of a social support boosting intervention on stress, coping, and social support in caregivers of children with HIV/AIDS. *Nursing Research, 47*(2), 79–86.

Herbert, R. S., Weinstein, E., Martire, L. M., & Schulz, R. (2006) Religion, spirituality and the well-being of informal care-givers: a review, critique, and the research prospectus. *Ageing and Mental Health, 10*, 497–520.

Herbst, J. H., Kay, L. S., Passin, W. F., Lyles, C. F., Crepaz, M., & Marin, B. V. (2007). A systematic review and meta analysis of behavioral interventions to reduce HIV risk behaviors among Hispanics in the United States and Puerto Rico. *AIDS Behavior, 11*, 25–47.

Herman, D. S., Bishop, D., Anthony, J. L., Chase, W., Trisvan, E., Lopez, R., et al. (2006). Feasibility of a telephone intervention for HIV patients and their informal caregivers. *Journal of Clinical Psychology in Medical Settings, 13*(1), 81–91.

Kmita, G., Baranska, M., & Niemiec, T. (2002). Psychosocial intervention in the process of empowering families with children living with HIV/AIDS: A descriptive study. *AIDS Care: Psychological and Social-Medical Aspects of AIDS/HIV, 14*(2), 279–284.

Knight, B., & Sayegh, P. (2010). Cultural values and caregiving: The updated sociocultural stress and coping model. *Journal of Gerontology: Psychological Sciences, 65B*(1), 5–13.

Knowleton, K. (2003). Informal caregiving in a vulnerable population: Toward a network resource framework. *Social Science and Medicine, 56*, 1307–1320.

Land, H. (2010). HIV affected caregiver. In C. C. Poindexter (Ed.), *Handbook of HIV and Social Work* (pp. 311–326). New York: Wiley.

Land, H., & Hudson, S. (2002). HIV serostatus and factors related to physical and mental well-being in Latina family AIDS caregivers. *Social Science and Medicine, 54*(1), 147–159.

Land, H., & Hudson, S. (2004). Stress, coping, and depressive symptomatology in Latina and Anglo AIDS caregivers. *Psychology and Health, 19*(5), 643–666.

Land, H., Hudson, S., & Stefiel, B. (2003). Stress and depression among HIV-positive and HIV-negative gay and bisexual AIDS caregivers. *AIDS and Behavior, 7*(1), 41–53.

Le Blanc, A. J., & Wight, R. G. (2000). Reciprocity and depression in AIDS care giving. *Sociological Perspectives, 43*(4), 631–649.

Li, L., Ji, G., Liang, L., Ding, Y., Tian, J., & Xiao, Y. (2011). A multilevel intervention for HIV affected families in China: Together for empowerment activities. *Social Science Medicine, 73*(8), 1214–1221.

Linsk, N., & Mason, S. (2004). Stresses on grandparents and other relatives caring for children affected by HIV/AIDS. *Health and Social Work, 29*(2), 127–136.

Magana, S. (2007). Psychological distress among Latino family caregivers of adults with schizophrenia: The roles of burden and stigma. *Psychiatric Services, 58*(3), 378–384.

McAdoo, J. L. (1993) The roles of African American fathers: An ecological perspective. *Families in Society, 74*(1), 28–35.

Meier, A., Galinsky, M. J., Rounds, K. A. (1995). Telephone support groups for caregivers of persons with AIDS. *Social Work and Groups, 18*(1), 99–108.

Miller, I. W., Bishop, D. S., Herman, D. S., & Stein, M. D. (2007). Relationship quality among HIV patients and their caregivers. *AIDS Care, 19*(2), 203–211.

Mitchell, M., & Knowlton, A. (2009). Stigma, disclosure, and depressive symptoms among informal caregivers of people living with HIV/AIDS. *AIDS Patient Care STDs, 23*(8), 611–617.

Mitchell, M., & Knowlton, A. (2012) Caregiver role overload and network support in a sample of predominantly low-income, African-American caregivers of persons living with HIV/AIDS: A structural equation modeling analysis. *AIDS and Behavior, 16*(2), 278–287.

Mukherjee, J. (2010). Psychosocial functioning among HIV-affected youth and their caregivers in Haiti: Implications for family-focused service provision in high HIV burden settings. *AIDS Patient Care and STDs, 24*(3), 147–158.

Muraco, A., Fredriksen-Goldsen K. (2011). "That's what friends do": Informal caregiving for chronically ill midlife and older lesbian, gay, and bisexual adults. *Journal of Social and Personal Relationships, 28*(8), 1073–1092. [Originally published March 23, 2011.]

Neff, J. A., Amodei, N., Valescu, S., & Pomeroy, E. C. (2003). Psychological adaptation and distress among HIV+ Latina women: Adaptation to HIV in a Mexican American cultural context. *Social Work in Health Care, 37*, 55–74.

Oliveros, C. (2008). The Latino caregiver experience among dementia and non-dementia caregivers: Can community based care management to improve caregiver health? *Dissertation Abstracts, 69*(4-B), 2275.

Pakenham, K. I., Dadds, M. R., & Lennon, H. V. (2002). The efficacy of a psychosocial intervention for HIV/AIDS caregiving dyads and individual caregivers: A controlled treatment outcome study. *AIDS Care: Psychological and Social-Medical Aspects of AIDS/HIV, 14*(6), 731–750.

Pearlin, L. I. (2010). The Life Course and the Stress Process: Some Conceptual Comparisons. *J Gerontol B Psychol Sci Soc Science, 65B*(2), 207–215.

Pearlin, L. I., Aneshensel, C. S., & Leblanc A. J. (1997). The forms and mechanisms of stress proliferation: The case of AIDS caregivers. *Journal of Health and Social Behavior, 38*(3), 223–236.

Pearlin, L. I., Mullan, J. T., Aneshensel, C. S., Wardlaw, L., Harrington, C. (1994). The structure and function of AIDS care giving relationships. *Psychosocial Rehabilitation Journal, 17*, 51–67.

Pomeroy, E. C., Rubin, A., & Walker, R. J. (1995). Effectiveness of a psychoeducational and task-centered group intervention for family members of people with AIDS. *Social Work Research, 19*(3), 142–152.

Pomeroy, E. C., Thompson, S., Gober, K., & Noel. L. (2006). Predictors of medication adherence among HIV positive clients. *Journal of HIV/AIDS and Social Services, 6*(1/2), 65–81.

Pomeroy, E. C., Green, D. L., & Van Laningham, L. (2002). Couples who care: The effectiveness of a psychoeducational group intervention for HIV serodiscordant couples. *Research on Social Work Practice, 12*(2), 238–252.

Pomeroy, E. C., Rubin, A., & Walker, R. J. (1996). A psychoeducational group intervention for family members of persons with HIV/AIDS. *Family Process, 35*(3), 299–312.

Redgrave, G., Swartz, A., & Romanoski, A. (2003). Alcohol misuse by women. *International Review of Psychiatry, 15*, 256–268.

Smith Fawzi, M.C., Eustache, E., Oswald, C., Surkan, P., Louis, E., Scanlan, F., Wong, R., Li, M., & Mukherjee, J. (2010). Psychosocial functioning among HIV-affected youth and their caregivers in Haiti: Implications for family-focused service provision in high HIV burden settings. *AIDS Patient Care and STDs, 24*(3), 147–158.

Stetz, K. M., & Brown, M. A. (2004). Physical and psychosocial health in family care giving: A comparison of AIDS and cancer caregivers. *Public Health Nursing, 21*(6), 533–540.

Stewart, M. J., Hart, G., Mann, K., Jackson, S., Langille, L, & Reidy, M. (2001). Telephone support group intervention for persons with hemophilia and HIV/AIDS and family caregivers. *International Journal of Nursing Studies, 38*, 209–225.

Strug, D., Rabb, L., & Nanton, R. (2002). Provider views of the support service needs of male primary caretakers of HIV/AIDS-infected and affected children: A needs assessment. *Families in Society, 83*(3), 303–313.

Wight, R. G. (2000). Precursive depression among HIV infected AIDS caregivers over time. *Social Science and Medicine, 51*, 759–770.

Wingood, G. (2003). The feminization of the HIV Epidemic Journal of Urban Health, iii67–iii76.

Wyatt, G., Carmona, J., Loeb, T., & Williams, J. (2005). HIV-positive black women with histories of childhood sexual abuse: Patterns of substance use and barriers to health care. *Journal of Health Care for the Poor and Underserved, 16*, 9–23.

6

Caring for Individuals Near the End of Life

REBECCA S. ALLEN, HYUNJIN NOH,
LISA N. BECK, AND LAURA JANE SMITH ■

MULTIMORBIDITY, PROGNOSTICATION, AND DIVERSITY IN PALLIATIVE CAREGIVING

Family members are intimately involved in decisions regarding care near the end of life, and they face both stressors and opportunities for growth in witnessing and providing relief for the suffering of their loved ones (Allen & Shuster, 2002; Haley et al., 2002; Hilgeman, Allen, DeCoster, & Burgio, 2007; Monin & Schulz, 2009). The prevalence of angina/coronary heart disease, arthritis, cancer, diabetes, heart attack, hypertension, and stroke increase across the life span (Pearson, Bhat-Schelbert, & Probst, 2012), and older adults represent the fastest growing segment of the U.S. population. According to the Center for Disease Control and Prevention (http://www.cdc.gov/nchs/fastats/older-american-health.htm), as of 2013 there were 44.7 million adults age 65 years and older, and the number of those older than 85 is increasing at a rapid rate. Discussions regarding goals of care and the potential of death often occur very late during the disease process or not at all (Bailey et al., 2012; Guo et al., 2010; The SUPPORT Principal Investigators, 1995; Tschann, Kaufman, & Micco, 2003). Notably, medical providers are not accurate with prognostication regarding the disease trajectory of chronic illness, sometimes misestimating an individual's time left to live by a factor of as much as five (Chow et al., 2011; Christakis & Lamont, 2000; Stiel et al., 2009). Chen and colleagues found that about 20% of patients with advanced cancer reported that hospice care was first suggested by a family caregiver, although healthcare providers initiated more than half of such discussions (Chen, Haley, Robinson, & Schonwetter, 2003).

The World Health Organization defines hospice and palliative care as meeting the physical, psychosocial, and spiritual needs of patients with life-limiting and advanced chronic illness and their families through an interprofessional approach that improves comfort and quality of life (Campbell & Amin, 2012). The focus of palliative care is on the prevention and relief of suffering through early identification and treatment of physical, psychosocial, and spiritual problems. Certainly, then, the goals of palliative care are antithetical to the most readily available treatment settings for older adults near the end of their lives and those caring for them: primary care clinics focus largely on treating the symptoms of acute illness and, perhaps, the prevention of disease. According to Wagner (1998) and Bodenheimer and colleagues (Bodenheimer, Wagner, & Grumbach, 2002), problems in the implementation of the current primary care system in the United States limit the ability to meet the needs of family caregivers and individuals with advanced chronic illness.

Wagner (1998) outlines the problems with primary care relative to chronic illness—for example, the primary care system has been developed to treat acute disorders and not those arising from chronic illness. As a new medical profession, palliative care is often misunderstood and underused by referring physicians in primary care clinics, and perhaps more so by the general public (Koffman et al., 2007). Further complicating hospice and palliative care use is the issue of health disparities. The ability to achieve optimal health outcomes may be greatly reduced among minority groups, including individuals of color, women, those with low education and income, and members of stigmatized groups. A particularly neglected area of palliative caregiving involves the lesbian, gay, bisexual, transgender, and queer (LGBTQ) community.

This chapter presents information regarding the characteristics of caregivers and care recipients in need of palliative and hospice care resulting from the progression of a variety of chronic illnesses and/or multimorbidity. We highlight disparities in receipt of such care among racial/ethnic and sexual minorities. Given that most of the literature concerning sexual and gender-variant elders and their caregivers is focused on HIV/AIDS (see Chapter 5), our focus is other LGBTQ issues in palliative caregiving. Evidence regarding the efficacy of interventions targeting palliative caregivers are reviewed thoroughly and illustrated with two case examples. We then describe research efforts to translate palliative caregiver interventions for use in primary care and community settings. We also provide a table of evidence that supports the efficacy of community-based interventions to reduce the suffering of palliative caregivers.

Racial/Ethnic Disparities in the Use of End-of-Life Care

Serving as the primary caregiver for a loved one is undoubtedly a formidable responsibility (Aneshensel, Pearlin, Mullan, Zarit, & Whitlatch, 1995; Dilworth-Anderson, Williams, & Gibson, 2002; Family Caregiver Alliance, 2006; Monin & Schulz, 2009; Pinquart & Sörensen, 2005; Zarit, Todd, & Zarit, 1986). Despite the rapid increase in the proportion of racial or ethnic minority individuals in the United States, racial/ethnic disparities in receiving palliative and hospice care have been identified persistently. To gain an understanding of such disparities, researchers have explored possible *barriers* that may prevent racial/ethnic minority groups from accessing palliative and hospice care, and *preferences* that may discourage them from seeking such care even when they have access to the service. Such barriers and preferences make it difficult for family caregivers of racial/ethnic minority patients to consider palliative and hospice care as an end-of-life care option for their dying family member.

Structural Barriers in Accessing Palliative and Hospice Care

Lack of health insurance and limited income are structural barriers to minority groups' access to hospice care. According to the National Hospice and Palliative Care Organization's 2012 report, the Medicare Hospice Benefit[1] (Centers for Medicare and Medicaid Services, 2007) has been the biggest payment source of hospice care, covering 84% of patients in 2010 (National Hospice and Palliative Care Organization, 2014). Compared with non-Hispanic whites, minority groups are less likely to have health insurance[2] and more likely to have limited income, which makes it difficult for them to gain access to hospice care if they have to pay out of pocket (Reese, Melton, & Ciaravino, 2004). Moreover, lack of knowledge of hospice care also presents a barrier to minority groups' consideration and discussion of—and therefore access to—the service.

Previous studies conducting interviews or focus groups with minority community members, their religious leaders, and healthcare providers found that their level of awareness of hospice care was low and their knowledge of this service was often misinformed (Born, Greiner, Sylvia, Butler, & Ahluwalia, 2004; Jackson, Schim, Seeley, Grunow, & Baker, 2000; Jenkins, Zapka, Kurent, & Lapelle, 2005). In her focus group study, Jackson and colleagues (2000) found that blacks without prior experience and those with hospice experience (i.e., family caregivers of deceased hospice patients) identified lack of knowledge about where to get information about hospice services as a major barrier. Some blacks without prior hospice caregiving experience were not aware that hospice care existed and wished that such care had been recommended as an alternative to the care their loved ones received near the end of life. Even black family caregivers with hospice experience reported lack of information regarding hospice and wished more information had been given to them about the scope of benefits and services available for their loved ones and themselves.

In her interviews with black hospice patients, Noh (2012) reported that some study participants had misconceptions toward hospice care as a place to die, which was clarified only after talking in detail with their physicians or hospice admissions staff. Considering that physicians are the primary source of information for both patients and their family caregivers regarding a patient's condition and available care options, lack of a relationship with a primary care physician among minority groups (Reese et al., 2004) may be one of the reasons for lack of knowledge about hospice care among patients and family caregivers. In addition, physicians make fewer hospice referrals for minority patients than for their non-Hispanic white counterparts, and hospice and palliative care providers view lack of hospice referrals by physicians as one of the barriers in accessing hospice care among minority groups (Crawley, 2000; Reese et al., 2004; Winston, Leshner, Kramer, & Allen, 2004). Physicians' low hospice referral rates for minority groups can also be attributed to minority physicians' *own* attitude toward end-of-life care being more supportive of aggressive treatment than that of non-Hispanic white physicians, and thus recommend hospice care to their minority patients and family caregivers less frequently than non-Hispanic white physicians (Winston et al., 2004). Last, some researchers (Lorenz et al., 2004; O'Mahony et al., 2008; Reese et al., 2004) have pointed out insufficient outreach efforts as a possible reason for lack of knowledge of hospice care in minority communities. Even when the patient has health insurance with hospice care coverage, such lack of knowledge about hospice care prevents family caregivers of minority patients from considering the service as an alternative to end-of-life care for their dying family member and, therefore, prevents them from benefiting from services that may reduce their caregiving burden significantly.

End-of-Life Healthcare Preferences and Cultural Preferences among Minority Groups

Researchers argue that minority groups' cultural, spiritual, or religious beliefs influence their preferences for chronic and end-of-life health care (Bullock, 2006; Harris, Allen, Dunn, & Parmelee, 2013; Hilgeman et al., 2009; Kwak & Haley, 2005). Most often discussed is the belief of fatalism among black and Hispanic populations, which Damron-Rodriguez and colleagues described as reliance on God or fate to determine one's health outcome (Damron-Rodriguez, Wallace, & Kington, 1994). This fatalism brings about the attitude that perceives life and death to be determined by God or fate rather than medical care (Winston et al., 2004). Furthermore, in black culture, pain and suffering may be viewed as a spiritual commitment to faith, rather than something to be avoided using medical care (Crawley, 2005), and life, even in a dire condition, is preferred to death (Hallenbeck, Goldstein, & Mebane, 1996).

These beliefs toward health/illness and pain/suffering at the end of life lead to minority groups' attitude toward end-of-life healthcare choices. In general, minority groups are significantly less supportive of any measures that may shorten life, such as physician-assisted hastened death or withholding or withdrawing life-sustaining treatment (Bayer, Mallinger, Krishnan, & Shields, 2006; Gessert, Curry, & Robinson, 2001; Kwak & Haley, 2005; Werth, Blevins, Toussaint, & Durham, 2002). Minority populations also show a lower completion rate of advance directives and do not resuscitate (DNR) orders compared with non-Hispanic whites (Braun, Onaka, & Horiuchi, 2001; Carr, 2011; Degenholtz,

Arnold, Meisel, & Lave, 2002; Johnson, Kuchibhatla, & Tulsky, 2008), which may be attributed to minority groups' unwillingness to talk about the taboo topic of death and dying, as well as their assumption they may receive lower quality care when compared to a non-Hispanic white person if they sign a living will. Such an attitude was exemplified in Bullock's study (2006), in which one participant commented, "As a black man, I am subject to receive less care and attention than a white man, and if I had a living will, they might not care for me at all" (p. 192). Researchers argue that this attitude toward end-of-life health care among minority groups has been influenced by the medical racism deeply rooted in the history of the United States and a resulting mistrust in the mainstream healthcare system (Bullock, 2006; Pullis, 2011; Winston et al., 2004).

Another end-of-life care preference often found among minority groups is a family-centered culture of care. Previous studies on the family-centered culture of care have two themes: preference for family-centered decision making and family-centered caregiving. Searight and Gafford (2005) pointed out that nondisclosure of terminal diagnosis to the patient is accepted in many minority communities to protect the patient from getting distressed hearing "bad news." The terminal diagnosis, therefore, is often disclosed to family members only, who take the responsibility to make treatment decisions. Because accepting hospice care implies that the patient cannot be cured, curative or life-sustaining treatment may be chosen over hospice care by minority family members who perceive withholding or withdrawing treatment as "giving up hope" (Jackson et al., 2000, p. 70) and who have a strong faith in God's "miraculous power" for healing (Winston et al., 2004, p. 153). Asian families, strongly influenced by cultural norms based on filial piety, also may feel obligated to choose curative or life-sustaining treatment for their older parents or relatives over other alternatives such as hospice care (Searight & Gafford, 2005).

Along with family-centered decision making, the culture of family-centered caregiving may also discourage family caregivers in minority communities from choosing hospice care for their dying family members. In Hispanic cultures, family members are expected to provide care at the patient's end of life and to share caregiving responsibility. In this culture, receiving formal care from those outside the family, such as hospice care, may be seen as the family's lack of caregiving ability, which could embarrass the family (Gelfand, Balcazar, Parzuchowski, & Lenox, 2001). Black families also show hesitance in accessing formal service providers when their family member is dying because of their desire for privacy and their reluctance to expose information or issues related to their family and their dying family member to outsiders (Winston et al., 2004). As a result of changes in the family structure and economic burden in many minority families, however, many cannot care for their dying family members to the extent traditional families did (Torrez, 1998). Therefore, although the existence of strong supportive family care systems may mitigate minority groups' need for formal healthcare services, providers should not underestimate minority patients' and their families' need for such support (Damron-Rodriguez et al., 1994). Even when minority patients' and their families' end-of-life care preferences are in favor of hospice care, they may be troubled by a lack of diversity among hospice care providers and a lack of staff knowledge regarding cultural diversity. Lack of minority staff at local hospice agencies may result in minority patients and family caregivers' inability to identify with the hospice staff, and may lead them to view hospice care as part of the mainstream healthcare system for which they have mistrust and fear (Burrs, 1995; Cort, 2004). End-of-life care preferences and cultural preferences held by minority patients and their family caregivers influence their attitudes toward hospice care and may serve as barriers to their actual use of such care.

SEXUAL MINORITY DISPARITIES IN PALLIATIVE CAREGIVING

Further difficulties are encountered by LGBTQ caregivers as a result of stigma and ongoing legal and political backlash for the historic June 26, 2015 ruling by the Supreme Court of the United States (SCOTUS) guaranteeing the right to same sex marriage. Both this recent ruling and the June 2013 SCOTUS case (*U.S. v. Windsor*, 570 U.S. 12-307, 2013) that declared the Defense of Marriage Act as unconstitutional were rooted in issues of palliative caregiving. For example, Edie Windsor retired early to become primary caregiver for her partner Thea Spyer, who was diagnosed with multiple sclerosis at the age of 45 in 1977. When the care recipient's physician gave the prognosis that she had less than a year to live in 2007, the couple traveled to Toronto to wed legally. Less than two years after they were married, Thea Spyer died. Currently, disparities for same-sex couples include experiencing discrimination and prejudice from providers and with regard to housing or public accommodations, including nursing homes. Moreover, in many geographic areas same sex couples have difficulty finding culturally appropriate programs and services.

LGBTQ Caregivers: To Be or Not to Be … Out

In a 1999 survey of almost 1,466 gay and lesbian individuals, just more than 27% (n = 400) of respondents were providing care for adults with an illness or disability. Their relationship to the care recipient varied, with a majority caring for friends (61%) and others caring for parents (16%), partners (13%), and other family members (10%). Respondents who served as a caregiver for another adult were more likely to be out than noncaregivers, and a majority (62%) were out to their medical service providers. The heterogeneous nature of the community of LGBTQ caregivers makes it vital that service providers be familiar with the unique challenges faced by these individuals as well as the resources available to them (Fredriksen-Goldsen, Kim, Muraco, & Mincer, 2009).

In a recent qualitative study, Price (2010) conducted semistructured interviews with 10 gay and 11 lesbian-identified individuals who had or were providing care for a person with dementia to explore their experiences of coming out to healthcare service providers. The results suggested that the respondents' decision to come out was based on their previous "experiences with negative reactions to their sexual orientation, their perceived feelings of discrimination, and ... their anticipation of negative responses" (Price, 2010, p. 166). Although these three factors proved to be common, the decisions made subsequently were heterogeneous: some chose not to come out at all, some were "outed" by the individual for whom they were caring, whereas others decided to be open about their sexual orientation to avoid confusion. Provider responses varied from openly homophobic to heterosexist to a disregard for the unique needs of this community of caregivers.

Discrimination Affects LGBTQ Caregivers

Discrimination against LGBTQ individuals also affects the perceived effectiveness of advance directives and alternative care provision facilities, and is associated with increased mental health concerns within caregiving dyads. Although advance directives are completed to ensure a person's wishes are respected, the participants in one study (Hash & Netting, 2007) were fearful that family members who were not supportive of the care recipient's sexual orientation would attempt to interfere in their preferred care despite an advance directive. A majority of respondents preferred care to be provided at home because of fear of harassment and discrimination from staff in long-term care facilities based on their sexual orientation. Although respondents were more prepared in terms of executed advance directives and financial planning compared with the general population, they remained unsure whether their care guidelines would be honored.

After a thorough review of the research relating to sexual minorities and palliative care, Harding and colleagues concluded that the "paucity of literature" (Harding et al., 2012, p. 609) overall is an issue, but that there is, especially, a shortage of information about sexual minority caregivers. They recommend further research concerning caregiver outcomes, the definition of family, and the policies and legislation that create disparities for members of the LGBTQ community. They also suggest the development of intervention and education programs for healthcare service providers to reduce discrimination and provide better holistic care. Although the research concerning sexual minority caregivers is scarce, there is greater dearth of literature regarding transidentified caregivers. Williams and Freeman (2005) point to the complete absence of research regarding transidentified caregivers at any stage of caregiving and speculate that issues may exist as a result of social isolation, lack of familial support, fear of discrimination, and difficulty finding sources of assistance that are affirming and respectful of the individual's transidentity. Last, Harding and colleagues highlight that most of the existing data are from "white, middle class, and well-educated individuals" (Harding et al., 2012, p. 609). Individuals are often complex and assume several intersecting identities. A caregiver that identifies as a sexual/gender minority and also as a racial/ethnic minority has the potential to face a "triple jeopardy" of sorts that can be complicated even further by socioeconomic status and geographic location.

Proposed SURE 2 Intervention for Sexual Minority Caregivers

To our knowledge, there are currently no published studies of randomized clinical trials of interventions that are LGBTQ caregiver specific. However, one model (SURE 2 [Coon, 2007]) has been developed that suggests merging aspects of a support group with cognitive–behavioral therapy (CBT) to assist LGBTQ caregivers to access services more readily and to cope with issues inherent to being a caregiver and a member of a marginalized population. The SURE 2 acronym stands for sharing and support, unhelpful thoughts/behaviors and understanding, reframes and referrals, and education and exploration. Within the "sharing and support" component, members of the group are encouraged to discuss experiences and ideas with others who are in similar roles. The "unhelpful thoughts/behaviors and understanding" and "reframes and referrals" elements incorporate a variety of CBT techniques, such as identifying maladaptive patterns and coping mechanisms, brainstorming and creating plans for implementation of more adaptive skills to reduce stress, cognitive restructuring and positive reframing, basic problem solving, enhancing communication skills, learning time management, and scheduling enjoyable activities.

The primary goal of SURE 2 is to acknowledge the sociocultural context in which one might serve as a caregiver that is often hostile or dismissive towards an LGBTQ identity. Originally developed as a support group for dementia caregivers, SURE 2's open-ended framework allows it to be adapted easily to a wide array of other potential modalities and circumstances. Other resources that can provide information and recommendations for LGBTQ-identified caregivers include Services and Advocacy for Gay, Lesbian, Bisexual, & Transgender Elders (SAGE; http://www.sageusa.org/), the Human Rights Campaign (HRC; http://www.hrc.org/), the Family Caregiver Alliance (FCA; http://www.caregiver.org/), and the National LGBT Cancer Network (http://www.cancer-network.org/).

CAREGIVER SUPPORT INTERVENTIONS

This section is broken into two components: (a) interventions designed to increase the completion of written advance directives by patients and communication of healthcare wishes between patients and their family caregivers, and (b) interventions to reduce the stress of palliative caregiving. Studies reviewed in this section are organized alphabetically within each separate topic area in an evidence table (Table 6.1).

Table 6.1. INTERVENTION STUDIES FOR FAMILY CAREGIVERS OF PATIENTS NEAR THE END OF LIFE

Author (Year)	Design/Sampling	Subject Characteristics	Methods/Interventions	Data/Measures	Findings/Outcomes	Limitations
			ADVANCE CARE PLANNING			
Briggs et al., 2004	Heart failure, renal dialysis and cardiovascular surgery unit patients from one community hospital selected to meet established criteria for high-risk, life-threatening complications; random assignment	27 patient–surrogate pairs participated; mean age, 68.7 years; 71% of surrogates in both groups were women; PC-ACP group, 76.9% adult children; 50% spouses in control group	1-hour patient-centered advance care planning interview (five stages) delivered by an experienced advance care planning facilitator versus usual care; intervention based on the interactive decision-making model and the representational approach to patient education.	Treatment decision-making role preference (not an outcome measure), patient–proxy congruence, knowledge of advance care planning, satisfaction with decision-making process, O'Connor decisional conflict scale, quality of patient–clinician communication	Pre-/posttreatment assessment. Greater patient–proxy congruence in the PC-ACP intervention. There were no group differences in knowledge of advance care planning. However, there was greater satisfaction with the decision-making process and less decisional conflict in the PC-ACP intervention. There were no group differences in perceptions of quality of patient–clinician communication.	Race/ethnicity of participants NR. Only pre-/postchange measured without longitudinal follow-up.
Ditto et al., 2001	RCT; five experimental conditions: no intervention, instructional advance directive and discussion, instructional advance directive alone, values-based advance directive and discussion, values-based advance directive alone	401 outpatients and their self-designated surrogate decision makers (62% spouses, 29% adult children); participants: 92% non-Hispanic whites, predominantly Protestant with relatively high socioeconomic status	Three 1- to 2-hour in-home interviews over 2 years.	Life-Support Preferences/ Predictions Questionnaire; five questions assessing perceived benefits of advance directive completion using 5-point Likert-type scales (questions included proxy's general understanding of patient preferences, confidence in proxy's ability to predict patient preferences accurately, proxy's likelihood of honoring patient's preferences, proxy's comfort in making medical decisions for the patient, and the perceived importance of having an advance directive	t-Tests were used for continuous variables; chi-square tests of independence were used for categorical variables. Two multivariate analyses of covariance were conducted to test the effects of the intervention on perceived benefits of advance directive completion. None of the interventions produced significant improvements in the accuracy of proxy-substituted judgment. Interventions improved perceived proxy understanding and comfort for patient–proxy pairs in which the patient had not completed an advance directive before study participation.	Impact of intervention was small. Participants included 92% non-Hispanic whites, predominantly Protestant, with relatively high socioeconomic status (homogeneous sample).

Song et al., 2009	RCT, pre-/posttest design, social workers at the dialysis clinics recruited blacks from six out-patient dialysis clinics in western Pennsylvania	58 dyads participated; patients were 57% male, surrogates were 24% male; surrogate relationship to patient was 31% spouse or partner, 19% parent, 24% sibling, 7% child, 19% other	The experimental group was given the SPIRIT intervention (a 1-hour, single-session, interview with a patient-proxy dyad, delivered by a trained nurse interventionist). The control group was administered usual care. Obtained measures at baseline, 1 week, and 3 months; when death occurred. Medical record reviews and a semistructured interview were conducted with the bereaved surrogate within 2 weeks.	Patient–Clinician Interaction Index, quality of patient–clinician communication, *Goals of Care*, Decisional Conflict Scale (Song & Sereika, 2006), decision-making confidence scale, 28-item Self-Perception and Relationship Tool, 30-item Dialysis Symptom Index, SF-12, medical record review, semistructured interview	Changes among baseline, 1 week, and 3 months were compared between the two groups using t-tests. Dichotomized variables were analyzed using Fisher's exact tests. The intervention patient's quality of communication was significantly greater than the control group at times 2 and 3. SPIRIT was effective in improving dyad congruence regarding goals of care and surrogate decision making confidence over time. Choices expressed in the *Goals of Care* document did not shift supporting that patients end-of-life treatment preferences are stable over time.	A small number of dyads was studied. Lack of intervention effect on decisional conflict could be the result of a one-time rather than a more than a one-time intervention. There is a need for further evaluation of the instrument's validity when used with black populations. A possible ceiling effect was noted.
The SUPPORT Principal Investigators, 1995	A 2-year RCT (N = 4,804) that followed a prospective observational study, patients/ physicians randomized by specialty to the intervention group (n = 2,652) or the control group (n = 2,152), participants recruited from 5 teaching hospitals in the United States	In both groups, the patient's median age was 65 years. The control group was 43% female and the intervention group was 45.4% female. The control group was 82.1% non-Hispanic white and the intervention group was 77% non-Hispanic white.	Physicians in the intervention group received survival estimates of the likelihood of 6-month survival for every day up to 6 months, outcomes of cardiopulmonary resuscitation (CPR), and functional disability at 2 months. A specially trained nurse had multiple contacts with the patient, family, physician, and hospital staff to elicit preferences, improve understanding of outcomes, encourage attention to pain control, and facilitate advance care planning and patient–physician communication. A total of 95% of the intervention group received one or more patient-specific components of the intervention with the SUPPORT nurse.	Medical records data were captured, including timing of written DNR orders, patient–physician agreement on treatment preferences, days spent in intensive care, frequency and severity of pain, and hospital resource use	Patients experienced no improvement in patient–physician communication (e.g., 37% of control patients and 40% of intervention patients discussed CPR preferences) or in the five targeted outcomes (incidence or timing of written DNR orders, physicians' knowledge of their patients' preferences, number of days spent in an intensive care unit receiving mechanical ventilation or comatose before death, or level of reported pain). The intervention also did not reduce use of hospital resources.	The patient's proximity to death varied. A large percentage of participants were non-Hispanic white.

(continued)

Table 6.1. CONTINUED

Author (Year)	Design/Sampling	Subject Characteristics	Methods/Interventions	Data/Measures	Findings/Outcomes	Limitations
			PSYCHOSOCIAL PALLIATIVE CAREGIVING			
Addington-Hall et al., 1992	RCT	203 participants consisting of terminally ill cancer patients and their families; 104 in coordination group, 99 in control group; of caregivers, 84% lived with and 65% were married to the patient, 30% of caregivers were male	Both the control and coordination group received regularly available services. The coordination group also received assistance from two nurse coordinators, whose purpose was to make sure the patients were receiving coordinating services that met their individual needs.	Spitzer Quality of Life Index, Hospital Anxiety and Depression Scale, Leeds Depression and Anxiety Scale	Few statistically significant results were observed. The coordination group patients were less likely to experience vomiting or to be concerned about having itchy skin; they were more likely to report effective treatment for vomiting and to have seen a specialist. Coordination group caregivers were less likely to feel angry about the patient's death and reported that during the patient's last week of life, they received effective treatment for anxiety.	The effect of intervention was small. Only families of cancer patients participated.
Allen et al., 2008	RCT; sample recruited from community and healthcare agencies, including hospitals and dialysis centers	31 families; control group, 14; 11 female, 11 black; intervention group, 17; 12 females, 11 black	Intervention delivered in three in home visits scheduled approximately weekly, during which the patient and caregiver found a common memory and made a Legacy project. Control group was contacted via telephone weekly and provided minimal nonspecific support.	Mini-Mental State Examination; activities of daily living; instrumental activities of daily living; modified Edmonton Symptom Assessment Scale; Brief Multidimensional Measure of Religion and Spirituality; Subjective Well-being; Center for Epidemiological Studies: depression scale, Caregiver Stressor Scale–Revised, Project Evaluation Survey	A two (group)-by-two (time of assessment) mixed-model analysis of variance for each of the primary outcomes was conducted. Caregivers in the intervention group showed reduced caregiving stress across time. Intervention caregivers reported that patients were more talkative across time. Patients in the intervention group were engaged more socially with their family caregivers and reported an increased sense of religious meaning whereas control group patients reported a decreased sense of meaning.	The sample was primarily black, Protestant, and urban. The longevity of Legacy treatment effects was not examined. Patients' proximity to death varied.

| Carter, 2006 | Repeated-measures experimental design, recruitment from community oncology clinics in the central Texas area (flyers/ newsletters and online advertisements) | 30 adult caregivers of patients with advanced-stage cancer; 15 in intervention group, 15 in control group; 80% white, 63% female, 57% spouse or partner of patient | Data collected from both groups at baseline, at 3 weeks and 5 weeks, and at 2, 3, and 4 months postbaseline. The intervention group also received the Caregiver Sleep Intervention, a 1-hour session that specializes treatments for insomnia for caregivers. | PSQI, CES-D, Caregiver Quality of Life–Cancer Scale | All caregivers showed improvement in sleep quality, depressive symptoms, and quality of life throughout the course of the study. Intervention caregivers showed greater improvement in PSQI and CES-D scores. | Small sample size, homogenous sample (cancer patients), 80% non-Hispanic white. |
| Chochinov et al., 2011 | RCT, participants assigned randomly in 1:1:1 ratio to one of three groups: dignity therapy, standard palliative care, or client-centered care | 326 participants; 108 in dignity therapy group, 111 in standard palliative care, 107 in client-centered care; 161 men; 291 whites; mean age, 65 years; participant life expectancy ≤6 months received palliative care in a hospital or community setting | During dignity therapy, patients were recorded talking about their hopes, wishes for loved ones, lessons learned, and things they wanted remembered. These recordings were transcribed then edited by the participant, and a final version was printed and given to the participant. The client-centered care group discussed here-and-now issues. Both groups participated in three meetings, all of which lasted about the same time. The standard palliative care group was given access to all the palliative care support services that were available to all study patients. | Palliative Performance Scale, Functional Assessment of Chronic Illness Therapy Spiritual Well-Being Scale, Patient Dignity Inventory, Hospital Anxiety and Depression Scale, items from the Structured Interview for Symptoms and Concerns, two-item Quality-of-Life Scale, modified Edmonton Symptom Assessment Scale | t-tests or Mann–Whitney U tests, analysis of variance, or Kruskal–Wallis tests. Patients given dignity therapy were significantly more likely than were those in either of the other two groups to report that treatment was helpful to them, improved their quality of life, and gave them a sense of dignity. They reported that the study treatment changed how their family saw and appreciated them, and that it had or would be of help to their family. Dignity therapy was significantly better than client-centered care in improving spiritual well-being and was significantly better than standard palliative care in terms of lessening sadness or depression. Significantly more patients who received dignity therapy reported that the study group was satisfactory, as opposed to those who received standard palliative care. | 89% non-Hispanic white. There was no screening of patients' baseline critical distress. |

(continued)

Table 6.1. CONTINUED

Author (Year)	Design/Sampling	Subject Characteristics	Methods/Interventions	Data/Measures	Findings/Outcomes	Limitations
Hudson et al., 2005	RCT	106 primary caregivers of someone with advanced cancer admitted to a home-based palliative care service; 54 in control group, 52 in intervention	Both groups received standard home-based palliative care services. The intervention group also received two home visits by a nurse, one phone call, a guidebook about caring for a dying person, and an audiotape of reflections from caregivers, including relaxation exercises. Data were collected at baseline, 5 weeks after baseline, and 8 weeks after the patient's death.	Preparedness for Caregiving Scale, Caregiver Competence Scale, Rewards of Caregiving Scale, The Hospital Anxiety and Depression Scale	No intervention effects were identified with respect to preparedness to care, self-efficacy, competence, and anxiety. Participants who received the intervention reported a significantly more positive caregiver experience.	This study had insufficient power to detect differences based on a simultaneous comparison of data obtained at all three assessment times. Caregivers were highly functioning. Ceiling and floor effects were noted on the Likert-type scales.
Ingersoll-Dayton et al., 2013	Structured life review, recruitment by contacting several organizations related to Alzheimer's care	20 completed intervention; mean caregiver age, 72.2 years; mean care recipient age, 74.0; caregivers were 35% men, care recipients were 70% men; all participants were white	Five one-hour sessions, each of which included an explanation of a new communication skill and reviewed a section of the couple's life together: early years, middle years, later years, the future, and review.	Questionnaires that had open-ended question about their responses to the Couples' Life Story Approach	Dyads used words such as *we* and *partners* toward the end of the intervention. Most had a positive reaction, but a few participants felt a sense of loss over what they had. Sessions were most productive when they occurred weekly.	Homogenous sample of families in which one individual had dementia, 100% non-Hispanic white.
Keefe et al., 2005	RCT; recruitment from hospices and clinics of the Duke Comprehensive Cancer Center and Dartmouth–Hitchcock Medical Center	78 advanced cancer patients and partners; 37 in control, 41 received intervention: patient mean age, 60.49 years; 43.9% female, 78% white; partner mean age, 58.48 years; 61.8% female, 79% white	The intervention was a partner-guided pain management training protocol, which included three sessions at the patients' home. These sessions integrated information about cancer pain and trained patients and partners about cognitive and behavioral pain coping skills.	Brief Pain Inventory; FACT-G, version 4; Chronic Pain Self-Efficacy Scale; Caregiver Strain Index; condensed version of the Profile of Mood States–B	Intervention produced significant increases in partners' ratings of their self-efficacy for helping the patient control pain and self-efficacy for controlling other symptoms; also reported improvements in their levels of caregiver strain.	Small sample size, only families of cancer patients participated, 78% non-Hispanic white.

| Kissane et al., 2006 | RCT | 81 families of patients dying from cancer; 53 families (233 individuals) received family-focused grief therapy, 28 families (130 individuals) in control | Family-focused grief therapy attempts to prevent the complications of bereavement by enhancing the functioning of the family. Families in the control group did not receive any formal psychological treatment beyond standard palliative care. Data collection occurred at baseline, and 6 months and 13 months after the patient's death. | Family Environment Scale, Family Relationships Index, Family Assessment Device, Brief Symptom Inventory, Beck Depression Inventory, Social Adjustment Scale, Bereavement Phenomenology Questionnaire | Significant improvements in distress and depression occurred among individuals with high baseline scores on the Brief Symptom Inventory and Beck Depression Inventory. Sullen and intermediate-functioning families tended to improve overall. Depression was unchanged in hostile families and there was increased conflict at 13 months in the intervention group (steady improvement in the control group). | Impact of intervention was small, only families of cancer patients participated. |
| McClement et a., 2007 | | Family members of people who had completed dignity therapy and had agreed previously to participate in the follow-up portion of the study were contacted 9 to 12 months after the death of the patient | 60 family members of deceased, terminally ill patients who previously took part in dignity therapy; 70% female, mostly spouses (53.3%) or daughters (31.7%) of the deceased | Depending on participant preference, questionnaires were completed face-to-face with a research nurse, or returned by mail. | Completed an evaluation consisting of Likert scales and open- and close-ended questions to elicit feedback about the effect of dignity therapy on both the dying patient and the caregiver | A total of 95% of participants reported that dignity therapy helped the patient, 78% reported it heightened the patient's sense of dignity, 72% reported it heighted the patient's sense of purpose, 65% reported it helped the patient prepare for death, 65% reported it was as important as any other aspect of the patient's care, and 43% reported it reduced the patient's suffering. Regarding family members, 78% reported the generativity document helped them during their time of grief, 77% reported the document would continue to be a source of comfort for their families, and 95% reported they would recommend dignity therapy to others. | Respondents were mostly elderly female spouses or adult-children of the deceased. Only families of cancer patients participated. Participants were mostly non-Hispanic white, Anglo-Saxon, and Protestant. |

(continued)

Table 6.1. CONTINUED

Author (Year)	Design/Sampling	Subject Characteristics	Methods/Interventions	Data/Measures	Findings/Outcomes	Limitations
McMillian et al., 2006	Three-group RCT; sample from consecutive admissions to a large, nonprofit community-based hospice in the southeastern United States	354 family caregivers of community-dwelling hospice patients with advanced cancer; 109 in group 1, 109 in group 2, 111 in group 3	Group 1, the control group, received standard hospice care. Group 2 received standard hospice care and three supportive visits that matched the duration and frequency of group 3's intervention. Group 3 received standard care and three visits to teach a coping skills intervention, from the Family COPE model, which matched the duration and frequency of Group 2.	Caregiver Quality of Life Index–Cancer, Memorial Symptom Assessment Scale, Caregiver Demands Scale, Brief COPE Scale, Short Portable Mental Status Questionnaire	The COPE intervention was uniquely effective in improving caregivers' overall quality of life and in decreasing burden related to patients' symptoms and caregiving tasks. Burden was also significantly improved by the intervention. Group 2 (emotional support visits plus hospice care) showed no significant effects on any of the dependent measures compared with group 1 (hospice care alone).	High rate of attrition resulting from the patient's decline or death and the caregiver feeling overwhelmed.
Northouse et al., 2005	Longitudinal RCT	132 patient–caregiver dyads; 66 dyads in experimental group, 65 dyads in the control group; mean patient age, 54 years; mean caregiver age, 52 years; 77% white; 62% of caregivers were husbands	Control group received standard care. Experimental group received standard care and the FOCUS Program.	Appraisal of Illness Scale; Appraisal of Caregiving Scale; Mishel Uncertainty in Illness Scale; Beck Hopelessness Scale; Brief COPE; FACT, version 3; SF-36 Health Survey	Experimental group patients reported significantly less hopelessness and less negative appraisal of illness. Experimental group caregivers reported significantly less negative appraisal of caregiving. Intervention effects were not sustained at 6 months.	Possibility of type 1 error. Variables that could have affected the family intervention may have been excluded. No cost-effectiveness measures were included.

Study	Design	Sample	Intervention	Measures	Results	Limitations
Northouse et al., 2007	RCT	235; 123 in control, 112 in experimental; mean patient age in the final sample, 63 years; mean spouse age, 59 years; 84% of dyads non-Hispanic white; 65% in newly diagnosed phase	Couples in control group received standard clinic care. Experimental group received standard clinic care plus a version of the FOCUS Program modified to address the needs of prostate cancer patients and their spouses. The intervention included three 90-minute home visits and two 30-minute telephone sessions spaced 2 weeks apart and delivered between baseline and 4 months.	Medical Outcomes Study 12-item short form, version 2; FACT-G, version 4; Appraisal of Illness or Appraisal of Caregiving Scales; Mishel Uncertainty in Illness Scale; Beck Hopelessness Scale; Brief Coping Orientations to Problems Experienced scale; Lewis Cancer Self-efficacy Scale; Lewis Mutuality and Interpersonal Sensitivity Scale; Symptom Scale of the Omega Screening Questionnaire; Expanded Prostate Cancer Index Composite; Omega Screening Questionnaire developed by Mood and Bickes	Patients in experimental group reported less uncertainty and better communication with spouses than those in the control group. Spouses in the experimental group reported higher quality of life, more self-efficacy, better communication, and less negative appraisal of caregiving, uncertainty, hopelessness, and symptom distress.	Possibility of type 1 error. Numbers of patients in the biochemical and advanced phases were small. All patients had partners.
Walsh et al., 2007	RCT	271 informal caregivers; 134 in control group, 137 in experimental group; 21% male; mean age, 56.3 years; 86% white	Control group received usual palliative care. Experimental group received usual care plus a caregiver advisor intervention, which was delivered in six visits over a 6-week period.	GHQ-28	In both the intervention and the control groups, scores on the GHQ-28 fell below the recruitment threshold of 5 of 6 points at any follow-up. There were no significant differences in the mean scores at any time and there were no observed differences in primary outcomes.	Recruitment may have been influenced by gatekeeping. External validity may have been lowered by inclusion criteria. Missing data because of the death of a patient.

NOTE: CES-D, Center for Epidemiological Studies–Depression scale; COPE, Coping Orientations to Problems Experienced; CPR, cardiopulmonary resuscitation; DNR, do not resuscitate; FACT, Functional Assessment of Cancer Therapy; FACT-G, Functional Assessment of Cancer Therapy–General; FOCUS, Family involvement, Optimistic attitude, Coping effectiveness, Uncertainty reduction, and Symptom management; GHQ-28, General Health Questionnaire; NR, not reported; PC-ACP, patient-centered advance care planning; PSQI, Pittsburgh Sleep Quality Index; RCT, randomized controlled trial; SF-12, 12-Item Short Form Health Survey; SF-36, 36-Item Short Form Health Survey; SPIRIT, Sharing Patients' Illness Representations to Increase Trust.

INTERVENTIONS TO INCREASE COMPLETION
OF ADVANCE DIRECTIVES AND COMMUNICATION
OF HEALTH CARE PREFERENCES

The Patient Self-Determination Act (PSDA) required that healthcare institutions receiving federal funds such as Medicare must "educate" potential patients about their rights to make decisions about their own health care. The specific requirements of the PSDA are that individuals have the right to facilitate their own healthcare decisions, to accept or refuse medical treatments, and to execute an advance directive. The PSDA also requires that healthcare institutions inquire whether the individual has an advance directive and make note of such documents in the medical records, as well as educate staff members about an individual's right to engage in advance care planning and to execute advance directives. In the absence of such documentation, hospitals and courts look to the closest biological family member of individuals who are (or are not) considered to be married to make such decisions (Haley et al., 2002; Hopp & Duffy, 2000). Thus, advance directives are often especially crucial for sexual minorities, because the suffering person's closest relationship may be stigmatized in majority society.

Schmid and colleagues found racial/ethnic differences in naturally occurring treatment preference agreement, with black dyads (primarily older adults and their adult children) showing greater treatment preference agreement (Schmid, Allen, Haley, & DeCoster, 2010). Only prior participation in advance care planning discussions facilitated dyadic agreement; black family members tended to make undertreatment errors in the absence of such discussions whereas non-Hispanic white families tended to make overtreatment errors.

Multiple interventions seek to improve communication of treatment preferences and documentation of these preferences in advance directives. The Study to Understand Prognoses and Preferences for Outcomes and Risks of Treatment (SUPPORT) examined the effectiveness of a nurse as a discussion facilitator promoting completion of advance directives among hospitalized patients (The SUPPORT Principal Investigators, 1995). The results of SUPPORT indicated there was no difference in rates of recorded, formal discussions pertaining to treatment preferences, DNR orders, or attempted resuscitations at the end of life. In an elegant study with four separate intervention conditions compared with a control condition, Ditto and colleagues examined whether advance directives paired with informal discussion increased the accuracy of proxy end-of-life decision making (Ditto et al., 2001). Participants were randomized into one of five groups; intervention participants were instructed to complete one of two types of advance directive (instructional or values based) either with or without an accompanying discussion with their proxy (directive [instructional or values based] and discussion, directive only, discussion only). These groups were compared with dyads that did not complete either type of directive and did not discuss treatment preferences. Across intervention groups, proxy decision making did not improve relative to the "patient." However, the interventions helped individuals feel better about advance care planning. Proxies reported more understanding, confidence, and a stronger belief in the importance of advance planning whereas patients reported a significant increase in their belief that their proxy understood their wishes and comfort with the decision-making process.

Similarly, Briggs and colleagues reported a successful, education-based patient-centered advance care planning (PC-ACP) approach (Briggs, Kirchhoff, Hammes, Song, & Colvin, 2004). By educating potential patients and family members about the progression of the patient's medical condition, potential complications, and benefits and burdens of available treatments, this intervention improved patient–proxy treatment preference agreement. The intervention entails a one-time, 1-hour interview with the goal of increasing dyadic congruence and advance care planning knowledge, and decreasing decisional conflict. The success of the intervention was attributed to the involvement of the proxy throughout the intervention, and realistic scenarios specific to each family's medical situation.

One intervention targeted black individuals with end-stage renal disease and their chosen family proxy: the Sharing Patients' Illness Representations to Increase Trust (SPIRIT) project (Song et al., 2009). This 1-hour, nurse-facilitated intervention increased patient–proxy treatment congruence in end-of-life decision making and incorporated a discussion of spirituality and values in the internal representations about the illness held by both the patient and the proxy. SPIRIT also succeeded in increasing the proxies' confidence in their decision-making abilities.

Case Study 1: "Planning for Future Care"

Lenora is a 72-year-old woman who resides in a rural area in Mississippi with her partner of almost 45 years, Ray. Ray is 67 years old and was diagnosed with amyotrophic lateral sclerosis (ALS; Lou Gehrig's disease) just 2 years previously. As expected with ALS, his physical condition has deteriorated rapidly and he is now bound to a wheelchair throughout the day. Lenora is Ray's primary caregiver; his only living relative is a sister who refused contact with Ray after he came out as a transgendered man (female-to-male transgendered individual) when he was 25 years old. Although Ray has never had access to the information and resources necessary to have transition surgeries or to change his gender on his driver's license, he is consistent with his hormone replacement therapy and presentation as a masculine gender.

Both Lenora and Ray feel discriminated against by service providers, including Ray's primary care physician and the nurses and aides who provide him with home health care. Healthcare professionals who at first seem warm and genuinely concerned and willing to discuss ALS with the couple quickly become distant and reserved when learning of Ray's trans identity. Answers to Lenora's questions about what they should expect next or resources available to them are met with terse responses and minimal eye contact, as it seems providers are writing quickly whatever is necessary to be out of the couple's presence as soon as possible. For these reasons, Ray often attempts to not reveal his identity as a transgendered man when visiting doctors' offices, but this is nearly impossible given the physicality required during routine exams. Similarly, when nurses or aides are in the home to help Ray shower and dress, they often treat him with disdain and cast looks of disgust toward what they view as incongruities between Ray's physical body and gender presentation. All of this is hurtful to Ray and makes him feel some sense of shame, although he has been comfortable with his identity as a transgendered man for decades. Lenora often finds herself angry, with elevated blood pressure, because of the poor treatment of the person she loves and with whom she has built and shared her life.

In addition to the prejudice felt from those who are supposed to be helping Lenora take care of her partner, she often experiences great difficulty just trying to retrieve Ray's medication from the pharmacy, a problem that typically would not exist for most couples that have been together for more than four decades. Without a marriage license, available in the US to same-sex couples only since June 26, 2015, it is unlikely that Lenora will be allowed to make decisions for Ray based on his wishes when he becomes unable to communicate.

PSYCHOSOCIAL INTERVENTIONS TO REDUCE THE STRESS OF PALLIATIVE CAREGIVING

A Cochrane review of 11 diverse interventions targeting palliative caregivers found weak evidence for any therapeutic effect and highlighted the need for greater methodological rigor in future studies (Candy, Jones, Drake, Laurent, & King, 2011). Interventions to reduce the stress of palliative caregiving and to improve the lives of palliative care patients often use reminiscence as a therapeutic tool (Allen, 2009; Allen, Hilgeman, Ege, Shuster, & Burgio, 2008; Ando, Morita, Akechi, & Okamoto, 2009; Chochinov, 2012; Chochinov et al., 2011; McClement et al., 2007). The most widely studied of these interventions is Chochinov's Dignity Therapy (Chochinov, 2012; Chochinov et al., 2011), during which a healthcare professional helps the palliative care patient and, potentially, family members, complete a dignity-preserving interview consisting largely of a review of the patient's life story. McClement and colleagues (2007) reported that 95% of bereaved family members perceived their loved one's participation in dignity therapy as beneficial, 78% reported that the "generativity document" helped their grief process, and 95% would recommend dignity therapy to others. In a randomized controlled trial (RCT), Chochinov and colleagues (2011) found that dignity therapy improved spiritual well-being and was perceived as more helpful than standard palliative or client-centered care.

Addington-Hall and colleagues conducted an RCT comparing the coordination of care by two nurses whose role was to ensure that patients received appropriate and well-coordinated services tailored to their own needs in comparison with usual care at baseline, near death, and with family caregivers after bereavement (Addington-Hall et al., 1992). They found few differences between groups. Coordination group caregivers were more likely to report the patient had a cough during the last week of life and had ineffective treatment for anxiety but effective physical symptom control. They were also less likely to report feeling angry about the death of the patient than caregivers whose patients received usual care.

Many additional palliative caregiver-focused interventions describe the experience of caring for someone with cancer (see Chapter 4). Carter (2006) tested the effectiveness of a brief behavioral sleep intervention (e.g., stimulus control, relaxation, cognitive therapy, sleep hygiene) for family caregivers of individuals with advanced cancer. Results indicated that caregivers in the intervention group showed greater improvement than control caregivers across time in subjective sleep quality and indicated reduced symptoms of depression. Hudson, Aranda, and Haymen-White (2005) conducted an RCT with palliative caregivers providing care to a relative dying of cancer at home. The psychoeducational intervention bundled with standard home-based palliative care services was compared with usual treatment. Results indicated that the intervention group caregivers reported a more positive caregiving experience than control caregivers; there were no group differences in preparedness to care, self-efficacy, competence, or anxiety. These results coincide with findings among dementia caregivers that experiencing positive aspects of caregiving moderates treatment efficacy (Hilgeman et al., 2007).

Keefe and colleagues tested a partner-guided cancer pain management protocol in comparison with usual care among cancer patient–caregiver dyads near the end of life (Keefe et al., 2005). The three-session home-based intervention integrated education with CBT techniques to improve pain coping skills. Results showed significant increases in caregiver self-efficacy for controlling patient pain and other symptoms among those in the intervention group. Intervention caregivers also demonstrated a trend toward improved caregiver strain relative to the control group.

Kissane and colleagues conducted a two-group RCT to examine the effect of family-focused grief therapy on the level of distress and depression of family members of terminally ill cancer patients (Kissane et al., 2006). Family-focused grief therapy aims to prevent morbid effects of bereavement and grief among families at risk for poor psychosocial outcomes, and is composed of four to eight 90-minute sessions across 9 to 18 months. Levels of distress and depression among participants were assessed at baseline and 6 and 13 months after the patient's death. Overall reduction in general distress was reported at 13 months, and significant improvement in distress and depression was found among family members with greater baseline scores. Intermediate-functioning families showed improvement whereas hostile families did not and were affected negatively by therapy. Hostile family members may be better helped individually.

McMillan and colleagues (2006) conducted a three-group RCT with advanced cancer patients and their family caregivers and compared standard hospice care, standard hospice care plus three supportive visits by research staff, and standard hospice care plus three coping skills training visits by research staff. Results indicated the coping skills training intervention produced significantly greater improvement in caregiver quality of life, burden of patient symptoms, and caregiver task-related burden in comparison with the other conditions. No group differences were found in caregiver mastery (general or task specific), or problem-focused or emotion-focused coping.

Northouse and colleagues conducted a two-group RCT with recurrent breast cancer patients and their family caregivers to examine the effect of a family-based intervention (the Family involvement, Optimistic attitude, Coping effectiveness, Uncertainty reduction, and Symptom management [FOCUS] Program) (Northouse, Kershaw, Mood, & Schafenacker, 2005). The intervention was designed to provide information and support to the patients and their family caregivers that addressed five content areas: family involvement, optimistic attitude, coping effectiveness, uncertainty reduction, and symptom management. The intervention group, which received both usual care and intervention, reported significantly less hopelessness and less negative appraisal of illness than the control group, which received usual care only. Family caregivers in the intervention group reported significantly less negative appraisal of caregiving than those in the control group. Such effects for patients and family caregivers were evident at 3 months; however, they did not last to 6 months. There was no difference between the intervention group and the control group with regard to quality of life.

Northouse and colleagues (2007) evaluated the effect of the FOCUS Program intervention in a two-group RCT with prostate cancer patients and their spouses, comparing standard care only and standard care plus the FOCUS intervention. Findings showed that less uncertainly and better communication with one's spouse were apparent at 4 months by the patients in the intervention group in comparison with those in the control group. Higher quality of life, more self-efficacy, better communication, and less negative appraisal of caregiving, uncertainty, hopelessness, and symptom distress were reported at 4 months by intervention spouses in comparison with those in the control group. Some of the effects reported by spouses were sustained at 8 and 12 months.

Walsh and colleagues conducted an RCT in which the experimental group received usual care plus an informal caregiver advisor intervention delivered in six visits during a 6-week period (Walsh et al, 2007). The relationship between informal caregivers and palliative care patients was not specifically defined (e.g., family relation, volunteer). Usual care comprised the comparison condition. The intervention consisted of eight domains: patient care, physical health needs, need for time away from the patient in the short or long term, need to plan for the future, psychological health, relationships and social networks, relationships with health and social service providers, and finances. Using the General Health Questionaire-28 (Goldberg & Hillier, 1979), there were no significant group differences at any time point observed in primary outcomes.

Our prior work (Allen, 2009; Allen & Hilgeman, 2009; Allen et al., 2008) differs from the aforementioned interventions in taking a general rather than cancer-specific approach to palliative caregiver stress reduction. Social work and psychology graduate students with bachelor's or master's degrees delivered a three-session, home-based reminiscence and creative activity intervention to palliative care patients and their family caregivers. In contrast with dignity therapy, the Legacy Project was created by the family with assistance from the interventionist. Results indicate the intervention improved family caregivers' levels of stress and improved palliative patients' sense of meaning and reduced their physical symptom burden relative to a control group. Fidelity data revealed accuracy of treatment delivery averaged 91.55% (Allen et al., 2008).

Ingersoll-Dayton and colleagues created a dyadic intervention for couples in which one individual had been diagnosed with dementia (Ingersoll-Dayton et al., 2013). They based their social worker-driven intervention on the prior work of Allen and colleagues (Allen et al., 2008). Social workers delivered a 5-week intervention using life review and communication skills techniques. Qualitative results of this small study ($N = 20$) suggest that couples who created a "couples life story" album by working together with an interventionist reported improved mood and communication. Both participants with dementia and their spouses reported benefit from the intervention in terms of meaningful engagement and enhanced interaction.

Case Study 2: "Palliative Caregiver Distress and Suffering"

Na-mi is a 48-year-old Korean American woman who immigrated to the United States with her husband and their two children 12 years ago. Na-mi and her family settled in a community heavily populated by Korean immigrants, where her brother, Sung (52 years old), and his family moved a couple of years earlier. After both Na-mi and Sung settled down in the new environment, Sung invited their mother, Jin, to the United States to live with him and his family. Jin, now a 73-year-old widow, sold all her assets in Korea and left her home country to live with her children in the United States, where she has lived for 5 years. During those years, Jin helped Sung financially to a great degree. She worked part-time jobs babysitting and cooking for other Korean families in the community to provide extra income for her son and his family. She experienced pain in her pelvic area for almost a year but did not discuss it with any of her children because she did not want to worry them. However, recently the pain has gotten worse—to the degree she cannot keep it to herself any longer. She talked to her daughter, Na-mi, about her pain and asked if Na-mi could get some medicine to relieve her pain. Na-mi was frustrated to find out that her elderly mother kept such pain to herself and that her brother and his wife did not notice any change in their mother's health even when living in the same house.

When Na-mi discussed their mother's need to be seen by a doctor and get an exam, Sung and his wife were hesitant to take her to a doctor's office and wanted to try some painkillers first. Sung expressed concerns regarding the expense, because Jin did not have any health insurance and was not eligible for Medicare as a result of her immigration status. Sung has serious financial difficulties and does not have health insurance for himself and his wife. Sung was also concerned that his congregation and neighbors might believe he was not taking care of his mother's health if they saw he and Jin in doctors' offices and learned about Jin's health condition. Jin did not want to upset her only son, so she refused to see a doctor and just wanted to try strong painkillers and rest as her son recommended.

It took Na-mi 2 weeks to persuade Jin and Sung to see a doctor. They finally agreed, and Na-mi took Jin to a doctor's office, with Jin lying in the back of her van because she could not sit or walk because of the pain. After a series of exams, Jin was diagnosed with terminal stage uterine cancer with metastasis in her colon. The doctor, who was also a Korean, shared the diagnosis with Na-mi and Sung alone and left them to decide whether to tell their mother. He also added there was really no available curative treatment and that there was a local hospice agency with Korean staff, if they were interested in getting some help taking care of their mother at home. Na-mi consulted with her friend, who was a nurse, and learned about the services provided by hospice care. Na-mi did not tell her mother about her diagnosis but assured her, saying she would get a nurse who would come home and help with pain management. Then, Na-mi discussed the option of hospice care with Sung; however, Sung neither wanted to accept Jin's terminality nor consider hospice care. He blamed Na-mi for lack of faith in God's healing power and was concerned also about the medical expense for potential treatments. After a few days and nights of heated discussions with Na-mi, Sung declared that it would be best for Jin to go back to Korea and to seek medical care there because she was still eligible for health insurance in her home country. Also, he did not want his community members to know about his mother's terminal diagnosis because he was afraid that people might blame him for his mother's ill health.

Knowing there was no family caregiver available and no place for Jin to live in Korea, Na-mi insisted that Jin stay in the States and receive care from the Korean staff at the local hospice agency. Sung and his wife got very upset with Na-mi and eventually did not let her in their house or answer her telephone calls. Na-mi was able to see her mother again only after Jin fell into a coma and was admitted to an intensive care unit on life support. Na-mi is paying for Jin's hospital expenses, not knowing what her mother's end-of-life wishes are. Despite his inability to afford his mother's medical expenses, Sung wants Jin to receive life-sustaining treatment.

EFFORTS IN TRANSLATING PALLIATIVE
CAREGIVING INTERVENTIONS

Although hospice and palliative care social workers frequently use reminiscence and creative activities with their patients (Csikai & Weisenfluh, 2012), such interventions need to be more accessible to patients and families transitioning through primary care to hospital and palliative care settings. Kazdin and Blase (2011) strongly suggest the need for new modes of intervention delivery targeting prevention and treatment to alleviate suffering. Few such studies, however, have been completed and published.

In a demonstration project, Lukas and colleagues studied the effects of an intervention using a before-and-after single-patient group design (Lukas, Foltz, & Paxton, 2013). The intervention included a home-based palliative care consultation on hospitalization, emergency department visits, and admission cost for patients with advanced chronic illness. The intervention also provided palliative care consultation on symptom management, advance care planning, goal-directed care, and care coordination for patients and their families. Direct care was provided by nurse practitioners, and psychospiritual needs were met by psychiatric homecare nurses, network chaplains, or behavioral health physicians, all of whom collaborated with the patient's primary care physician. After the 1- to 2-hour initial consultation with multidimensional assessment, goals of treatment were prepared and added to the patient's hospital record for reference during future hospital admissions. Advance directive forms were provided, and completion of the forms was encouraged. The frequency of follow-up consultation visits varied from weekly to every 3 months, depending on the severity of symptoms and the need for ongoing advance care planning. A significant reduction was found in the number of hospitalizations, hospital days, cost for admissions, and the probability of 30-day readmissions.

If hospice or palliative care is not chosen as a treatment option, few means of delivering therapeutic reminiscence-based interventions exist. This represents a significant gap in practice and in the psychosocial palliative care intervention literature. Recently, our research team completed an RCT (Allen et al., 2014) to evaluate the effectiveness of retired senior volunteers (RSVs) available through the National Senior Corp Program to deliver the manualized, three-session Legacy (e.g., reminiscence and creative activity) intervention previously found effective in improving palliative care patient and caregiver outcomes (Allen, 2009; Allen et al., 2008). If successful, this mode of treatment delivery (e.g., RSV intervention) would represent a significant step toward translation and greater access at earlier disease stages of therapeutic psychosocial interventions for individuals near the end of life and for their family members.

Of the 45 dyads that completed the baseline, 28 completed postintervention and 24 completed follow-up. The intervention group received three home visits by RSVs; control group families received three supportive telephone calls by research staff. Patients in the intervention group reported a significantly greater reduction in frequency of emotional symptoms and emotional symptom bother than the control group, as well as improved spiritual functioning. Family caregivers in the intervention group were more likely than control caregivers to endorse experiencing meaning in life. Only improvement in intervention patients' emotional symptom bother maintained at the 3-month follow-up after discontinuing RSV contact.

CONCLUSION

At some point in the life span, it is probable that most, if not every individual, will become a palliative caregiver to a loved one with an advanced, chronic illness. Viewed through the lens of the chronic care model (Koffman et al., 2007; Wagner, 1998), effective interventions must prepare caregivers to communicate with care recipients and healthcare professionals across the disease trajectory—from planning for future care and discussing advance directives, to provision of direct care near the end of life, to preserving the care recipient's dignity. Regarding future planning, one issue that requires greater clinical and scientific attention involves the need for effective and culturally sensitive patient-centered education about advance directives and end-of-life treatment approaches to reduce and, eventually, to eliminate health disparities. There is a particular need for attention to cultural sensitivity within the LGBTQ community.

With regard to the stress of palliative caregiving, we understand why the Cochrane review (Candy et al., 2011) found weak evidence of therapeutic effect and the need for rigorous scientific methodology in future studies. Palliative caregiving shares common themes such as witnessing the suffering of a family member (Monin & Schulz, 2009), yet the literature tends to focus on particular diseases such as cancer or dementia. Methodologically rigorous research that applies generally applicable techniques such as reminiscence or mindfulness and acceptance-based approaches (Baer, 2006) may show reductions in caregiver stress and improvements in positive affect or quality of life across disease categories. Future research should focus on carefully measuring disease burden and pursue enrollment of individuals and families presenting at palliative care centers that provide care to individuals with a myriad of specific chronic diseases in the advanced stage. These interprofessional treatment centers prioritize improvement of comfort and quality of life rather than "cure" of the advanced chronic illness (Campbell & Amin, 2012) and address the needs of individuals and families.

Notably, translation of effective interventions to improve advance care planning at the front-end of the chronic illness trajectory (e.g., PC-ACP [Briggs et al., 2004], SPIRIT [Song et al., 2009]) and well-being of caregivers in the latter days of a loved one's life (e.g., dignity therapy [Chochinov, 2012; Chochinov et al., 2011]; reminiscence and creative activity [Allen, 2009; Allen et al., 2014; Allen et al., 2008]) may proceed in concert with expansion of the evidence base of treatments. At the least, demonstration projects administered by palliative care or hospice staff or by RSVs could examine effectiveness of treatments with initial and growing evidence of efficacy. Such an approach would answer the call of Kazdin and Blase (2011) to address unmet mental health needs of stressed individuals and their families in the context of advanced, chronic illness.

NOTES

1. To receive the Medicare Hospice Benefit, patients must have Medicare Part A (Hospital Insurance), and the patients' doctor and the hospice medical director must certify the patient is terminally ill, with 6 months or less to live.
2. Minority groups are less likely than non-Hispanic whites to have a stable work history or to have Medicare-covered employment that would provide Medicare eligibility (Feldman, 1999).

REFERENCES

Addington-Hall, J. M., MacDonald, L. D., Anderson, H. R., Chamberlain, J., Freeling, P., Bland, J. M., et al. (1992). Randomised controlled trial of effects of coordinating care for terminally ill cancer patients. *British Medical Journal, 305,* 1317–1322.

Allen, R. S. (2009). The Legacy Project intervention to enhance meaningful family interactions: Case examples. *Clinical Gerontologist, 32*(2), 164–176.

Allen, R. S., Harris, G. M., Burgio, L. D., Azuero, C. B., Miller, L. A., Shin, H., et al. (2014). Can senior volunteers deliver reminiscence and creative activity interventions? Results of the Legacy Intervention Family Enactment randomized controlled trial. *Journal of Pain and Symptom Management, 48*(4), 590–601. doi: 10.1016/j.jpainsymman.2013.11.012.

Allen, R. S., & Hilgeman, M. M. (2009). Helping people with dementia approach the end of life: Issues for families: Finding, reinforcing and preserving identity. *Generations, 33*(1), 74–77.

Allen, R. S., Hilgeman, M. M., Ege, M. A., Shuster, J. L., Jr., & Burgio, L. D. (2008). Legacy activities as interventions approaching the end of life. *Journal of Palliative Medicine, 11*(7), 1029–1038.

Allen, R. S., & Shuster, J. L. (2002). The role of proxies in treatment decisions: Evaluating functional capacity to consent to end-of-life treatments within a family context. *Behavioral Sciences and the Law, 20,* 235–252.

Ando, M., Morita, T., Akechi, T., Okamoto, T. (2009). Efficacy of short-term life-review interviews on the spiritual well-being of terminally ill cancer patients. *Journal of Pain and Symptom Management, 9*(6), 993–1002.

Aneshensel, C. S., Pearlin, L. I., Mullan, J. T., Zarit, S. H., & Whitlatch, C. J. (1995). *Profiles in caregiving: The unexpected career.* San Diego, CA: Academic Press.

Baer, R. A. (2006). *Mindfulness-based treatment approaches: Clinician's guide to evidence base and treatment approaches.* Burlington, MA: Elsevier.

Bailey, F. A., Allen, R. S., Williams, B. R., Goode, P. S., Granstaff, S., Redden, D. T., et al. (2012). Do-not-resuscitate orders in the last days of life. *Journal of Palliative Medicine, 15*(7), 751–759.

Bayer, W., Mallinger, J., Krishnan, A., & Shields, C. (2006). Attitudes toward life-sustaining interventions among ambulatory black and white patients. *Ethnicity & Disease, 16*(4), 914–919.

Bodenheimer, T., Wagner, E. H., Grumbach, K. (2002). Improving primary care for patients with chronic illness: The chronic care model, part 2. *Journal of the American Medical Association, 288*(15), 1909–1914.

Born, W., Greiner, K. A., Sylvia, E., Butler, J., & Ahluwalia, J. S. (2004). Knowledge, attitudes, and beliefs about end-of-life care among inner-city African Americans and Latinos. *Journal of Palliative Medicine, 7*(2), 247–256.

Braun, K. L., Onaka, A. T., & Horiuchi, B. Y. (2001). Advance directive completion rates and end-of-life preferences in Hawaii. *Journal of the American Geriatrics Society, 49*(12), 1708–1713.

Briggs, L. A., Kirchhoff, K. T., Hammes, B. J., Song, M. K., & Colvin, E. R. (2004). Patient-centered advance care planning in special patient populations: A pilot study. *Journal of Professional Nursing, 20*(1), 47–58.

Bullock, K. (2006). Promoting advance directives among African Americans: A faith-based model. *Journal of Palliative Medicine, 9*(1), 183–195.

Burrs, F. A. (1995). The African American experience: Breaking the barriers to hospices. *Hospice Journal, 10*(2), 15–18.

Campbell, L. M., & Amin, N. (2012). A poststructural glimpse at the World Health Organization's palliative care discourse in rural South Africa. *Rural and Remote Health, 12*, 1–8.

Candy, B., Jones, L., Drake, R., Leurent, B., & King, M. (2011). Interventions for supporting informal caregivers of patients in the terminal phase of a disease (review). *The Cochrane Database of Systematic Reviews, 7*. John Wiley & Sons, LTD, 1–75. CD007617.

Carr, D. (2011). Racial differences in end-of-life planning: Why don't blacks and Latinos prepare for the inevitable? *Omega: Journal of Death and Dying, 63*(1), 1–20.

Carter, P. A. (2006). A brief behavioral sleep intervention for family caregivers of persons with cancer. *Cancer Nursing, 29*, 95–103.

Chen, H., Haley, W. E., Robinson, B. E., & Schonwetter, R. S. (2003). Decisions for hospice care in patients with advanced cancer. *Journal of the American Geriatrics Society, 51*, 789–797.

Chochinov, H. M. (2012). *Dignity therapy: Final words for final days.* New York: Oxford University Press.

Chochinov, H. M., Kristjanson, L. J., Breitbart, W., McClement, S., Hack, T. F., Hassard, T. et al. (2011). Effect of dignity therapy on distress and end-of-life experience in terminally ill patients: A randomised controlled trial. *The Lancet Oncology, 12*(8), 753–762.

Chow, E., Harth, E. T., Hruby, G., Finkelstein, J., Wu, J., & Danjoux, C. (2011). How accurate are physicians' clinical predictions of survival and the available prognostic tools in estimating survival times in terminally ill cancer patients? A systematic review. *Clinical Oncology, 13*, 209–218.

Christakis, N. A., & Lamont, E. B. (2000). Extent and determinants of error in doctors' prognoses in terminally ill patients: Prospective cohort study. *British Medical Journal, 320*, 469–472.

Centers for Medicare and Medicaid Services. (2007). *Medicare hospice benefits.* http://www.cms.gov/Regulations-and-Guidance/Guidance/Manuals/downloads/bp102c09.pdf.

Coon, D. W. (2007). Exploring interventions for LGBT caregivers: Issues and examples. *Journal of Gay & Lesbian Social Services: Issues in Practice, Policy & Research, 18*(3–4), 109–128.

Cort, M. A. (2004). Cultural mistrust and use of hospice care: Challenges and remedies. *Journal of Palliative Medicine, 7*(1), 63–71.

Crawley, L. (2000). Palliative and end-of-life care in the African American community. *Journal of American Medical Association, 284*(19), 2518–2521.

Crawley, L. (2005). Racial, cultural, and ethnic factors influencing end-of-life care. *Journal of Palliative Medicine, 8*(Suppl 1), S58–S69.

Csikai, E. L., & Weisenfluh, S. (2012). Hospice and palliative social workers' engagement in life review interventions. *The American Journal of Hospice & Palliative Care, 30*(3), 257–263.

Damron-Rodriguez, J., Wallace, S. P., & Kington, R. (1994). Service utilization and minority elderly: Appropriateness, accessibility and acceptability. *Gerontology & Geriatrics Education, 15*(1), 45–63.

Degenholtz, H. B., Arnold, R. A., Meisel, A., & Lave, J. R. (2002). Persistence of racial/ethnic disparities in advance care plan documents among nursing home residents. *Journal of the American Geriatrics Society, 50*, 378–381.

Dilworth-Anderson, P., Williams, I. C., & Gibson, B. E. (2002). Issues of race, ethnicity, and culture in caregiving research: A 20-year review (1980–2000). *The Gerontologist, 42*, 237–272.

Ditto, P. H., Danks, J. H., Smucker, W. D., Bookwala, J., Coppola, K. M., Dresser, R., et al. (2001). Advance directives as acts of communication: Randomized controlled trial. *Archives of Internal Medicine, 161*, 421–430.

Family Caregiver Alliance. (2006). *Caregiver assessment: Voices and views from the field*. Report from a National Consensus Development Conference, vol. II. San Francisco, CA: Author.

Feldman, R. S. (1999). *The psychology of adversity*. Amherst, MA: University of Massachusetts Press.

Fredriksen-Goldsen, K. I., Kim, H., Muraco, A., & Mincer, S. (2009). Chronically ill midlife and older lesbians, gay men, and bisexuals and their informal caregivers: The impact of the social context. *Sexuality Research & Social Policy: A Journal of the NSRC, 6*(4), 52–64.

Gelfand, D. E., Balcazar, H., Parzuchowski, J., & Lenox, S. (2001). Mexicans and care for the terminally ill: Family, hospice, and the church. *American Journal of Hospice & Palliative Care, 18*(6), 391–396.

Gessert, C. E., Curry, N. M., & Robinson, A. (2001). Ethnicity and end-of-life care: The use of feeding tubes. *Ethnicity and Disease, 11*, 97–106.

Goldberg, D. P., & Hillier, V. F. (1979). A scaled version of the General Health Questionnaire. *Psychological Medicine, 9*(1), 139–145.

Guo, Y., Palmer, J. L., Bianti, J., Konzen, B., Shin, K., & Bruera, E. (2010). Advance directives and do-not-resuscitate orders in patients with cancer with metastatic spinal cord compression: Advanced care planning implications. *Journal of Palliative Medicine, 13*, 513–517.

Haley, W. E., Allen, R. S., Reynolds, S., Chen, H., Burton, A., & Gallagher-Thompson, D. (2002). Family issues in end-of-life decision making and end-of-life care. *American Behavioral Scientist, 46*, 284–298.

Hallenbeck, J., Goldstein, M. K., & Mebane, E. W. (1996). Cultural considerations of death and dying in the United States. *Clinics in Geriatric Medicine, 12*, 393–406.

Harding, R., Epiphaniou, E., & Chidgey-Clark, J. (2012). Needs, experiences, and preferences of sexual minorities for end-of-life care and palliative care: A systematic review. *Journal of Palliative Medicine, 15*(5), 602–611.

Harris, G. M., Allen, R. S., Dunn, L., & Parmelee, P. (2013). "Trouble won't last always": Religious coping and meaning in the stress process. *Qualitative Health Research, 23*(6), 773–781.

Hash, K., & Netting, F. E. (2007). Long-term planning and decision-making among midlife and older gay men and lesbians. *Journal of Social Work in End-of-Life and Palliative Care, 3*(2), 59–77.

Hilgeman, M. M., Allen, R. S., DeCoster, J., & Burgio, L. D. (2007). Positive aspects of caregiving as a moderator of treatment outcome over 12 months. *Psychology and Aging, 22*, 361–371.

Hilgeman, M. M., Durkin, D. W., Sun, F., DeCoster, J., Allen, R. S., Gallagher-Thompson, D., et al. (2009). Testing a theoretical model of the stress process in Alzheimer's caregivers with race as a moderator. *The Gerontologist, 49*(2), 248–261.

Hopp, F. P., & Duffy, S. A. (2000). Racial variations in end-of-life care. *Journal of the American Geriatrics Society, 48*, 658–663.

Hudson, P. L., Aranda, S., Hayman-White, K. (2005). A psychoeducational intervention for family caregivers of patients receiving palliative care: A randomised controlled trial. *Journal of Pain and Symptom Management, 30*, 329–341.

Ingersoll-Dayton, B., Spencer, B., Kwak, M., Sherrer, K., Allen, R. S., & Campbell, R. (2013). The couples life story approach: A dyadic intervention for dementia. *Journal of Gerontological Social Work, 56*(3), 237–254.

Jackson, F., Schim, S. M., Seeley, S., Grunow, K., & Baker, J. (2000). Barriers to hospice care for African Americans: Problems and solutions. *Journal of Hospice & Palliative Nursing, 2*(2), 65–72.

Jenkins, C., Zapka, J. G., Kurent, J. E., & Lapelle, N. (2005). End-of-life care and African Americans: Voices from the community. *Journal of Palliative Medicine, 8*(3), 585–592.

Johnson, K. S., Kuchibhatla, M., & Tulsky, J. A. (2008). What explains racial differences in the use of advance directives and attitudes toward hospice care? *Journal of the American Geriatrics Society, 56*(10), 1953–1958.

Kazdin, A. E., & Blase S. L. (2011). Rebooting psychotherapy research and practice to reduce the burden of mental illness. *Perspectives on Psychological Science, 6*(1), 21–37.

Keefe, F. J., Ahles, T. A., Sutton, L., Dalton, J. A., Baucom, D., Pope, M. S., et al. (2005). Partner-guided cancer pain management at the end of life: A preliminary study. *Journal of Pain and Symptom Management, 29*, 263–272.

Kissane, D. W., McKenzie, M., Bloch, S., Moskowitz, C., McKenzie, D. P., & O'Neill, I. (2006). Family focused grief therapy: A randomised controlled trial in palliative care and bereavement. *American Journal of Psychiatry, 163*, 1208–1218.

Koffman, J., Burke, G., Dias, A., Raval, B., Byrne, J., Gonzales, J., et al. (2007). Demographic factors and awareness of palliative care and related services. *Palliative Medicine, 21*, 145–153.

Kwak, J., & Haley, W. E. (2005). Current research findings on end-of-life decision making among racially or ethnically diverse groups. *The Gerontologist, 45*, 634–641.

Lorenz, K. A., Ettner, S. L., Rosenfeld, K. E., Carlisle, D., Liu, H., & Asch, S. M. (2004). Accommodating ethnic diversity: A study of California hospice programs. *Medical Care, 42*(9), 871–874.

Lukas, L., Foltz, C., & Paxton, H. (2013). Hospital outcomes for a home-based palliative medicine consulting service. *Journal of Palliative Medicine, 16*(2), 179–184.

McClement, S., Chochinov, H. M., Hack, T., Hassard, T., Kristjanson, L. J., & Harlos, M. (2007). Dignity therapy: Family member perspectives. *Journal of Palliative Medicine, 10*(5), 1076–1082.

McMillan, S. C., Small, B. J., Weitzner, M., Schonwetter, R., Tittle, M., Moody, L., et al. (2006). Impact of coping skills intervention with family caregivers of hospice patients with cancer. *Cancer, 106*, 214–222.

Monin, J. K., & Schulz, R. (2009). Interpersonal effects of suffering in older adult caregiving relationships. *Psychology and Aging, 24*(3), 681–695.

Mood, D., & Bickels, J. (1989). Strategies to enhance self-care in radiation therapy. *Oncology Nursing Forum, 16*, 143.

National Hospice and Palliative Care Organization. (2014). NHPCO's facts and figures: 2005 Findings. http://www.nhpco.org/sites/default/files/public/Statistics_Research/2014_Facts_Figures.pdf

Noh, H. (2012). *Terminally ill black elders: Making the choice to receive hospice care.* Doctoral dissertation [Online]. Available: http://depot.library.wisc.edu/repository/fedora/1711.dl:YYXFLEKMS6KC58K/datastreams/REF/content.

Northouse, L., Kershaw, T., Mood, D., & Shafenacker, A. (2005). Effects of a family intervention on the quality of life of women with recurrent breast cancer and their family caregivers. *Psycho-Oncology, 14*, 478–491.

Northouse, L. L., Mood, D. W., Schafenacker, A., Montie, J. E., Sandler, H. M., Forman, J. D., et al. (2007). Randomised clinical trial of a family intervention for prostate cancer patients and their spouses. *Cancer, 110*, 2809–2818.

O'Mahony, S., McHenry, J., Snow, D., Cassin, C., Schumacher, D., & Selwyn, P. A. (2008). A review of barriers to utilization of the Medicare hospice benefits in urban populations and strategies for enhanced access. *Journal of Urban Health, 85*(2), 281–290.

Pearson, W. S., Bhat-Schelbert, K., & Probst, J. C. (2012). Multiple chronic conditions and the aging of America. *Journal of Primary Care & Community Health, 3*(1), 51–56.

Pinquart, M., & Sörensen, S. (2005). Ethnic differences in stressors, resources, and psychological outcomes of family caregiving: A meta-analysis. *The Gerontologist, 45*, 90–106.

Price, E. (2010). Coming out to care: Gay and lesbian carers' experiences of dementia services. *Health & Social Care in the Community, 18*(2), 160–168.

Pullis, B. (2011). Perceptions of hospice care among African Americans. *Journal of Hospice & Palliative Nursing, 13*(5), 281–287.

Reese, D. J., Melton, E., & Ciaravino, K. (2004). Programmatic barriers to providing culturally competent end-of-life care. *American Journal of Hospice & Palliative Care, 21*(5), 357–364.

Schmid, B., Allen, R. S., Haley, P. P., & DeCoster, J. (2010). Family matters: Dyadic agreement in end-of-life medical decision making. *The Gerontologist, 50*(2), 226–237.

Searight, H. R., & Gafford, J. (2005). Cultural diversity at the end of life: Issues and guidelines for family physicians. *American Family Physician, 71*(3), 515–522.

Song, M. K., & Sereika, S. M. (2006). An evaluation of the Decisional Conflict Scale for measuring the quality of end-of-life decision making. *Patient Education and Counseling, 61*(3), 397–404.

Song, M. K., Ward, S. E., Happ, M. B., Piraino, B., Donovan, H. S., Shields, A. M., et al. (2009). Randomized controlled trial of SPIRIT: An effective approach to preparing African American dialysis patients and families for end of life. *Research in Nursing and Health, 32*, 260–273.

Stiel, S., Bertram, L., Neuhaus, S., Nauck, F., Ostgathe, E., Elsner, F., et al. (2009). Evaluation and comparison of two prognostic scores and the physician's estimate of survival in terminally ill patients. *Support Care Cancer, 18*, 43–49.

The SUPPORT Principal Investigators. (1995). A controlled trial to improve care for seriously ill hospitalized patients: The Study to Understand Prognoses and Preferences for Outcome and Risks of Treatments (SUPPORT). *Journal of the American Medical Association, 274*, 1591–1598.

Torrez, D. (1998). Health and social service utilization patterns of Mexican American older adults. *Journal of Aging Studies, 12*(1), 83–99.

Tschann, J. M., Kaufman, S. R., & Micco, G. P. (2003). Family involvement in end-of-life hospital care. *Journal of the American Geriatrics Society, 51*, 835–840.

Wagner, E. H. (1998). Chronic disease management: What will it take to improve care for chronic illness? *Effective Clinical Practice, 1*(1), 2–4.

Walsh, K., Jones, L., Tookman, A., Mason, C., McLoughlin, J., Blizard, R., et al. (2007). Reducing emotional distress in people caring for patients receiving specialist palliative care. *British Journal of Psychiatry, 190*, 142–147.

Werth, J. L., Jr., Blevins, D., Toussaint, K. L., & Durham, M. R. (2002). The influence of cultural diversity on end-of-life care and decisions. *American Behavioral Scientist, 46*(2), 204–219.

Williams, M. E., & Freeman, P. A. (2005). Transgender health: Implications for aging and caregiving. *Journal of Gay & Lesbian Social Services: Issues in Practice, Policy & Research, 18*(3–4), 93–108.

Winston, C. A., Leshner, P., Kramer, J., & Allen, G. (2004). Overcoming barriers to access and utilization of hospice and palliative care services in African-American communities. *Omega: Journal of Death & Dying, 50*(2), 151–163.

Zarit, S. H., Todd, & Zarit, J. (1986). Subjective burden of husbands and wives as caregivers: A longitudinal study. *The Gerontologist, 26*(3), 260–266.

Caregiving for Individuals with Serious Mental Illness: A Life Cycle Perspective

HELLE THORNING AND LISA DIXON ■

Serious mental illness is associated with enormous economic, social, and personal costs for the person who has the illness, as well as his or her family and significant others. This chapter presents the experience of family caregivers who are in the unique situation of providing care to a loved one with serious mental illness for an extended period of time. We discuss interventions that have proved to be effective in facilitating positive outcomes for the person with illness and his or her family or natural supports. The discussion is informed by the emerging theoretical framework of recovery.

The concept of recovery took center stage in public mental health and policy with the publication of *Mental Health: A Report of the Surgeon General and the President's New Freedom Commission of Mental Health Final Report, Achieving the Promise: Transforming Mental Health Care in America* (Davidson, O'Connell, Tondora, Lawless, & Evans, 2005). The publication of the report of the New Freedom Commission signaled the adoption of a paradigm shift away from the traditional medical model to a consumer-based model grounded in the belief that consumers can recover from illness (Farone, 2006; Mechanic, 2008; Scheyett, DeLuca, & Morgan, 2013). Within this paradigm, the person is at the center, with the focus on harnessing individual strengths, and with the goal aimed toward recovery. This viewpoint moves away from the perspective of the traditional medical model that describes recovery as "cured from" all symptoms to "recovery in," which refers to the idea of living with symptoms in one's life. The chronic care model presented in an earlier chapter underscores the value of the continuous and integrated care in the community. This model supports the person challenged by a prolonged period of living with mental illness to build on personal strength, agency, and self-efficacy and to find meaningful ways to participate in life (Davidson, Chinman, Sells, & Rowe, 2006). Thus, the construct of "recovery in" refers to a life that is determined by the individual, reflecting that person's values, conditions, and goals (Deegan & Drake, 2006). This framework creates a space for the person with mental illness to explore opportunities for personal development and growth. The concept encompasses a renewed sense of a possibility to gain or *regain* competency, to connect or *reconnect* with society, and to move to a sense of "recover in life" (Padgett, Henwood, Abrams, & Drake, 2008).

Although family members and the natural support system carry a substantial weight in caring for persons with mental illness, they have, historically, been at the periphery of the discussion of impact of illness on their lives. Their experience has been seen separately from their ill family member. A recent systematic review of the literature about the role of family caregivers supporting a relative with serious mental illness and their relationship and engagement with providers revealed a clear tension between families and providers (Rowe, 2011). The review Rowe (2011) brought to light that family caregivers feel obligated to help support mental health care of their loved one but that the ability to carry this out is not endorsed or reinforced by mental healthcare providers. In his review, Rowe found that staff attitude toward family caregivers rendered them hidden, invisible, in narrowly defined roles, and with an expectation that the family caregivers *just cope*. When family caregivers attempted to share information about the individual with mental illness, they were seen as pushy and demanding. Thus, family members were excluded from the discussion of care planning, medication, and wellness management, but were expected to *pick up* the caregiving role after the family member was returned to their care. Family members' roles in providing care and support, as well as the direct impact of mental illness on the lives of caregivers, are seldom recognized. Instead, family members may be viewed as the source of the problem, rather than the solution. Thus, the absence of family participation in care represents a serious and ongoing gap in the provision of evidence-based practices and a lost opportunity to promote recovery and patient-centered care for all affected by illness (Dixon et al., 2010).

Keeping the families and/or the natural support system out of view not only misses an opportunity to help the individual with the illness achieve recovery, but also to address the negative consequences of prolonged caregiving. Family caregivers are at risk for developing primary and behavioral health conditions associated with the burden of providing prolonged caregiving. Throughout the course of the personal and family life cycle, caregiving demands may vary greatly as the individual's need changes. For example, a young woman who is challenged by a first-episode psychosis has needs or wishes for family support that are different from when, later in life, she may be a mother of young children. Consequently, caregiving needs are constantly shifting and are not predictable. The unpredictability and, hence, uncertainty of what may be needed at any given time is stressful and can overshadow family life. In the context of caring for other family members, family caregivers tend to neglect their own health and hide their concerns about their own health problems (Kauffman, Scogin, MacNeil, Leeper, & Wimberly, 2010; Ward-Griffin & McKeever, 2000). Worldwide studies report levels of caregiver burden and negative impacts on well-being as well as psychological and physical health. These studies are similar to those conducted in the United States despite differences in caregiving arrangement and governmental support (Chang, Chiou, & Chen, 2010; Gonçalves-Pereira et al., 2013; Hsiao & Van Riper, 2009; Weiman, Hedelin, Sällström, & Hall-Lord, 2010; ZamZam et al., 2011; Zegwaard, Aartsen, Grypdonck, & Cuijpers, 2013).

In this chapter we first discuss common effects of serious mental illness and the challenges of prolonged caregiving on the natural support system, family, and significant others. By serious mental illness, we mean psychotic disorders such as schizophrenia, schizoaffective disorder, and schizophrenia spectrum disorders. These conditions present challenges that can span a lifetime and, as such, we think of them as chronic conditions. However a chronic condition is not a *life sentence* that necessarily limits a person's opportunities in life. Rather, the notion of recovery in the context of the chronic model of care offers a perspective in which care and support are ongoing and supportive of the individual while life goals are pursued.

After the discussion of the effect of prolonged and chronic mental illness on family caregivers, we review research on family interventions, followed with two case studies that illustrate current family interventions. We acknowledge that mental illness affects both the person with the illness and his or her family and significant others. Thus, interventions should be flexible and adaptive at both the individual and family level to address each family member's challenges and opportunities for growth. Thus, this chapter seeks to demonstrate the importance of the inclusion of family caregivers who can provide support and advocacy for their family member as they journey toward recovery. The chronic care model represents a paradigm shift *from* a chronic disease care model *to* a collaborative and community-based model (Wagner, 1998). Family inclusion, in concert with a person-centered, recovery-based, and wellness focus, benefits not only the person with illness, but also can mediate stress inherent in providing prolonged family caregiving and, as such, provide hope in recovery.

MENTAL ILLNESS IS A FAMILY AFFAIR

When serious mental illness erupts in a family, it can have dire consequences not only for the person who develops a mental illness, but also for the family. Because mental illness is poorly understood and is still surrounded by great mystery, stigma, misunderstanding, and fear, it can have long-standing effects on all family members. Parents, siblings, and grandparents in immediate and extended family situations are greatly affected. Like an earthquake, the effect of mental illness often reverberates throughout the ill person's community of family and friends. With the shock of mental illness, the experience is that of the ground giving way, leaving the person with mental illness and the family shaken and unsettled. Having lost their footing, the psychological consequences can ripple through all areas of life. Mental illness is thus often experienced as a catastrophic and traumatic event producing a rupture in the fabric that interweaves family members' sense of self, family identity, and past and future directions.

For individuals faced with the illness of schizophrenia and schizoaffective disorders, the effect of illness can be pervasive and traumatic, and can interfere with the person's sense of self. Considered a disease of the brain that develops in response to a complex and intertwined set of biological, genetic, and environmental factors, the diagnosis is based on symptoms that may interfere with daily function and activities such as social, occupational, and school functioning (Lukens & Thorning, 2010). According to the *Diagnostic and Statistical Manual of Mental Disorders*, 5th edition (2013), schizophrenia is characterized by so-called positive symptoms of delusions, hallucinations, disorganized speech and behavior, diminished emotional expression and/or avolition also referred to as negative symptoms. For a diagnosis, symptoms must have been present for 6 months and must include at least 1 month of active symptoms.

ILLNESS IS VIEWED IN THE CONTEXT OF THE FAMILY LIFE CYCLE

During the early phases of schizophrenia or schizoaffective disorders that typically start in late adolescence or early adulthood, symptoms can be confused with behavior that is often ascribed to normal adolescent behavior. Hence, parents witness an interruption in their child's development and are uncertain whether their child will revert to "normal" development and developmental milestones. Guilt, rage, and self-blame create suffering in families, and major adjustments are needed within the family to accommodate the ill adolescent or young adult. This is both a similar and a different experience for parents who discover early in their child's life the presence of an irreversible disease or disability. Negative psychological consequences, such as disappointment, fear, and grief, are common reactions to such a trauma for parents in any situation when something goes wrong with their child. Although emotionally close relationships can be disrupted at any time during the life cycle, when a relationship of attachment is disrupted after the emergence of mental illness that renders a loved one forever changed from the hoped-for child or from the known person, recurrent sadness, or chronic sorrow, is a frequently encountered response (Struening et al., 1995; Struening et al., 2001; Teel, 1991; Thorning, 2004).

There is some evidence that grief experienced by parents of disabled or chronically ill children may never fully resolve (Fraley, 1990). The sadness that originates from a child's disability, which can occur at any age, has much to do with the disparity between the person who was known before the onset of illness or the imagined, hoped-for child and who the child has become. When the onset of an illness or disability occurs after relationships have been firmly established and a developmental path set, albeit uncertain for the future, parents face a particular challenge. This is true for serious mental illness as well.

Because serious mental illnesses typically begin during the early part of adult life, parents and siblings may at times be the only consistent sources of social and financial support (Horwitz, 1993; Judge, 1994; Kauffman et al., 2010). Historically, expectation for recovery was focused on stabilization of symptoms associated with illness and provision of formal community support such as day treatment programs; housing and employment was contingent on stabilization. The notion that persons with illness are estranged from their families is a stereotype that predates deinstitutionalization and has little relevance today (Hatfield, 1989; Semple et al., 1997). Moreover, social services alternatives offer little relief, as current housing needs for persons with mental illness grossly exceed availability. For example, this housing crisis is particularly evident in New York State, where for the past 15 years or more an estimated 20,000 additional community beds are needed to meet the needs of persons with mental illness (Stout, 1998). As many as 35% to 75% of persons with mental illness live with their relatives (Bengtsson-Topps & Hansson, 2001; Kauffman et al., 2010), and many more families are actively involved with caregiving even when the person with mental illness resides away from the family.

What seems clear from the accumulated literature on family burden is that living with and caring for a person with mental illness has a tremendous effect on the family (Johnson, 2000; Marsh et al., 1996). Family caregiving poses unique challenges for family caregivers over a lifetime. Caregiving can range from assisting with illness-related activities such as medication adherence and reactions to medication, the monitoring of fluctuations in symptoms (including attention to safety), to activities of daily living such as providing transportation, financial support, and guidance to accessing benefits regardless if the family member lives at home, in congregate housing, or independently. Demands for assistance may intensify with a change in symptoms or any other physical, psychiatric, or psychosocial crisis.

As aging parents or siblings care for a person with mental illness, they may also develop needs for care themselves as they face the adversities of aging. The significant decline in mortality, especially from heart disease, and a consequent shift from acute to chronic disease care management has resulted in an elderly population confronted with the task of negotiating a fragmented health system (Aschbrenner, Greenberg, Allen, & Seltzer, 2010; Biegel & Shultz, 1999; Greenberg, 1995). Thus, the demands associated with caregiving for a person with mental illness over a lifetime can be increasingly stressful as the needs of the aging family caregivers start to parallel those of the ill relative (Cox, 1993). The accumulated stress, disappointment, and lost opportunities experienced by the family caregivers for both themselves and the person with mental illness intensify the experience of grief and burden as family caregivers worry about what will happen when they are no longer able to provide care (Palmer, 1998). The episodic exacerbation of the illness coupled with the subsequent intensification of grief arising at unpredictable intervals during the course of family life therefore have a significant impact on the trajectory of the family's adaptation to living with mental illness and the changes it engenders.

In contrast to the negative outcomes associated with family caregiver burden, personal gains accompanying caregiving can be assessed when expanding the conversation to the experience of positive transformations as a result of being able to cope in the face of adversity. For instance, caring for a loved one with mental illness has led some parents and siblings to experience a deepening sense of self-awareness and inner strength, as well as greater empathy toward others in society (Zauszniewski, Beket, & Suresky, 2010). Parents and sibling caregivers have reported becoming stronger, more tolerant, less judgmental, and more sensitive and empathetic toward others (Lukens & Thorning, 2011; Lukens, Thorning, & Lohrer, 2004). Understanding family caregivers' experiences of hope, mastery, and self-efficacy, and the positive outcome for the person with illness promotes a sense of resiliency (Marsh et al., 1996). Embracing the family's experience of personal growth, and the role of the adult with mental illness in contributing to these gains, has taken on a new significance, with efforts to transform the mental health system care based on recovery principles (Aschbrenner et al., 2010).

DEFINING FAMILY CAREGIVING IN THE CONTEXT OF THE RELATIONSHIP BETWEEN THE CAREGIVER AND THE CARE RECEIVER

Because family caregiving is becoming an expected norm, the terms *caregiver* and *caregiving* have become part of everyday speech. Yet, few clear definitions that explicate the boundaries of these concepts exist (Lohrer, 2001; Lohrer, Lukens, & Thorning, 2006). Although providing support and assistance to family members is a normal part of family expectations and functioning, family caregiving can be understood as a situation that "represents an increment of extraordinary care that goes beyond the boundaries of normal or usual care" (Song, Biegel, & Miligan, 1997, p. 17). In the context of serious mental illness, caregiving most often refers to the relationship between two adult individuals who are typically related through kinship. One (the caregiver) assumes an unpaid and unanticipated responsibility for another (the person being cared for) whose mental health problems are prolonged, and recovery is a process of discovering new strengths. The person with mental illness may at times have difficulties fulfilling the reciprocal obligations associated with normative adult relationships, and the mental health problems are serious enough to require substantial amounts of care. What makes it burdensome is the addition of the caregiving role to the already existing family responsibilities, such as work, community involvement, and attending to other family members (Schene, Tessler, & Gamache, 1994).

Although there has been an increase in attention to families' experience of caregiving for a mentally ill relative, a major gap exists in the understanding of caregiving as an *interactional dynamic process* between the caregiver and the person being cared for. In David Karp's book *The Burden of Sympathy: How*

Families Cope with Mental Illness (2001), the author explores the personal, moral, and cultural dimensions inherent in the sense of obligation and duty reported by family members when taking on the caregiving role. His qualitative study consisted of in-depth interviews with family caregivers and found evidence for the notion that caregiving is not a singular role implying a consistency and uniformity of experience, but rather the caregiver's phenomenology shifts as clarity about the character of mental illness emerges over time. Consequently, Karp (2001) found evidence for the notion that caregiving is a "dialectical, processual, and emergent relationship between the sufferers of any illness and those who care for them" (p. 69). From this perspective, he suggests the moral boundaries of caregiving are constantly "under construction" and influenced by the meanings attributed to this interaction by both the caregiver and the person with the illness (Karp, 2001, p. 69). Thus, the caregiving dynamic is affected by the specific nature of the relationship between the caregiver and the ill person (Guberman, Maheu, & Maillé, 1992; Smith, Tobin, & Fullmer, 1995) as well as by the meaning caregiving holds for both the caregiver and the person receiving care. Increasing our understanding of this dialectic, and the meaning ascribed to caregiving and receiving, is critical for planning and delivering optimal services across cultures.

MUTUALITY AND RECIPROCITY BETWEEN THE FAMILY CAREGIVER AND THE PERSON RECEIVING CARE

In the general population, studies show that reciprocity is a critical factor in determining the amount and type of exchange among family members (Horwitz, Reinhard, & Howell-White, 1996). Reciprocity refers to a mutual exchange between two people that is experienced as beneficial to both partners—that is, it describes the normative obligations of a help-recipient to assist people who have provided help to him or her (Gouldner, 1960; Horwitz et al., 1996). In general, caregiving has been viewed as an unidirectional provision of support and assistance for the ill person, although more recent studies have sought to examine the effects of mutual support on the caregiving dynamic (Aschbrenner et al., 2010; Greenberg, 1995; Greenberg, Greenley, & Benedict, 1994; Horwitz, 1993; Horwitz et al., 1996; Kramer, 1997; Reinhard & Horwitz, 1995).

Common to the findings among these studies is that the burden of caregiving is reduced significantly when the family caregiver reports having a relationship that is recipical in nature. Furthermore, positive outcomes for the family caregiver were identified when reciprocity and mutuality were promoted in the interventions (Kramer, 1997; Zauszniewski et al., 2010). The ability to adjust and adapt to new responsibilities and expectations when a family member has mental health concerns, can result in caregivers reporting enhanced feelings of pride, self-worth, meaning, warmth, and pleasure in their ability to meet challenges (Kramer, 1997).

The family caregiver's evaluation of his or her relational and attitudinal ties to the person with serious and prolonged mental illness depends on what meaning the family caregiver bestows on the family member with illness and the overall caregiving experience. In this regard, all human experience is an ongoing exercise in sense-making (Karp, 2001). If addressed from a point of opportunity for growth, caregiving can increase feelings of resilience, improve the caregivers' sense of self-worth, enhance coping effectiveness, and provide caregivers with a greater sense of purpose and self-efficacy (Zauszniewski et al., 2010).

Family Interventions for Family Caregivers of Adults with Serious Mental Illness: Recommendations and Evidence

In 1992, The Agency for Health Care Policy and Research and the National Institute for Mental Health funded the Schizophrenia Patient Outcome Research Team (PORT) to review the scientific evidence and to develop and disseminate recommendations for the treatment of serious mental illness—in particular, schizophrenia (Lehman & Steinwachs, 1998). Twenty-nine recommendations were offered based on extensive reviews of outcome literature and addressed medication, adjunctive pharmacotherapies, electroconvulsive therapy, psychological intervention, vocational rehabilitation, assertive community treatment, and family interventions. Family interventions in particular were highlighted as pivotal to positive patient outcomes, but were inadequately provided across the United States. The PORT report provided two updates of these recommendations, and each included family psychoeducation as a recommended practice. We present the most recent PORT recommendation, which is a synthesis of the available evidence, followed by a summary of the studies contributing to the recommendation (Dixon et al., 2010). Table 7.1 presents an evidence table of family interventions discussed in the following section.

PORT 2009 Recommendations for Family Interventions

Recommendation: Persons with schizophrenia who have ongoing contact with their families, including relatives and significant others, should be offered a family intervention that lasts at least 6 to 9 months. Interventions that last 6 to 9 months have been found to reduce rates of relapse and rehospitalization significantly. Although not as consistently observed, research has found other benefits for patients and families, such as increased medication adherence, reduced psychiatric symptoms, and reduced levels of perceived stress for patients. Family members have also been found to have lower levels of burden and distress, and improved family relationships. Key elements of effective family interventions include illness education, crisis intervention, emotional support, and training in how to cope with illness symptoms and related problems. Family interventions are typically conducted by mental health professionals such as social workers, psychiatrists, and psychiatric nurses. The interventions most often take place in community settings. The selection of a family

Table 7.1. Intervention Studies for Family Caregivers of Patients with Severe Mental Illness

Author (Year)	Design/Sampling	Subject Characteristics (cultural factors, diversity)	Methods/ Intervention	Data/Measures Used	Findings/Outcomes	Limitations
Rotondi et al., 2010	Random assignment to either online intervention treatment or "usual care" control group; recruitment through community mental health facilities and inpatient units	31 patients with schizophrenia and 24 support persons; random assignment to telehealth (online intervention) or treatment as usual; in schizophrenia group, 10 males and 21 females with an average age of 38 years, 48% white; in support persons group, 9 males and 15 females with an average age of 50 years, 46% white	Year-long intervention period, assessment of SOAR website use by schizophrenic patients and support persons, interviewer-administered assessments at 3, 6, and 12 months	Intention-to-treat analyses were used to compare severity of positive conditions and knowledge of schizophrenia in both study groups.	Significant reduction in positive symptoms ($p = .042$, $d = -.88$), significant increase in knowledge about prognosis ($p = .036$, $d = 1.94$)	Omission of discussion of limiting effects of low computer literacy
Lucksted et al., 2013	Randomized assignment to intervention and control groups; sample obtained through family members' expressions of interest in FTF, followed by individual screening for eligibility	318 family members or close friends of persons with SMI between the ages of 21 years and 80 years, 38 men and 120 women randomized to FTF, 64% white	FTF, a peer-run, community-based, education and support program conducted over 12 weekly sessions; study analyses with 6-month follow-up data on a NAMI-funded assessment on measures of distress, family functioning, coping and empowerment; control group (not assessed at 6 months)	Multilevel regression model to test for significant changes, Brief Symptom Inventory-18 to assess psychological distress in nonclinical settings, CES-D, Family Assessment Device, Family Problem-Solving Communication Scale, Family Empowerment Scale, COPE acceptance scale, Family Experience Interview Survey to assess subjective burden	At least 6-month reduction in family member distress and improvements in family problem-solving in family members of adults with mental illnesses	Control group not assessed at 6 months; 26% of individuals randomized to FTF were lost by the 9-month follow-up. No strict uniformity in participants' relationships to person with SMI (combination of immediate and removed family members, and friends).

(continued)

Table 7.1. CONTINUED

Author (Year)	Design/Sampling	Subject Characteristics (cultural factors, diversity)	Methods/Intervention	Data/Measures Used	Findings/Outcomes	Limitations
Perlick et al., 2010	Caregivers with demonstrated physical and mental health problems were recruited from three outpatient New York hospitals, random assignment to one of two study groups	Primary family caregivers of 43 patients with bipolar I or II disorder; 36 females and 7 males; among 40 patients with bipolar disorder, 25 females and 15 males	Two study groups: FFT-HPI, a cognitive–behavioral intervention, over 12 to 15 sessions; or 8 to 12 sessions of health education intervention delivered via videotapes, using a didactic approach	Double-blind treatment assignment by research assistants, Mini International Neuropsychiatric Interview used to evaluate caregivers' lifetime diagnosis, CES-D, Quick Inventory of Depressive Symptomatology, Hamilton Rating Scale for Depression, Young Mania Rating Scale, Structured Clinical Interview for DSM-IV Axis I disorders; health risks behavior assessment, adapted Ways of Coping Questionnaire	Decreases in caregivers' depression in FFT-HPI group and significant reductions in subjective burden, bipolar patients of caregivers in FFT-HPI group showed decreases in depression and mania	FFT-HPI group received nearly twice as many sessions as the health education control group; therefore, caregivers' improvements in the FFT-HPI group could also be attributed to frequency in dosage. Lack of ethnic and socioeconomic diversity; limited sample size
Perlick et al., 2011	Recruitment from urban mental health center and a family and consumer advocacy organization. selection of caregivers depended on at least a moderate level of perceived mental illness-related stigma (self-report), random assignment to one of two group interventions after being evaluated for self-stigma	122 caregivers of persons with schizophrenia; caregivers more than 18 years of age; in caregiver assessment, 90 females and 32 males, 83% white; in consumer assessment, 36 females and 86 males, 81% white	IOOV-FC, a peer-led intervention consisting of a 15-minute video followed by a 60-minute group discussion versus a clinician-based intervention consisting of a 75-minute educational video (both interventions were conducted in one session and were aimed at lessening self-stigma in caregivers)	Devaluation of Consumer Families Scale	Significant reduction in self-stigma in caregivers in the IOOV-FC group whose pretreatment self-stigma assessments were low to moderate, less of a reduction was observed in caregivers in the IOOV-FC with high self-stigma	Lack of ethnic diversity
Kaufman et al., 2010	Aging parental caregivers of adult children with schizophrenia	Five aging caregivers in intervention group, 10 aging caregivers in control group	Home-delivered, multidimensional problem-solving intervention	Mini-Mental State Examination, Zarit Burden Interview, Family Burden Interview Schedule–Short Form, QOLI, SCL-90-R	Positive effect on emotional well-being, life satisfaction, and feelings of caregiver burden	Very small sample size, issues with recruitment for study

Hazel et al., 2004	Consumers with schizophrenia or other psychotic disorders and their family caregivers recruited from large community mental health centers, random assignment to one of two study groups	Two study groups over 2 years: standard psychiatric care or, in addition to standard psychiatric care, multiple-family group treatment, consisting of six to eight families and two clinicians using the multiple-family group treatment manual from (Dyck et al., 2002), with bimonthly meetings during the first year, and monthly meetings the second year, each lasting 90 minutes	14-Item Perceived Stress Scale used to assess caregiver distress, 40-item Interpersonal Support Evaluation List, and the Social Support Questionnaire were used to assess caregiver resources; and Structured Clinical Interview for DSM-IV, Psychotic Disorders version, the BPRS, and mSANS were used to assess consumer clinical status	Controlling for clinical status and baseline caregiver distress and resources, multiple-family group treatment reduced caregiver distress, but did not increase caregivers' resources compared with standard psychiatric care.	Lack of ethnic diversity, lack of age diversity, lack of representation of nonparent caregivers, baseline resources of intervention group was higher than standard group, limited sample size resulting from attrition
	97 consumers with schizophrenia or other psychotic disorder, 74 male, 21 female, 88% white; caregivers, 16 male, 87 female, 87% white; caregivers primarily mothers with mean age of 51.3 years				
Dyck et al., 2002	Outpatients with schizophrenia or schizoaffective disorder and all their available family members, random assignment to one of two study groups, recruited from a large community mental health clinic	Two study groups over 2 years: standard psychiatric care or, in addition to standard psychiatric care, multiple-family system group treatment, consisting of weekly group sessions run by two clinicians using a standardized protocol	Intention-to-treat analyses were used to compare outpatient services and inpatient services for 1 year after random assignment date. The Structured Clinical Interview for DSM-IV, the BPRS, and mSANS were used to assess patient diagnosis.	Multiple-family group treatment associated with lower rate of psychiatric hospitalizations than standard care during the year after random assignment date. Marginally associated with lowered crisis services usage; not associated with outpatient service time.	No discussion of demographics of participants. Only the first year of the study is reported, because it was ongoing at the time of publication. Other interventions, such as criminal justice system involvement or chemical dependence, are not considered in the outcomes. Intensity and expectations of studied interventions are not considered in outcomes.
	106 outpatients; 82 male, 24 female; mean age, 32.7 years				

(continued)

Table 7.1. Continued

Author (Year)	Design/Sampling	Subject Characteristics (cultural factors, diversity)	Methods/Intervention	Data/Measures Used	Findings/Outcomes	Limitations
Bradley et al., 2006	People diagnosed with schizophrenia, and their caregivers, recruited from a community mental health program, outpatient continuing care setting	Study conducted in Australia; 59 consumers, 35 female, 15 male, and their caregivers; 34 pairs English-speaking; two of these caregivers were born overseas, had been in Australia for more than 25 years and were proficient in English, 25 pairs Vietnamese speaking, all born in Vietnam and arrived in Australia between 1978 and 1985	Multiple-family system group treatment along with standard case management, 26 sessions over 12 months, compared with standard case management care	Assessments conducted with the Brief Psychotic Rating Scale, Scale for the Assessment of Negative Symptoms, the Health of the Nation Outcome Scale, and the Quality of Life Scale. Caregiver burden measured with the Family Burden Scale. Outcomes measured immediately after intervention, and again after 18 months. Blind treatment conducted by an experienced clinical psychologist and an experienced Vietnamese psychiatric–disability worker who is also qualified as an interpreter and translator.	Multiple-family group treatment extended time to relapse, treatment effects increase over time	Formal measure of acculturation not used, small sample size, full range of dependent measures not collected at follow-up because of funding constraints, lack of assessment of treatment fidelity

| Ran et al., 2003 | People diagnosed with schizophrenia and their caregivers, cluster randomized control trial | Study conducted in rural China (Xining County, Chengdu), in six townships; 326 consumers, 128 male, 198 female; 326 caregivers, 194 male, 132 female; most patients and caregivers had a low socioeconomic status | Three study groups over 9 months: family intervention and medication, medication alone, or control, where medication was neither encouraged nor discouraged; family intervention was modified to take into account the characteristics of Chinese rural areas, such as dispersed residences and a generally low level of education; family intervention conducted once per month and lasted 1.5 to 3 hours each visit; multiple family workshops held once every 3 months; family interventions conducted by trained psychiatrists and village doctors who assisted with the interventions | PSE-9 (Chinese translation) to assess relapse rate, General Psychiatric Interview Schedule and Summary Form, SDSS to assess mental disability, Relatives' Investigation Scale and Relatives' Beliefs Scale to determine relatives' characteristics and beliefs about mental illness, Schizophrenia diagnosed according to ICD-10 and CCMD-2-R, data recorded at baseline and at 9-month treatment phases by 15 independent researchers; rater training sessions held before each measurement to ensure interrater reliability | Psychoeducational family intervention improved the level of relatives' recognition of mental illness and enhanced treatment compliance, and the results demonstrated a positive change in relatives' caring attitudes toward the patient. The relapse rate for the family intervention group was half that of the drug-only group and just more than one quarter of that of the control group. Antipsychotic drug treatment and families' attitudes toward patients were associated significantly with clinical outcome. | Variation in duration of family intervention sessions; randomization done by township, not individual participant; lack of discussion regarding culture/ethnicity |

(continued)

Table 7.1. CONTINUED

Author (Year)	Design/Sampling	Subject Characteristics (cultural factors, diversity)	Methods/Intervention	Data/Measures Used	Findings/Outcomes	Limitations
Zhang et al., 1993	People diagnosed with schizophrenia, discharged from hospital and living in the community with their relatives; recruited from mental health centers; random cluster sampling method	Study conducted in the Chinese cities of Jinan, Hangzhou, Shengyang, Suzhou, and Shanghai; 3,092 consumers, 1,821 males, 1,261 females; majority, blue-collar families, single, and 6–12 education years; 3,092 caregivers, 1,323 male, 1,769 female	Two study groups over 1 year: family psychoeducation in addition to routine community mental health services and routine community mental health services alone. Psychoeducation consisted of 10 lectures and three discussions drafted by mental health workers at Shanghai Mental Health Center and delivered by psychiatrists to relatives.	Schizophrenia diagnosed according to CCMD-2; outcome measures: Family Burden Interview Schedule to assess the burden patient constituted for the family; DAS to assess social dysfunction of the patient; a patient questionnaire to assess sociodemographic, clinical, and historical information; a relatives' questionnaire to assess sociodemographic information, level of education, and knowledge of schizophrenia; data recorded at enrollment, 6 months, and 12 months	Family psychoeducation showed a greater rate of recovery or stabilization of condition; a greater reduction in exacerbation of symptoms, relapse rate, number institutionalized, duration of hospitalization, total score and factor score on DAS, and sick leave days; and an increase in proportion able to return to work and in the number seeking medical consultation and treatment compliance. Family psychoeducation decreased family burden of care significantly and also increased knowledge of schizophrenia.	Significant difference in the duration of present episode of schizophrenia between the two groups. Caregivers of patients in intervention group seemed more likely to be white collar and have a higher level of education. Randomization done by catchment area, not individual participant. Lack of discussion regarding culture/ethnicity.

| Pickett-Schenk et al., 2006 | Relatives of individuals with mental illness (schizophrenia, schizoaffective disorder, bipolar disorder, depression, and obsessive–compulsive disorder); recruited through media announcements, flyers at community agencies/buildings, and mental health referrals; random assignment to one of two study groups; randomization occurred within site and cohort | Study conducted at three sites in Louisiana: Baton Rouge, Lafayette, and New Orleans; broad definition of "family member" used to encompass parents, spouses, siblings, adult children, grandparents, and friends; 462 participants, 90 male, 372 female; 85% white, 11% black; 55% parent caregivers | Two study groups over 8 months: family-led education program called JOH, or control group consisting of patients assigned to a course waiting list; JOH an 8-week, manualized education course, meeting once a week for 1.5 to 2 hours; instructors trained volunteers who themselves have a relative with mental illness; treatment fidelity assessed after each class taught; attendance taken for each class; data collected at baseline (1 month before course start), at course completion, and 6 months after course completion | Participant interviews for demographic and relatives' psychiatric characteristics; Caregiving Satisfaction Scale; two subscales from the Family Information Needs scale, the Problem Management subscale and Social Functioning subscale demographic and psychiatric illness characteristics | The JOH group showed significant improvement in caregiving satisfaction and information needs; gains maintained for another 6 months | Lack of gender diversity, lack of ethnic diversity. Unlike Lafayette and New Orleans sites, the Baton Rouge site had multiple instructors. Improvements were somewhat modest. Caregiver level of motivation and use of outside resources were not assessed/ There was a lack of long-term follow-up assessment. |

(continued)

Table 7.1. Continued

Author (Year)	Design/Sampling	Subject Characteristics (cultural factors, diversity)	Methods/Intervention	Data/Measures Used	Findings/Outcomes	Limitations
Pickett-Schenk, Cook, et al., 2006	Relatives of individuals with mental illness (schizophrenia, schizoaffective disorder, bipolar disorder, depression, and obsessive–compulsive disorder); recruited through media announcements, flyers at community agencies/buildings, and mental health referrals; random assignment to one of two study groups; randomization occurred within site and cohort	Study conducted at three sites in Louisiana: Baton Rouge, Lafayette, and New Orleans; broad definition of "family member" used to encompass parents, spouses, siblings, adult children, grandparents, and friends; 462 participants, 90 male, 372 female; 85% white, 11% black; 55% parent caregivers	Two study groups over 8 months: family-led education program called JOH, or control group consisting of patients assigned to a course waiting list; JOH an 8-week, manualized education course, meeting once a week for 1.5 to 2 hours; instructors trained volunteers who themselves have a relative with mental illness; treatment fidelity assessed after each class taught; attendance taken for each class; data collected at baseline (1 month before course start), at course completion, and 6 months after course completion	Participant interviews for demographic and relatives' psychiatric characteristics; CES-D and depression subscale of the Brief Symptom Inventory to assess participant level of depression; medical and social functioning subscales of the Medical Outcomes Study 36-Item Short-Form Health Survey to assess participant overall mental health, social relationships, energy and activity, and role limitations resulting from emotional problems; negative relationship subscale from the You and Your Family Scale to assess participants' rating of their relationships' with their ill relatives	JOH participants reported fewer depressive symptoms, greater emotional role functioning and vitality, and fewer negative views of their relationships with their ill relatives; outcomes maintained at 6 months post-JOH completion	Lack of gender diversity, ethnic diversity, long-term follow-up assessment, and formal assessment of change in relationship. Use of outside resources not assessed.

Pickett-Schenk et al., 2008	Relatives of individuals with mental illness (schizophrenia, schizoaffective disorder, bipolar disorder, depression, and obsessive–compulsive disorder); recruited through media announcements, flyers at community agencies/buildings, and mental health referrals; random assignment to one of two study groups; randomization occurred within site and cohort	Study conducted at three sites in Louisiana: Baton Rouge, Lafayette, and New Orleans; broad definition of "family member" used to encompass parents, spouses, siblings, adult children, grandparents, and friends; 462 participants, 90 male, 372 female; 85% white, 11% black; 55% parent caregivers	Two study groups over 8 months: family led education program called JOH, or control group consisting of patients assigned to a course waiting list; JOH an 8-week, manualized education course, meeting once a week for 1.5 to 2 hours; instructors trained volunteers who themselves have a relative with mental illness; treatment fidelity assessed after each class taught; attendance taken for each class; data collected at baseline (1 month before course start), at course completion, and 6 months after course completion	Family Knowledge scale, consisting of 40 multiple-choice items to assess knowledge regarding topics covered in the JOH course and knowledge of problem-solving skills; Family Information Needs scale, assessing interest in learning about 45 specific topics regarding mental health treatment and care	JOH participants reported greater knowledge gains and fewer needs for information on coping with positive and negative symptoms, problem management, basic facts about mental illness and treatment, and community resources at course end, and the 6-month follow-up.	Lack of gender diversity, ethnic diversity, and long-term follow-up assessment. Use of outside resources and caregiver level of motivation not assessed.

(continued)

Table 7.1. CONTINUED

Author (Year)	Design/Sampling	Subject Characteristics (cultural factors, diversity)	Methods/Intervention	Data/Measures Used	Findings/Outcomes	Limitations
Solomon et al., 1996	Relatives of individuals with serious mental illness; random assignment to one of three groups; recruited through support groups, hospital social service departments, information programs for family members of psychiatric patients, and media outreach	Study conducted in large East Coast city; 225 family members; 188 female, 37 male; 84% white; mean age, 55.7 years, 76.4% parent caregivers	Three study groups, with study ongoing at time of publication: individualized consultation consisting of at least 6 hours and no more than 15 hours of educational assistance over 3 months, group psychoeducation consisting of weekly 2-hour sessions over 10 weeks, or control group consisting of a 9-month wait list; both interventions administered by the Training and Education Center Network; data collected at baseline and at 3 months	Participant interviews for demographics, relative's psychiatric illness history, and personal history with ill relative; adaptation of interview developed by Pai and Kapur (1981) used to assess burden; Norbeck Social Support Questionnaire used to assess social support; Scherer et al.'s (1982) self-efficacy scale; Texas Inventory of Grief; stress assessed through Greene et al.'s (1982) scale; self-efficacy scale for coping skills; satisfaction with the two psychoeducation interventions assessed with a nine- question inventory	Group psychoeducation was helpful in increasing self-efficacy of family members who had never participated in a support or advocacy group for mentally ill relatives.	Lack of gender diversity, ethnic diversity, and long-term follow-up assessment.
Xiang et al., 1994	Individuals with schizophrenia and affective psychoses; random assignment into one of two study groups	Study conducted in rural China, three townships in Xinjin County, Sichuan Province; 77 patients	Two study groups: drug treatment plus psychoeducational family intervention, or drug treatment only	Drug treatment compliance, understanding of and changing attitude toward mental illness, adaptation of an appropriate method of caring for the patient, effectiveness of clinical treatment, improvement of the patients' working ability, rate of social disturbance assessed through medical records, PSE, and SDSS	Psychoeducational family intervention improved treatment compliance, increased family recognition of mental disorders, and decreased insufficient care and maltreatment by family members.	Lack of discussion of culture/ethnicity. Caregiver motivation was not assessed. Lack of discussion regarding method of psychoeducational family intervention. Wide variation in illness duration.

Study	Sample	Location/Demographics	Study design	Measures	Results	Limitations
Spiegel & Wissler, 1987	Families of schizophrenic patients from a Veterans Affairs hospital, patients lived with family	Study conducted in Palo Alto, California; 36 patients; mean age, 36.7 years	Two study groups: periodic consultation in home from members of clinical team, or no periodic home consultation; data collection at baseline, 3 months, and 1 year after discharge from hospital	Vets Adjustment Scale, Personal Adjustment Scale, Family Environment Scale	At 3-month follow-up, periodic consultation in home decreased number of days spent in hospital. Difference not significant at 1-year follow-up. Families rated selves higher on the Vets Adjustment scale at both the 3-month and 1-year follow-ups.	Lack of discussion regarding gender and lack of discussion regarding culture/ethnicity. No assessment of use of outside resources by control group. Vets Adjustment Scale is self-report; small sample.
Merinder et al., 1999	Individuals with schizophrenia and their family; block randomized, stratified for gender and illness duration, into one of two groups; recruited from community psychiatric centers	Study conducted in Denmark; 46 patients, 24 male, 22 female; median age, 35.9 years	Two study groups: eight-session family psychoeducation program, or usual treatment	Schizophrenia diagnosed according to ICD-10, Danish version; OPCRIT 3.31 used to validate clinical diagnosis; BPRS; GAF; Insight Scale; Versona Service Satisfaction Scale; knowledge of schizophrenia	Increase of knowledge of schizophrenia in both patients and relatives at 3 months; nonsignificant trend at 1 year. Changes in satisfaction with relatives involvement for both patient and relatives.	Lack of discussion of culture/ethnicity. Unclear whether intervention group received usual treatment along with intervention; small sample.
Pitschel-Walz et al., 2006	Individuals with schizophrenia or schizoaffective disorder who had regular contact with at least one relative, block randomization into one of two study groups, recruited from three psychiatric hospitals	Study conducted in Germany; 236 patients, 54% female	Two study groups: encouragement to attend eight session-length psychoeducational groups over 4 to 5 months in addition to routine care, or routine care; psychoeducation group for patients and one for relatives; data collected at baseline, at discharge, and at 6, 12, 18, and 24 months; interventionists were nine psychiatrists and one clinical psychologist, all trained in psychoeducation	Diagnosed according to DSM-III-R/ICD-9, compliance assessed by treating psychiatrist and plasma drug level measurements, BPRS, GAF	Increased compliance in patient intervention group; reduced hospitalization rate in patient intervention group	Attrition at follow-up; no discussion of culture/ethnicity

(continued)

Table 7.1. CONTINUED

Author (Year)	Design/Sampling	Subject Characteristics (cultural factors, diversity)	Methods/Intervention	Data/Measures Used	Findings/Outcomes	Limitations
Cuijpers, 1999	Studies of family interventions that have positive effect on the burden of relatives of psychiatric patients	16 studies	Meta-analysis; to be included, study had to investigate effects of an intervention for relatives of psychiatric patients, use one or more outcome measures, and report pretest and posttest data	Meta-analysis of mean effect size on improvement from pretest to posttest, of mean effect size at posttest, of mean effect size at follow-up	Interventions with more than 12 sessions have larger effects than shorter interventions.	Limited number of studies
Posner et al., 1992	Family members of patients with schizophrenia, random assignment to one of two study groups, recruited by referrals from psychiatrists in four hospitals	Study conducted in Winnipeg, Canada; 55 patients, 39 male, 16 female; mean age, 29 years; 55 family members, 28 mothers, 11 fathers, 7 spouses, 8 siblings, and 1 in-law	Two study groups: psycho-educational support group with ongoing treatment, or ongoing treatment alone; psychoeducational support groups only for family members, both target family member and other family members; eight group sessions lasting 90 minutes led by two experienced therapists and supplemented by other professionals; data collected at pretest, posttest, and 6-month follow-up	Diagnosis confirmed with DSM-III-R as well as with referring psychiatrists and other available clinical personnel, Schizophrenia Knowledge Test, Consumer Satisfaction Questionnaire, Family Satisfaction Scale, Ways of Coping, Negative feelings for patient, General Health Questionnaire, hospital records used to assess rate of relapse and rehospitalization	Support group participants showed greater knowledge of schizophrenia and greater satisfactions with healthcare services	Complete data available for 39 of the 55 family members. Measures are self-reported. no discussion of culture/ ethnicity; small sample resulting from attrition

Pilling et al., 2002	Studies of social skills training and cognitive remediation for the treatment of negative symptoms of schizophrenia	13 studies total; 9 social skills trainings, 4 cognitive remediation trainings	Meta-analysis; randomized control trials that met strict criteria: for skills training, treatment was structured psychosocial intervention intended to enhance social performance and reduce distress and difficulty in social situations, behaviorally based assessments of social and interpersonal skills; for cognitive remediation, program focused on improving cognitive function using a procedure implemented with the intention of bringing about an improvement in the level of that specified cognitive function	Intention-to-treat analyses performed on all data; analysis of social skills training on relapse, treatment compliance, global adjustment, social functioning, and quality of life; analysis of cognitive remediation on attention, verbal memory, visual memory, mental state, and executive functioning	No reliable evidence that social skills training affects relapse rate, global adjustment, social functioning, quality of life, or treatment compliance, or that cognitive remediation provides benefit to attention, verbal memory, visual memory, planning, cognitive flexibility, or mental state.	Limited number of studies
Sellwood et al., 2007	Patients diagnosed with schizophrenia, schizoaffective disorder, or delusional disorder	60 patients; had participated in a randomized controlled effectiveness trial 5 years earlier	Case notes of patients examined to determine relapse rates over a 5-year period; patients had received a 24-week, needs-based cognitive-behavior-oriented family intervention along with routine care, or routine care alone	Standardized pro forma used to identify two types of relapse	Patients less likely to have relapsed if received needs-based family intervention.	Clinical practice changed during period of study, resulting in additional psychosocial services in routine care as well as fewer admission beds; attrition rate; trial therapist involved in data collection; not possible to interview and reassess participants at follow-up

(continued)

Table 7.1. CONTINUED

Author (Year)	Design/Sampling	Subject Characteristics (cultural factors, diversity)	Methods/Intervention	Data/Measures Used	Findings/Outcomes	Limitations
Tarrier et al., 1989	Patients diagnosed with schizophrenia and their families	71 patients; 2 years prior had participated in a controlled trial of a 9-month behavioral family intervention based on the expressed emotions status of patient	Admission records and case notes of patients examined to determine relapse rates over a 2-year period; original study consisted of six treatment groups, but were condensed to three for this follow-up: one behavioral intervention group (enactive and symbolic groups combined), one high-EE control group (patients either received short education with routine care, or routine care alone), and one low-EE group	Chi-square analyses	Patients from behavioral family intervention group had lower rates of relapse than patients from high-EE homes who received short educational program or routine care; relapse rate of behavioral family intervention group same as low-EE group, and lower than nonintervention high-EE group	Readmission rates used for relapse rates; not possible to reassess EE at follow-up
Xiong et al., 1994	Patients with schizophrenia living with family members, recruited from psychiatric hospital at admission, random assignment to one of two study groups	Study conducted at Shashi Psychiatric Hospital in China; patients from cities Shashi Jingzhou; 63 patients, 43 male, 20 female; mean age, 31 years	Two study groups: standard care, or family-based intervention consisting of monthly 45-minute counseling sessions; data collected at baseline and at 6, 12, and 18 months of follow-up	Diagnosis according to DSM-III-R; Scale for Assessment of Negative Symptoms, Chinese version; BPRS, Chinese version; GAF; Social Disability Assessment Schedule	Intervention group showed lower rate of rehospitalization, lower duration of rehospitalization, and longer duration of employment. Lower levels of burden associated with family intervention.	Small sample; treatment limited to Chinese culture

| Barrowclough et al., 1999 | Outpatients with schizophrenia and their family; random assignment to one of two study groups | Study conducted in England; 77 patient–caregiver pairs; of patients, 50 male, 27 female; majority white | Two study groups over 24 weeks: family support alone, or along with systematic psychosocial interventions based on assessment of need; data collected at pretest and posttest by psychology graduate research assistants | Need assessed by relatives' version of the Cardinal Needs Schedule, Positive and Negative Syndrome Scale, Social Functioning Scale, Global Assessment Scale, Beck Depression Inventory, Social Behavior Assessment Schedule (Section D only), expressed emotion assessed using 5-minute speech samples, medication compliance assessed from patient interviews, frequency and duration of relapse assessed through hospital record systems and case notes | Intervention group showed lowered relapse rates. | Lack of discussion of gender and ethnicity/culture of caregivers, reliance on hospital records for relapse rates, using patient report for medication compliance, lack of cultural diversity |

NOTE: BPRS, Brief Psychiatric Rating Scale; CCMD-2-R, Chinese Classification and Diagnostic Criteria of Mental Disorder; CES-D, Center for Epidemiological Studies–Depression scale; DAS, Psychiatric Disability Assessment Scale; DSM-IV, *Diagnostic and Statistical Manual of Mental Disorders*, 4th edition; EE, Expressed Emotions; FFT-HPI, Family-Focused Treatment–Health Promoting Intervention; FTF, family-to-family; GAF, Global Assessment of Functioning; ICD, International Classification of Diseases; IOOV-FC, In Our Own Voice–Family Companion; JOH, Journey of Hope; mSANS, modified Scale for the Assessment of Negative Symptoms; PSE, Present State Examination; SDSS, Social Disability Screening Schedule; SMI, serious mental illness.

intervention should be guided by collaborative decision making among the patient, family, and clinician. In addition, a family intervention that is shorter than 6 months, but is at least four sessions in length, should be offered to persons with schizophrenia who have ongoing contact with their families, including relatives and significant others, and for whom a longer intervention is not feasible or acceptable. Characteristics of the briefer interventions include education, training, and support. Possible benefits for patients include reduced psychiatric symptoms, improved treatment adherence, improved functional and vocational status, and greater satisfaction with treatment. Positive family outcomes include reduced family burden and increased satisfaction with family relationships.

2009 PORT Study Report of Evidence

Research demonstrating the effectiveness of family psychoeducation for individuals with schizophrenia dates back to the late 1970s and 1980s, and was reflected in the first set of PORT recommendations (Lehman & Steinwachs, 1998). Family intervention is grounded in psychoeducation, which is the synergy of educational and therapeutic theory, and a process that seeks to address the previously mentioned areas by increasing awareness of risk and preventive factors, building on formal and natural supports, and enhancing resiliency among all family members (Lukens & Thorning, 2010; Lukens, Thorning, & Herman, 1999). Psychoeducation most often is delivered in a group format. Mental health professionals impart up-to-date information about serious mental illness and how it may affect individuals and families, including providing information about diagnosis, medication, wellness management, crisis management though anticipatory planning, stigma busting, care coordination, community resources, and steps toward community integration. Participants contribute with their knowledge from living with serious mental illness. The core element of the intervention includes building a community of support within and among families, enhancing communication and problem-solving skills, encouraging advocacy and involvement in self-help, and instilling hope toward recovery (Lukens & Thorning, 2010).

Most investigations focused on family psychoeducation interventions that were 6 months or longer and included individuals who had a recent illness exacerbation. The studies demonstrated lower rates of relapse and rehospitalization among individuals receiving family psychoeducation relative to those in the control condition (de Jesus Mari & Streiner, 1994; Lenior, Dingemans, Linszen, de Haan, & Schene, 2001; Sellwood et al., 2001; Sellwood, Wittkowski, Tarrier, & Barrowclough, 2007; Tarrier et al., 1989; Xiong et al., 1994). Meta-analyses support the conclusion that a longer family intervention (i.e., an intervention lasting 6–9 months or longer) is necessary to reduce rates of relapse and rehospitalization significantly relative to a control condition (Falloon, Boyd, & McGill, 1985; Kurtz & Mueser, 2008; Pilling et al., 2002; Pitschel-Walz et al., 2001; Zhang,

Wang, Li, & Phillips, 1994). Family psychoeducation interventions that are 6 months or longer have also been shown to contribute to other positive patient and family outcomes among individuals who have had a recent illness exacerbation. Specifically, individuals who received family psychoeducation reported improved treatment adherence (Mueser et al., 2001), lower levels of perceived stress (Dyck, Short, & Hendryx, 2000), and better vocational outcome (Zhang et al., 1994) relative to individuals in the control condition. In terms of family member outcomes, family members of individuals who received family psychoeducation reported lower levels of burden and distress (Sellwood et al., 2007; Zhang et al., 1994) and improved family relationships (Dyck et al., 2000) relative to family members in the control condition.

As the effectiveness of family psychoeducation was established, more recent studies began to include patients who did not have a recent illness exacerbation. One set of studies includes only individuals without a recent exacerbation; a second set includes both individuals with a recent exacerbation and those without a recent exacerbation. Valencia and colleagues compared psychosocial skills training combined with family therapy with treatment as usual (TAU) among individuals without a recent illness exacerbation and found a reduction in hospitalization and relapse rates in the experimental condition, but it is not possible to attribute the success of the program to family psychoeducation alone (Valencia, Rascon, Juarez, & Murow, 2007). Neither Dyck and colleagues (2000) nor Magliano and colleagues (Magliano et al., 2000) observed differences in rates of relapse and/or rehospitalization between the family intervention and the control groups. However, they did report other positive outcomes associated with family psychoeducation, including fewer psychiatric symptoms (Magliano, Fiorillo, Malangone, De Rosa, & Maj, 2006; Magliano et al., 2000) and improved social and vocational outcomes (Hazel et al., 2004) relative to individuals in standard care. In terms of positive family outcomes, Magliano and colleagues (2006) found that family members receiving the family psychoeducation intervention reported increased perceptions of professional and social support. Hazel and colleagues (2004) reported caregiver outcomes from the study conducted by Dyck and colleagues (2000) and found that caregivers involved in the multiple-family group intervention reported lower levels of distress relative to those involved in standard outpatient treatment. Standard and usual care for family involvement most often consists of family meetings during the initial phase of admission to an inpatient unit to provide historical information about psychosocial development, symptoms, and past hospitalization as well as meetings around care planning after discharge.

Several studies included samples of both patients with and without a recent illness exacerbation, as well as their family members. Dyck and colleagues found that family psychoeducation reduced rates of hospitalization in the following year relative to a control condition (Dyck, Hendryx, Short, Voss, & McFarlane, 2002). Bradley and colleagues found an overall reduction in relapse among individuals receiving a multiple-family group intervention relative to those receiving standard case management (Bradley et al., 2006). Notably, this study also included a substantial group of poorly acculturated recent immigrants from Vietnam to Australia. Ran and colleagues compared family psychoeducation plus antipsychotic drug treatment with antipsychotic drug treatment alone, and with no intervention, and found that individuals who received both family therapy and antipsychotic drugs showed reduced relapse relative to individuals in the other two conditions (Ran et al., 2003). However, this study was conducted in rural China, in which the service context is not comparable with that observed in the United States. Another very large study of a family psychoeducation program conducted in China also included individuals who were characterized as stable, recovered, or remitted, and found reduced hospitalization and relapse among individuals involved in family psychoeducation. This study was conducted in five urban areas among patients who were living with a relative. As with the study by Ran and colleagues (2003), the generalizability of these findings to the United States is questionable. When considering other positive patient outcomes, relevant studies found that individuals involved in family psychoeducation reported fewer psychiatric symptoms (Bradley et al., 2006; Zhang, Yan, Yao, & Ye, 1993), improved treatment adherence (Ran et al., 2003; Zhang et al., 1993), and improved social, functional, and vocational outcomes (Bradley et al., 2006; Zhang et al., 1993) relative to individuals in the control condition. In terms of positive outcomes for family members, family members involved in the family psychoeducation condition reported greater knowledge of schizophrenia and improved family relationships compared with those in the control condition (Ran et al., 2003).

Overall, the evidence for the effectiveness of a 6- to 9-month family psychoeducation intervention for reduction of relapse and other outcomes among patients who have not had a recent illness exacerbation is not nearly as strong as the evidence for 6- to 9-month family psychoeducation for individuals who have had a recent illness exacerbation. Two relevant studies include only stable patients, although they both found benefits. The studies that include both stable and recently ill patients found benefit, but for several of these studies, their relevance to the U.S. health system is questionable. Nevertheless, given the data, and that the stability of patients fluctuates, the weight of evidence supports offering 6- to 9-month family psychoeducation to patients who are stable.

Family psychoeducation interventions that are shorter than 6 months (but are four sessions at a minimum) have been shown to contribute to positive patient and family outcomes among both individuals who are psychiatrically stable and those who have had a recent relapse. Notably, these studies show a benefit among a range of outcomes, although no single patient outcome is observed in all, or the majority, of studies. Also, more than half of these interventions are designed for family members only and do not include patients in the treatment sessions (Pickett-Schenk et al., 2006a; Pickett-Schenk et al., 2006b; Pickett-Schenk, Lippincott, Bennett, & Steigman, 2008; Posner, Wilson, Kral, Lander, & McLlwraith, 1992; Solomon, Draine, Mannion, & Meisel, 1996; Xiang, Ran, & Li, 1994). However, shorter interventions that include the patient have also been tested (Merinder et al., 1999; Pitschel-Walz et al., 2006; Speigel & Wissler,

1987). The inclusion of family members only permits families to participate in a program during circumstances when the patient is uninterested or unwilling to participate.

In terms of specific outcomes, Posner and colleagues (1992) conducted a study in which family members were assigned to an 8-week family psychoeducation group or a control group. Family members involved in the family psychoeducation group reported significantly greater knowledge of schizophrenia and satisfaction with medical care relative to those in the control group. Results of a study by Merinder and colleagues (1999) mirror those of Posner and colleagues (1992) in that Merinder compared patient and family outcomes between patients and families involved in an eight-session family psychoeducation group relative to those in a TAU group ($N = 46$) (Merinder et al., 1999). Families involved in the family psychoeducation intervention reported significantly greater increases in knowledge and greater satisfaction with their involvement in their relative's care. Patients involved in family psychoeducation also reported significant increases in knowledge and involvement in their care, as well as significantly fewer psychiatric symptoms and a longer time to relapse. Xiang and colleagues (1994) conducted a study comparing 4-month family psychoeducation and drug treatment with drug treatment alone condition in rural China. Although the applicability of conditions in rural China is subject to question, within the family psychoeducation and drug treatment group, patients reported greater levels of treatment adherence and higher levels of functioning relative to the drug-only condition. Family members also reported significantly better care of their ill relatives in the family psychoeducation and drug condition relative to the drug-only condition. A study by Speigel and Wissler (1987) compared a family psychoeducation treatment that involved a consultation team coming to the family's home for 4 to 6 weeks after the patient was discharged from the hospital with a control condition. The consultation team provided psychoeducation, problem solving, and crisis intervention to the family and patient. When considering patients with schizophrenia spectrum disorders only, patients in the family psychoeducation treatment group ($n = 14$) spent fewer days in the hospital, used more outpatient services, and rated their adjustment greater relative to those in the control group ($n = 22$) who did not receive family consultation. Likewise, Pitschel-Walz and colleagues (2006) found that individuals involved in an 8 session family psychoeducation intervention (over the course of 4–5 months) had lower rates of rehospitalization and better treatment adherence relative to individuals who received TAU. This study included patients with schizophrenia spectrum disorders who had been hospitalized recently. Solomon and colleagues (1996) compared individualized family consultation with group family psychoeducation, and also with a third arm that was a waiting list control for relatives of individuals diagnosed with mental disorders with 295 (schizophrenia spectrum, 64%) or 296 (mood disorder, 36%) codes.

Self-efficacy was significantly greater for the persons receiving individual consultation and those in group psychoeducation who had not previously attended a family support group relative to the wait-list control. Results of a meta-analysis by Cuijpers (1999) support positive outcomes, including reduced burden and distress, and improved relationships among family members receiving the family psychoeducation intervention. It is important to note that some studies did not show benefit of brief family psychoeducation interventions, but the weight of evidence suggests that shorter interventions can be beneficial, especially for family members (Vaughn et al., 1992).

An additional set of studies led by Pickett-Schenk compared families receiving the Journey of Hope (JOH), an 8-week family-led psychoeducation course, with a wait-list control group (Pickett-Schenk et al., 2006a; Pickett-Schenk et al., 2006b; Pickett-Schenk et al., 2008). Families involved in the family-led course reported significantly greater levels of knowledge about schizophrenia, improved information needs, lower levels of depression, improved family relationships, and improved satisfaction in their caregiver role. This program was delivered in the community, so even families in which the patient was not receiving services could participate. Their findings are consistent with the results of other briefer family-based models.

Following the recommendations of the PORT review (Dixon et al., 2009/2010), a few shorter studies of family education models have been conducted. A randomized trial of the National Alliance on Mental Illness–sponsored Family-to-Family Education Program (FFEP) found that participants had increased family functioning and coping as well as reduced distress. Participating family members also had increased knowledge and empowerment in the family, community, and service system domains (Dixon et al., 2011). The follow-up report by Lucksted and colleagues found that FFEP benefits were sustained 6 months after program completion (Lucksted et al., 2013). Furthermore, Marcus and colleagues showed that the benefits of FFEP observed in the randomized trial generalized to those who refused to participate in the randomized portion of the trial (Marcus et al., 2012).

Moreover, studies are emerging using online learning approaches to provide family psychoeducation. In a year-long study conducted by Rotondi and colleagues, 31 patients with schizophrenia and 24 support persons were assigned randomly to an online intervention (telehealth) or TAU (Rotondi et al., 2010). Participants accessed a website with resources focused on illness education, and participated in online therapy forums facilitated by clinicians, with emphasis on solving problems, alleviating stress, and interacting with peers. Participants in the telehealth approach increased their illness knowledge significantly; persons with illness showed a significant decrease in positive symptoms. Innovation in educational technology expands our possibility of reaching persons with serious mental illness and their families who live at a distance from each other, from the treatment facility, or from family support and advocacy groups.

CASE STUDIES

In the following sections, two case studies are presented. Each of the cases illustrate different family interventions that reflect variation of need, given different points in time of the family life cycle and involvement with the formal mental health system.

Case Study 1: "This Is Not the Way We Expected Parenting to be: Parents of a Young Adult Adjust to Living with Their Son's Serious Mental Illness"

Michael is a 25-year-old man who describes a difficult adolescence as a result of intense anxiety and periods of drug use. Despite his difficulties, Michael was able to complete high school and attend a nearby state university. Michael is the younger of two children. His older sister Susan attended college in a different state and is now employed and living on her own. Michael opted to live at home while attending college. In addition to school, he held a part-time position in a restaurant owned by a family friend. During the second semester of college, Michael's behavior shifted abruptly from being an outgoing young man with a strong social life to someone who was withdrawn from friends and family. At the beginning of the second semester of college, he quit his job because he felt that his boss was talking about him behind his back. Shortly thereafter, he missed classes as a result of an inability to leave the house. His parents reacted initially with concern and worry. When he expressed intense suspiciousness related to feeling watched and targeted by the Central Intelligence Agency, Michael's parents reached out to their primary care physician, who referred Michael to a psychiatrist. The psychiatrist prescribed antipsychotic medication and rest. Michael took a medical leave from college and, during the next few months, he continued to isolate himself in his room, in bed and under the covers. When Michael was unable to attend his appointments with his psychiatrist, hospitalization was recommended. Michael was hospitalized three times during the next 2 years. He was diagnosed with schizophrenia. After each hospitalization, he attended outpatient treatment and returned to live with his parents, who were able to provide financial support.

Michael has tried a host of different medications with limited success and a multitude of distressing side effects. Medications and their side effects have been a major source of complaints and worry for Michael and his family. The inpatient unit had a family education program in the form of a multiple-family group. The group met every other week and they attended regularly. Here they learned more about Michael's diagnosis of schizophrenia, medication, communication, coping with symptoms, and problem solving. They found it very helpful while Michael was in the hospital and they tried to follow what they had learned, but felt very alone when Michael was discharged from the hospital.

Michael lives with his parents in a suburban neighborhood. His parents are well established in their work and have strong ties to their religious community. Michael's illness had a significant impact on his parents,

Michael's sister, and the extended family. This was the first time the family had any encounter with the mental health system. They had to learn to navigate the complex mental health system, and they had to cope with immense changes and new experiences while maintaining or adapting their long-standing roles and responsibilities at work and at home. In addition, the parents felt a great deal of shame and uneasiness about reaching out to their community for support because of the fear of being stigmatized. As is often the situation, Michael's parents began to feel they were living a double life. They continued to work as usual and attend social activities with friends and at their place of worship. Without being able to seek support, they found themselves isolated emotionally from other relatives and friends whose adult children were following the expected life trajectory. This exacerbated their distress. Although they had received support, education, and learned some skills from the multiple-family group while Michael was in the hospital, at home they faced many difficulties as a family. They struggled with how much to expect of Michael and how much they should provide for him. Although it is currently not unusual for young adults to live with their parents, the stigma associated with severe mental illness remains a challenge for Michael and his family.

Things changed when the family's church hired a new young minister who was also a social worker. He developed programming about mental illness and wellness in addition to other educational initiatives that encouraged an atmosphere of acceptance for people in the community challenged by mental illness. Greatly relieved, this created an opportunity for Michael's parents to share their family situation with the minister. He recommended the family seek professional consultation with an expert on family psychoeducation to address daily issues and concerns.

Michael and his parents began to meet with a social worker every 2 to 3 weeks. Sometimes the three of them would come together, and sometimes just the parents would attend. The meetings gave the family a forum in which to address the impact of the illness on the family, and how to cope and manage the symptoms. When the parents met by themselves, they could talk about the profound sadness and grief they experience while witnessing their son's illness. Michael's illness had taken up much of their lives since he first began to have problems, leaving little time for them to pursue their own interests. Over time, they were able to invite friends to the house for dinner and to plan a few weekend getaways to nurture the marital relationship. As such, they began to reclaim their lives.

In one family meeting that took place around a holiday, Susan, the older daughter, also attended. Here she had an opportunity to express her experience with her brother's illness. She described feeling overwrought with guilt that she could go away to college and live an independent life. Like her parents, she also talked about the unease of leading a double life in which she kept her brother's struggle a secret from her friends and colleagues. Her parents and brother listened to her, expressed their pride in her accomplishments, and together they offered each other support. When hearing about how the parents sought support, she was able to seek out a support group for siblings of persons with serious mental illness when she returned home. Susan's renewed involvement with the family, despite at a distance, became another turning point for the family's journey toward recovery.

In time, the parents, too, were able to attend meetings at their local chapter of the National Alliance on Mental Illness (NAMI) and eventually enrolled in a family-to-family course. This proved to be immensely helpful for not just the parents, but also for Michael. With some starts and stops, Michael finished college and was accepted into a professional program in the medical field. Michael had previously declined to attend any programs with other people faced with mental illness. However, when he was introduced to a peer specialist who provided individual couching, he finally connected with someone who was dealing with similar experiences. He has since tackled a host of concerns that he had not been able to discuss with anyone before.

Over time, Michael and his family used a variety of different opportunities to educate themselves about mental illness and about how best to cope and manage individually and as a family through the different stages.

Case Study 2: "What Is Going to Happen to My Daughter When I Am No Longer Here? A Mother Struggles with Her Fear of Getting Older and Not Being Able to Care for Her Adult Daughter"

Marilyn is a 79-year-old black, single, retired woman and the mother of a 42-year-old daughter, Annette. They live together in a small apartment in a major city because Annette is unable to support herself. Annette received a diagnosis of schizoaffective disorder by a psychiatrist that she saw for a brief period during her early 20s, but has not sought treatment since. Marilyn describes having a tumultuous relationship with her daughter, leading to daily fights that at times become violent. Marilyn has been unable to convince her daughter to get help for her condition. According to Marilyn, Annette feels ashamed that she is not working and that she is single. Furthermore, Annette blames her mother for the way her life has turned out.

Marilyn has always been in good health, financially secure, and able to take care of herself and her daughter. Recently, she had major dental work completed. This ordeal made her acutely aware of her own mortality. Fueled by this crisis, Marilyn began looking for support and resources on the Internet, and she found her way to a NAMI meeting with a lawyer that provided estate planning for families of persons with serious mental health concerns. At the event, she gained relevant information and relief as a result of having found help. She also learned about other resources for families and subsequently joined a support group. Marilyn's participation in the group provides her with a great deal of support and guidance. She now has a community of older people who experience similar situations with their adult children. Marilyn describes a fresh sense of calm that allows her to step back from the negative interactions with her daughter. In the support group she is gaining a deeper understanding of mental illness. Marilyn is finding ways to begin a productive planning process with her daughter with the help and support from her NAMI support group, and she now engages in more constructive interactions with her daughter. Marilyn and Annette are beginning to talk about future planning and strategies that address Annette's goals for herself, and ways to meet her needs as her mother ages. Advancing old age can create a role reversal; children who once required a nurturing parent must now nurture their parents. Interestingly enough, Annette is beginning to see herself in a new light with renewed purpose. This is a healing process in its own right—for both mother and daughter.

Although Annette has yet to seek help from the formal treatment system, Marilyn and her daughter have become less isolated and more engaged with natural support systems. Family interventions in the community are particularly critical to people when the loved one is not involved with the formal treatment system. Marilyn's involvement with NAMI may provide her with familiarity and access to services for herself, such as the family-to-family group and other educational events relevant to her and her daughter's situation. This will have a positive impact on her relationship with her daughter going forward.

CONCLUSION

As Frank (2002) eloquently stated, "Caregivers are the other half of illness experiences" (p. 6). In this chapter, we presented the importance of having the two halves of the illness experience come together and be viewed as a whole. Involvement of family and the natural support system in the mental health care of individuals with serious mental illness opens up opportunities for accessing support, collaboration, care coordination, and integration, which in turn can foster recovery. Possible benefits for patients include reduced psychiatric symptoms, improved treatment adherence, improved functional and vocational status, and greater satisfaction with treatment. Positive family outcomes include reduced family burden and increased satisfaction with family relationships and the possibility of *recovering in illness together*. Much like the individual for which recovery is a personal journey, family members and significant others must find their own journey in creating meaning and finding hope. Family interventions encompass the idea of creating spaces in which families can find a *re*newed sense of possibility, can *re*gain competency as family caregivers, can *re*connect with society to counter stigma and isolation, and to move toward *re*conciliation and *re*claim life. A recent pilot study conducted by McNeil and Jaggers (2013) offers a new approach that uses cognitive–behavioral skills training for families to develop and maintain an emotional reserve to enable them to sustain effective caregiving over time. The intervention, Banking Positives, shows promise in improving emotional well-being and life satisfaction, and in reducing the feelings of burden reported by family caregivers.

Another large, important newly published study that collected data systematically about whether persons with serious mental illness prefer to have family involved in their treatment reported that many consumers are open to involving their families when offered a range of involvement types. The intervention, Recovery-Oriented Decisions for Relative's Support for Family Involvement (REORDER), is a "manualized" protocol that uses a shared decision-making process to facilitate a dialogue with the person with mental illness about the pros and cons of family involvement in the treatment. At the end of the session, a decision of types of involvement is agreed on. Family involvement ranges from providing the family with written information about the mental illness, giving the family permission to call the treatment team when concerns arise, providing family support, and promoting attendance at educational support groups (Cohen et al., 2013). Two hundred thirty-two persons with serious mental illness from outpatient mental health clinics in two Veterans Integrated Service Networks enrolled in the study. Seventy-eight percent (171 of 219) of the individuals with mental illness wanted family involvement in their treatment, and many wanted their family to be involved with several types of treatment offered. This underscores the importance of attending to patient and family preference when implementing evidence-based practices. The REORDER approach honors the person-centered component of the chronic care model and it extends the model by showing how to enhance family and community support—another core component of the chronic care model.

Caregivers must not be neglected when discussing *recovery in illness* for persons living with chronic illness. Mental health providers have an important opportunity to influence *living well with illness* when we include the family or the natural support system in our work. Involving family members of significant others connected with the person with schizophrenia or other serious mental illness early on is preventive in nature. Increasing understanding and enhancing coping skills mitigate the risk factors associated with caregiver burden. We should remain mindful that need varies from person to person, and that family interventions should be flexible in nature to address differences in needs over time and in the context of family, community, and culture.

The principles inherent in the chronic care model introduced in this book recognize the importance of mobilizing community resources outside, yet in collaboration with the formal treatment system, to meet the needs of people with long-term conditions, thereby creating a culture in organizations that promote safe and high-quality care. Family and natural support systems can play a significant role in empowering and preparing people to manage their health and health care. In collaboration with persons with serious mental illness and their natural supports, providers will be able deliver effective, efficient care and self-management support; promote care that is consistent with research evidence and patient preferences; and organize patient and population data to facilitate efficient and effective care (Wagner, 1998).

REFERENCES

American Psychiatric Association. (2013). *Diagnostic and statistical manual of mental disorders* (5th ed.). Washington, DC: Author.

Aschbrenner, K. A., Greenberg, J. S., Allen, S. M., & Seltzer, M. M. (2010). Subjective burden and personal gains among older parents of adults with serious mental illness. *Psychiatric Services, 61*(6), 605–611.

Bengtsson-Topps, A., & Hansson, L. (2001). Quantitative and qualitative aspect of the social network in schizophrenic patients living in the community: Relationship to socio-demographic characteristics and clinical factors and subjective quality of life. *International Journal of Social Psychiatry, 47*(3), 67–77.

Biegel, D. E., & Shultz, R. (1999). Caregiving and caregiver interventions in aging and mental illness. *Family Relations, 48*(4), 345–354.

Bradley, G. M., Couchman, G. M., Perlesz, A., Nguyen, A. T., Singh, B., & Riess, C. (2006). Multiple family group treatment for English- and Vietnamese-speaking families living with schizophrenia. *Psychiatric Services, 57*(4), 521–530.

Chang, H., Chiou, C., & Chen, N. (2010). Impact of mental health and caregiver burden on family caregivers' physical health. *Archives of Gerontology and Geriatrics, 50*(3), 267–271.

Cohen, A. N., Drapalski, A. L., Glynn, S. M., Medoff, D., Fang, L. J., & Dixon, L. B. (2013). Preferences for family involvement in care among consumers with serious mental illness. *Psychiatric Services, 64*(3), 257–263.

Cox, C. (1993). *The frail elderly: Problems, needs, and community responses.* Westport, CT: Auburn House.

Cuijpers, P. (1999). The effects of family interventions on relatives' burden: A meta-analysis. *Journal of Mental Health, 8*(3), 275–285.

Davidson, L., Chinman, M., Sells, D., & Rowe, M. (2006). Peer support among adults with serious mental illness: A report from the field. *Schizophrenia Bulletin, 32*(3), 443–450.

Davidson, L., O'Connell, M. J., Tondora, J., Lawless, M., & Evans, A. C. (2005). Recovery in serious mental illness: A new wine or just a new bottle? *Professional Psychology: Research and Practice, 36*(5), 480–487.

Deegan, P. E., & Drake, R. E. (2006). Shared decisionmaking and medication management in the recovery process. *Psychiatric Services (Washington D.C.), 57*(11), 1636–1639.

de Jesus Mari, J., & Streiner, D. L. (1994). An overview of family interventions and relapse on schizophrenia: Meta-analysis of research findings. *Psychological Medicine, 24*(3), 565–578.

Dixon, L. B., Dickerson, F., Bellack, A. S., Bennett, M., Dickinson, D., Goldberg, R. W., ... Kreyenbuhl, J. (2010). The 2009 PORT psychosocial treatment recommendations. and summary statements. *Schizophrenia Bulletin, 36*(1), 48–70.

Dixon, L. B., Lucksted, A., Medoff, D. R., Burland, J., Stewart, B., Lehman, A. F., ... Murray-Swank, A. (2011). Outcomes of a randomized study of a peer-taught family-to-family education program for mental illness. *Psychiatric Services, 62*(6), 591–597.

Dyck, D. G., Hendryx, M. S., Short, R. A., Voss, W. D., & McFarlane, W. R. (2002). Service use among patients with schizophrenia in psychoeducational multiple-family group treatment. *Psychiatric Services, 53*(6), 749–754.

Dyck, D. G., Short, R. A., & Hendryx, M. S. (2000). Management of negative symptoms among patients with schizophrenia attending multiple-family groups. *Psychiatric Services, 51*(4), 513–519.

Falloon, I. R., Boyd, J. L., & McGill, C. W. (1985). Family management in the prevention of morbidity of schizophrenia: Clinical outcome of a two-year longitudinal study. *Archive of General Psychiatry, 42*(9), 887–896.

Farone, D. W. (2006). Schizophrenia, community integration, and recovery: Implications for social work practice. *Social Work in Mental Health, 4*(4), 21–36.

Fraley, A. M. (1990). Chronic sorrow: A parental response. *Journal of Pediatric Nursing, 5*(4), 268–273.

Frank, A. W. (2002). *At the will of the body: Reflections on illness.* Houghton Mifflin Harcourt.

Gonçalves-Pereira, M., Xavier, M., van Wijngaarden, B., Papoila, A. L., Schene, A. H., & Caldas-de-Almeida, J. M. (2013). Impact of psychosis on Portuguese caregivers: A cross-cultural exploration of burden, distress, positive aspects and clinical–functional correlates. *Social Psychiatry and Psychiatric Epidemiology, 48*(2), 325–335.

Gouldner, A. (1960). The norm of reciprocity: A preliminary statement. *American Sociological Review, 25*(2), 161–178.

Green, B. L. (1982). Assessing Levels of Psychological Impairment Following Disaster Consideration of Actual and Methodological Dimensions. *The Journal of nervous and mental disease, 170*(9), 544–552.

Greenberg, J. S. (1995). The other side of caring: Adult children with mental illness as supports to their mothers in later life. *Social Work, 40*(3), 414–423.

Greenberg, J. S., Greenley, J. R., & Benedict, P. (1994). Contributions of persons with serious mental illness to their families. *Hospital & Community Psychiatry, 45*(5), 475–480.

Guberman, N., Maheu, P., & Maillé, C. (1992). Women as family caregivers: Why do they care? *The Gerontologist, 32*(5), 607–617.

Hatfield, A. B. (1989). Patients' accounts of stress and coping in schizophrenia. *Hospital & Community Psychiatry, 40*(11), 1141–1145.

Hazel, N. A., McDonnell, M. G., Short, R. A., Berry, C. M., Voss, W. D., Rodgers, M. L., & Dyck, D. G. (2004). Impact of multiple-family groups for outpatients with schizophrenia on caregivers' distress and resources. *Psychiatric Services, 55*(1), 35–41.

Horwitz, A. V. (1993). Adult siblings as sources of social support for the seriously mentally ill: A test of the serial model. *Journal of Marriage & Family, 55*(3), 623–632.

Horwitz, A. V., Reinhard, S. C., & Howell-White, S. (1996). Caregiving as reciprocal exchange in families with seriously mentally ill members. *Journal of Health & Social Behavior, 37*(2), 149–162.

Hsiao, C., & Van Riper, M. (2009). Individual and family adaptation in Taiwanese families of individuals with severe and persistent mental illness (SPMI). *Research in Nursing & Health, 32*(3), 307–320.

Johnson, E. D. (2000). Differences among families coping with serious mental illness: A qualitative analysis. *American Journal of Orthopsychiatry, 70*(1), 126–134.

Judge, K. A. (1994). Serving Children, siblings and spouses: Understanding the Needs of Other Family Members. In H. P. Lefley & M. Wasow (Eds.), *Helping families cope with mental illness* (pp. 161–194). Chur, Switzerland: Harwood Academic Publishers.

Karp, D. A. (2001). *The burden of sympathy: How families cope with mental illness.* New York: Oxford University Press.

Kauffman, A., Scogin, F., MacNeil, G., Leeper, J., & Wimberly, J. (2010). Helping aging parents of adult children with serious mental illness. *Journal of Social Service Research, 36*(5), 445–459.

Kramer, B. J. (1997). Gain in the caregiving experience: Where are we? What next? *The Gerontologist, 37,* 218–232.

Kurtz, M. M., & Mueser, K. T. (2008). A meta-analysis of controlled research on social skills training for schizophrenia. *Journal of Consulting and Clinical Psychology, 76* (3), 491–504.

Lehman, A. F., Steinwachs, D. M., Dixon, L. B., Goldman, H. H., Osher, F., Postrado, L., ... Zito, J. (1998). Translating research into practice: The schizophrenia Patient Outcomes Research Team (PORT) treatment recommendations. *Schizophrenia Bulletin, 24*(1), 1–10.

Lenior, M. E., Dingemans P. M, Linszen, D. H., de Haan L., & Schene A. H. (2001). Social functioning and the course of early-onset schizophrenia: Five-year follow up of a psychosocial intervention. *The British Journal of Psychiatry, 179,* 53–58.

Lohrer, S. P. (2001). *What will happen when our parents are gone? Present and future roles of adult siblings of persons with mental illness in instrumental caregiving.* Doctoral dissertation, Columbia University, New York. (Retrieved from Ann Arbor, Michigan, UMI no. 3028556.)

Lohrer, S., Lukens, E., & Thorning, H. (2006). The costs of caring: Instrumental caregiving involvement among adult siblings of persons with mental illness. *Community Mental Health Journal, 3,* 1573–1589.

Lucksted, A., Medoff, A., Burland, J., Stewart, B., Fang, L. J., Brown, C., ... Dixon, L. B. (2013). Sustained outcomes of a peer-taught family education program on mental illness. *Acta Psychiatrica Scandinavica, 127*(4), 279–286.

Lukens, E., & Thorning, H. (2010). Psychoeducational family groups. In A. Rubin, D. W. Springer, & K. Trawver (Eds.), *Psychosocial treatment of schizophrenia* (pp. 89–144). Hoboken, NJ: John Wiley & Sons, Inc.

Lukens, E. P., & Thorning, H. (2011). Siblings in families with mental illness. In J. Caspi (Ed.), *Sibling development: Implications for mental health practitioners* (pp. 195–219). New York, NY: Springer Publishing Corporation, LLC.

Lukens, E., Thorning, H., & Herman, D. (1999). Family psychoeducation in schizophrenia: Emerging themes and challenges. *Journal of Practical Psychiatry & Behavioral Health, 9,* 314–325.

Lukens, E., Thorning, H., & Lohrer, S. (2004). Sibling perspectives on severe mental illness: Reflections on self and family. *American Journal of Orthopsychiatry, 74*(4), 489–501.

MacNeil, G., & Jaggers, J. (2013). Banking Positives: A Strengths-Based Intervention for Long-Term Family Caregivers. *Best Practice in Mental Health, 9*(2).

Magliano, L., Fadden, G., Economou, M., Held, T., Xavier, M., Guarneri, M., ... Maj, M. (2000). Family burden and coping strategies in schizophrenia: 1-Year follow-up data from the BIOMED I study. *Social Psychiatry Psychiatric Epidemiology, 35,* 109–115.

Magliano, L., Fiorillo, A., Malangone, C., De Rosa, C., & Maj, M. (2006). Patient functioning and family burden in a controlled, real-world trial of family education for schizophrenia. *Psychiatric Services, 57*(12), 1784–1791.

Marcus, S. M., Medoff, D., Fang, L. J., Weaver, J., Duan, N., Lucksted, A., & Dixon, L. B. (2012). Generalizability in the family–family education program randomized waitlist-control trial. *Psychiatric Services, 64*(8), 754–763.

Marsh, D. T., Lefley, H. P., Evans-Rhodes, D., Ansell, V. I., Doerzbacher, B. M., LaBarbera, L., & Paluzzi, J. E. (1996). The family experience of mental illness: Evidence for resilience. *Psychiatric Rehabilitation Journal, 20*(2), 3–12.

Mechanic, D. (2008). *Mental health and social policy: Beyond managed care* (5th ed.). New York, NY: Pearson Education.

Merinder, L. B., Viuff, A. G., Laugesen, H. D., Clemmensen, K., Misfelt, S., & Espensen, B. (1999). Patient and relative education in community psychiatry: A randomized controlled trial regarding its effectiveness. *Social Psychiatry and Psychiatric Epidemiology, 34*(6), 287–294.

Mueser, K. T., Sengupta, A., Schooler, N. R., Bellack, A. S., Xie, H., Glick, I. D., & Keith, S. J. (2001). Family treatment and medication dosage reduction in schizophrenia: Effects on patient social functioning, family attitudes and burden. *Journal of Consulting and Clinical Psychology, 69*(1), 3–12.

Padgett, D. K., Henwood, B., Abrams, C., & Drake, R. E. (2008). Social relationships among persons who have experienced serious mental illness, substance abuse, and homelessness: Implications for recovery. *American Journal of Orthopsychiatry, 78*(3), 333–339.

Pai, S., & Kapur, R. L. (1981). The burden on the family of a psychiatric patient: development of an interview schedule. *The British Journal of Psychiatry, 138*(4), 332–335.

Palmer, S. D. (1998). *Facing an uncertain future: The influence of coping resources and responses on caregivers' concerns about their relatives with a mental illness.* Doctoral dissertation, Columbia University, New York.

Pickett-Schenk, S. A., Bennett, C., Cook, J. A., Steigman, P., Lippincott, R., Villagracia, I., & Grey, D. (2006a). Changes in caregiving satisfaction and information needs among relatives of adults with mental illness: Results of a randomized evaluation of a family-led education intervention. *American Journal of Orthopsychiatry, 76*(4), 545–553.

Pickett-Schenk, S. A., Cook, J. A., Steigman, P., Lippincott, R., Bennett, C., & Grey, D. D. (2006b). Psychological well-being and relationship outcomes in a randomized study of family-led education. *Archive of General Psychiatry, 63*(9), 1043–1050.

Pickett-Schenk, S. A., Lippincott, R. C., Bennett, C., & Steigman, P. J. (2008). Improving knowledge about mental illness through family-led education: The Journey of Hope. *Psychiatric Services, 59*(1), 49–56.

Pilling, S., Bebbington, P., Kuipers, E., Garety, P., Geddes, J., Orbach, G., & Morgan, C. (2002). Psychological treatments in schizophrenia: I. Meta-analysis of family intervention and cognitive behaviour therapy. *Psychological Medicine, 32*(5), 763–782.

Pitschel-Walz, G., Bäuml, J., Bender, W., Engel, R. R., Wagner, M., & Kissling, W. (2006). Psychoeducation and compliance in the treatment of schizophrenia: Results of the Munich Psychosis Information Project Study. *Journal of Clinical Psychiatry, 67*(3), 443–452.

Pitschel-Walz, G., Leucht, S., Bäuml, J., Kissling, W., & Engel, R. R. (2001). The effect of family interventions on relapse and rehospitalization in schizophrenia: A meta-analysis. *Schizophrenia Bulletin, 27*(1), 73–92.

Posner, C. M., Wilson, K. G., Kral, M. J., Lander, S., & McLlwraith, R. D. (1992). Family psychoeducational support groups in schizophrenia. *American Journal of Orthopsychiatry, 62*(2), 206–218.

Ran, M., Xiang, M., Chan, C. L., Leff, J., Simpson, P., Huang, M., … Li, S. (2003). Effectiveness of psychoeducational intervention for rural Chinese families experiencing schizophrenia: A randomized controlled trial. *Social Psychiatry Psychiatric Epidemiology, 38*(2), 69–75.

Reinhard, S. C., & Horwitz, A. V. (1995). Caregiver burden: Differentiating the content and consequences of family caregiving. *Journal of Marriage and Family, 57*, 741–750.

Rotondi, A. J., Anderson, C. M., Haas, G. L., Eack, S. M., Spring, M. B., Ganguli, R., … Rosenstock, J. (2010). Web-based psychoeducational intervention for persons with schizophrenia and their supporters: One-year outcomes. *Psychiatric Services, 61*(11), 1099–1105.

Rowe, J. (2011). Great expectations: A systematic review of the literature on the role of family carers in severe mental illness, and their relationships and engagement with professionals. *Journal of Psychiatric and Mental Health Nursing, 19*(1), 70–82.

Schene, A. H., Tessler, R. C., & Gamache, G. M. (1994). Instruments measuring family or caregiver burden in severe mental illness. *Social Psychiatry and Psychiatric Epidemiology, 29*(5), 228–240.

Scheyett, A. DeLuca, J., &Morgan, C. (2013). Recovery in severe mental illnesses: A literature review of recovery measures. *Social Work Research, 37*(3), 286–303.

Sellwood, W., Barrowclough, C., Tarrier, N., Quinn, J., Mainwaring, J., & Lewis, S. (2001). Needs-based cognitive–behavioural family intervention for carers of patients suffering from schizophrenia: 12-month follow-up. *Acta Psychiatrica Scandinavica, 104*(5), 346–355.

Sellwood, W., Wittkowski, A., Tarrier, N., & Barrowclough, C. (2007). Needs-based cognitive–behavioural family intervention for patients suffering from schizophrenia: 5-Year follow- up of a randomized controlled effectiveness trial. *Acta Psychiatrica Scandinavica, 116*(6), 447–452.

Semple, S. J., Patterson, T. L., Shaw, W. S., Grant, I., Moscona, S., Koch, W., & Jeste, D. (1997). The social networks of older schizophrenia patients. *International Psychogeriatrics, 9*(1), 81–94.

Sherer, M., Maddux, J. E., Mercadante, B., Prentice-Dunn, S., Jacobs, B., & Rogers, R. W. (1982). The Self-Efficacy Scale: Construction and validation. *Psychological Reports, 51*, 663–671.

Smith, G. C., Tobin, S. S., & Fullmer, E. M. (1995). Elderly mothers caring at home for offspring with mental retardation: A model of permanency planning. *American Journal on Mental Retardation, 99*(5), 487–499.

Solomon, P., Draine, J., Mannion, E., & Meisel, M. (1996). Impact of brief family psychoeducation on self-efficacy. *Schizophrenia Bulletin, 22*(1), 41–50.

Song, L.- Y., Biegel, D. E., & Miligan, S. E. (1997). Predictors of depressive symptomatology among lower social class caregivers of persons with chronic mental illness. *Community Mental Health Journal, 33*(4), 269–286.

Speigel, D., & Wissler, T. (1987). Using family consultation as psychiatric aftercare for schizophrenic patients. *Hospital & Community Psychiatry, 38*(10), 1096–1099.

Stout, M. (1998). *Senate testimony: Special committee on aging in United State Senate* (press release). Washington, DC: National Alliance for the Mentally Ill.

Struening, E. L., Perlick, D. A., Link, B. G., Hellman, F., Herman, D., & Sirey, J. A. (2001). Stigma as a barrier to recovery:The extent to which caregivers believe most people devalue consumers and their families. *Psychiatric Services, 52*(12), 1633–1638.

Struening, E. L., Stueve, A., Vine, P., Kreisman, D. E., Link, B. G., & Herman, D. B. (1995). Factors associated with grief and depressive symptoms in people with serious mental Illness. In J. R. Greenley (Ed.), *Research in community and mental health* (pp. 91–124). Greenwich, CT: JAI Press.

Tarrier, N., Barrowclough, C., Vaughn, C., Bamrah, J. S., Porceddu, K., Watts, S.,& Freeman, H. (1989). Community management of schizophrenia: A two-year follow-up of behavioral intervention with families. *The British Journal of Psychiatry, 154*, 625–628.

Teel, C. S. (1991). Chronic sorrow: Analysis of the concept. *Journal of Advanced Nursing, 16*(11), 1311–1319.

Thorning, H. (2004). *Grief: The psychological consequence of the caregiving dynamic on family caregivers of persons with severe mental illness.* PhD dissertation, New York University, New York.

Valencia, M., Rascon, M. L., Juarez, F., & Murow, E. (2007). A psychosocial skills training approach in Mexican out-patients with schizophrenia. *Psychological Medicine, 37*(10), 1393–1402.

Vaughn, K., Doyle, M., McConaghy, N., Blaszczynski, A., Fox, A., & Tarrier, N. (1992). The Sydney intervention trial: A controlled trial of relatives' counselling to reduce schizophrenic relapse. *Social Psychiatry and Psychiatric Epidemiology, 27*(1), 16–21.

Wagner, E. (1998). Chronic disease management: What will it take to improve care for chronic illness? *Effective Clinical Practice, 1*(1), 2–4.

Ward-Griffin, C., & McKeever, P. (2000). Relationship between nurses and family caregivers: Partners in care? *Advances in Nursing Science, 22*(3), 89–103.

Weiman, B. M., Hedelin, B., Sällström, C., & Hall-Lord, M. (2010). Burden and health in relatives of persons with severe mental illness: A Norwegian cross-sectional study. *Issues in Mental Health Nursing, 31*(12), 804–815.

Xiang, M., Ran, M., & Li, S. (1994). A controlled evaluation of psychoeducational family intervention in a rural Chinese community. *The British Journal of Psychiatry, 165*(4), 544–548.

Xiong, W., Phillips, M. R., Wang, R., Dai, Q., Kleinman, J., & Kleinman, A. (1994). Family-based intervention for schizophrenic patients in China: A randomised controlled trial. *The British Journal of Psychiatry, 165*(2), 239–247.

ZamZam, R., Midin, M., Hooi, L. S., Yi, E. J., Ahmad, S. A., Azman, S. A., … Radzi R. S. (2011). Schizophrenia in Malaysian families: A study on factors associated with the quality of life of primary family caregivers. *International Journal of Mental Health Systems, 5*(1), 16–25.

Zauszniewski, J. A., Bekhet, A. K., & Suresky, M. J. (2010). Resilience in family members of persons with serious mental illness. *The Nursing Clinics of North America, 45*(4), 613.

Zegwaard, M. I., Aartsen, M. J., Grypdonck, M. H., & Cuijpers, P. (2013). Differences in impact of long term caregiving for mentally ill older adults on the daily life of informal caregivers: a qualitative study. *BMC Psychiatry, 13*, 103.

Zhang, M., Wang, M., Li, J., & Phillips, M. R. (1994). Randomised-control trial of family intervention for 78 first-episode male schizophrenic patients: An 18-month study in Suzhou, Jiangsu. *The British Journal of Psychiatry Supplementum*, 165(Suppl24), 96–102.

Zhang, M., Yan, H., Yao, C., & Ye, J. (1993). Effectiveness of psychoeducation of relatives of schizophrenic patients: A prospective cohort study in five cities of China. *International Journal of Mental Health, 22*(1), 47–59.

8
—

Caring for Individuals with Chronic Musculoskeletal Pain

CATHERINE RIFFIN, CARY REID, AND KARL PILLEMER ■

Persistent pain from musculoskeletal disease constitutes a major public health concern. This condition afflicts an estimated 43 million Americans, with the highest rate of prevalence found among older adults (Institute of Medicine, 2011). Chronic musculoskeletal pain (CMP) is characterized by uncertainty in diagnosis and unpredictability in course, and leads to significant impairments in individual and family functioning (Sperry, 2009). CMP suffering undeniably exacts a toll on caregiving relatives, conferring severe and often damaging consequences. Given the highly interactive nature of CMP, caregiver support interventions primarily target dyadic exchanges and mutual coping through family-based approaches, rather than addressing the needs of the caregiver explicitly.

Currently, the intervention research on patients with CMP and their family members remains limited, with a notable dearth of studies exploring whether family-oriented programs provide any benefits to family members themselves (Martire, 2013; Martire, Schultz, Helgeson, Small, & Saghafi, 2010; Riffin, Suitor, Reid, & Pillemer, 2012). In this chapter, we begin with a brief overview of CMP, emphasizing the social and interactive nature of the pain experience. We then describe the spectrum of interventions for CMP that incorporates various levels of family involvement. In particular, we focus on family-based interventions that assess both patient and caregiver outcomes. Last, we conclude with two case examples to illustrate ways in which family-based approaches have been used to address the physical, emotional and relational needs of patients and their relatives.

CHRONIC MUSCULOSKELETAL PAIN

CMP is a common, costly, and often disabling condition. According to the National Center for Chronic Disease Prevention and Health Promotion (2000), the United

States spends $65 billion each year for medical care and for lost productivity for individuals with CMP. At present, nearly half of all community-dwelling adults over the age of 65 suffer from CMP (Helme & Gibson, 2001), 20% of whom regularly take medications to ameliorate their symptoms (AGS Panel of Persistent Pain in Older Persons, 2002). By 2020, this condition is expected to affect 60 million people (National Center for Chronic Disease and Health Promotion, 2000). The deleterious effects of severe musculoskeletal pain are far-reaching. Consequences include diminished immune function and quality of life, problems sleeping, cognitive disability, emotional disturbance, social withdrawal (Jakobsson, Klevsgard, Westergren, & Hallberg, 2003; Karp et al., 2006; Reid, Williams, & Gill, 2005; Tan, Jensen, Thornby, & Sloan, 2008; Zhu, Devine, Dick, & Prince, 2007) as well as impairment in activities of daily living (Leveille, Fried, & Guralnik, 2002).

Although CMP is present in all racial, ethnic, and economic groups, it affects women and minorities disproportionately in terms of disease severity and number afflicted. More women than men suffer from osteoarthritis (OA), rheumatoid arthritis (RA), and osteoporosis, and report greater levels of pain regardless of condition (National Institute of Arthritis and Musculoskeletal and Skin Diseases, 2010). Black and Hispanic adults report more severe pain compared with non-Hispanic whites and are at greater risk of functional decline as a result of pain (National Institute of Arthritis and Musculoskeletal and Skin Diseases, 2010). After disease onset, demographic factors—including socioeconomic status, education level, and culture—may determine access to healthcare services that may further distinguish individual differences in disease progression and treatment response (National Institute of Arthritis and Musculoskeletal and Skin Diseases, 2010).

Although additional research is necessary to elucidate the specific genetic and biological markers associated with CMP, its underlying etiology has been attributed to the dynamic interplay of physiological, psychological, and social factors (AGS Panel on Pain in Older Persons, 2002). Unfortunately, the multifaceted nature and unpredictability of CMP challenges even seasoned clinicians when assessing and treating this condition. Especially among older adults, the common occurrence of sensory impairment and dementia hamper accurate diagnosis, and the presence of multiple sources of pain in an individual can present an additional challenge to treatment. Rarely do older adults exhibit a singular impairment or condition; rather, they are often afflicted with multiple ailments. This is complicated further by the variability in pain expression across and within individuals. Fluctuating pain levels and variability in symptoms require vigilant care and attention by health professionals and family members, particularly when affected individuals are unable to care for themselves (AGS Panel of Persistent Pain in Older Persons, 2002).

FAMILIES COPING WITH MUSCULOSKELETAL PAIN

Although CMP was formerly perceived as a unidimensional sensory issue (affecting only the patient's physical symptoms), it is now viewed within a socioenvironmental context in which patient disability and suffering are met by a variety of emotional reactions and responses by family members (Keefe & Somers, 2010; Martire, 2013; Wilson et al., 2013). Indeed, the interactions between the patient and his or her relatives have implications for the interpersonal and emotional outcomes of both parties. For instance, a substantive body of research reveals that severe pain contributes to destructive family environments and lower relationship qualities (Leonard, Cano, & Johansen, 2006; Matheson, Harcourt, & Hewlett, 2010). The reverse is also true; family member attitudes and responses affect the patient's own well-being and symptomatology. In the case of CMP, significantly lower family cohesion, greater family conflict, and poor marital functioning are all associated with increased pain and disease activity (Rosland, Heisler, & Piette, 2012).

In addition to diminished relationship quality, the psychological and emotional health of patients with CMP and their relatives also suffers. Depression is a frequent concomitant condition of arthritis pain (Keefe & Somers, 2010; Parmelee, Katz, & Lawton, 1991; Stephenson, DeLongis, Esdaile, & Lehman, 2013). Approximately 15% to 40% of patients with CMP exhibit depressive symptomatology (Wolfe & Michaud, 2009), and prevalence rates are equally high among spouses (Walsh, Blanchard, Kremer, & Blanchard, 1999). Indeed, caregiving relatives may experience poor mental health as a consequence of patients' emotional disturbance and pain expression (Stephens, Martire, Cremeans-Smith, Druley, & Wojno, 2006).

As the caregiver's psychological and interpersonal functioning deteriorates, so does the ability to maintain restorative health behaviors critical to combat stress and preserve overall well-being. In particular, patient pain affects spouses' sleep quality adversely (Martire, Keefe, Schulz, Parris Stephens, & Mogle, 2013). Notably, predictive models show the strongest impact of patient pain on spousal sleep for couples reporting high levels of closeness. Overall, providing care to a patient with CMP threatens multiple aspects of caregivers' functioning as a result of the high level of burden associated with caring for a loved one in pain. Undeniably, the chronic stress of caring for a patient with CMP holds severe ramifications for family members. Caregivers under high stress may be especially vulnerable to deleterious outcomes, including elevated mortality risk (Fredman, Cauley, Hochberg, Ensrud, & Doros, 2010).

FAMILY-BASED INTERVENTIONS FOR PATIENTS WITH CHRONIC MUSCULOSKELETAL PAIN

Confirming early theoretical models that highlighted the significant interdependence between patients with musculoskeletal pain and their relatives (Turk, Flor, & Rudy, 1987), recent clinical investigations and controlled trials have underscored the integral role family and relatives play in the management of CMP (Keefe & Somers, 2010; Martire et al., 2010; Martire et al.,

2004; Stephenson et al., 2013). As such, therapeutic interventions have incorporated family members into the clinical content of behavioral and education programs. The most common approach has been to involve relatives in cognitive–behavioral therapy or skills training, in which patients and family members engage in specific strategies for coping with pain or avoiding reinforcement of pain behaviors (Martire, 2005). Educational programs have also solicited family member attendance. Patients and their relatives receive instruction regarding the etiology and treatment of the condition, and are taught stress management and/or communication skills. Both types of family-oriented interventions (cognitive–behavioral or educational) vary in the extent to which they consider interpersonal issues between the patient and family member (Martire, 2005). Although some interventions enlist a family member simply to provide assistance in altering the patient's pain and health behaviors, others are aimed at the dyadic relationship and reciprocal interactions between the family member and patient. Interventions in the second category also address the effect of illness on the relative.

Unfortunately, intervention research on patients with CMP and their family members remains underdeveloped, with a paucity of studies exploring whether participation provides advantages to family members themselves. Most interventions for CMP have focused almost exclusively on treatment gains for the patient, with far less attention paid to family members' well-being, quality of life, or ability to provide quality care and assistance (Martire, 2005; Martire et al., 2010). Results of these trials have demonstrated that family participation in psychosocial and behavioral treatment yields measurable benefits to the patient, including enhanced emotional well-being (Bradley et al., 1987; Keefe et al., 1996; Keefe et al., 1999; Keefe et al., 2004; Martire et al., 2003; Martire, Schulz, Keefe, Rudy, & Starz, 2007; Martire, Schulz, Keefe, Rudy, & Starz, 2008), positive health behaviors (Keefe et al., 1996; Keefe et al., 1999; Martire et al., 2003), and reduced symptomatology (Bradley et al., 1987; Keefe et al., 1996; Keefe et al., 1999; Keefe et al., 2004; Martire et al., 2007; Radojevic, Nicassio, & Weisman, 1992; Turner, Clancy, McQuade, & Cardenas, 1990; van Lankveld, van Helmond, Naring, de Rooij, & van den Hoogen, 2004).

A significant gap in the intervention literature for CMP is whether family-oriented approaches confer any benefit to the family member. In the following section, we describe this small but expanding body of research and the preliminary findings that have emerged to date. Specifically, we focus our discussion on interventions that assess and report outcomes for both patients with CMP and their caregivers. To facilitate ease of interpretation, all studies described within the following section are also reported in the accompanying evidence table (Table 8.1). More explicitly, studies presented in the table are family-based interventions for patients with CMP and their family members, conducted to date, that assess and report both caregiver and patient outcomes. Because of the relative dearth of research in this area, no other exclusion criteria were imposed.

Table 8.1. Family-Based Interventions for CMP (Caregiver Outcomes Examined)

Author (Year)	Design and Sampling	Subject Characteristics	Methods/Intervention	Data/Measures	Findings/Outcomes	Limitations
			COGNITIVE–BEHAVIORAL OR SKILLS TRAINING			
Keefe et al., 1996; Keefe et al., 1999	Random assignment to one of three conditions	88 OA patients with knee pain (54 women, 34 men; mean age, 63 years) and their spouses. Group 1: patient cognitive–behavioral coping skills training (n = 29) Group 2: dyad cognitive–behavioral coping skills training (n = 30) Group 3: dyad education and social support (n = 29)	Patient coping skills training: taught attention diversion skills, activity-based skills, cognitive coping strategies, and progressive relaxation. Dyad coping skills: same protocol as the patient coping skills condition, but also targeted couples' communication, behaviors, and mutual goal setting. Dyad education and support: basic information about OA, and methods of diagnosis and treatment All conditions: 10 weekly group sessions, each lasting 2 hours	Caregiver self-report process measures: Dyadic Adjustment Scale Patient self-report process measures: Dyadic Adjustment Scale, Arthritis Self-Efficacy Scale Patient self-report pre/post measures: Arthritis Impact Measurement Scales Coping Strategies Questionnaire Observer-rated patient pain behavior by trained observers. Medication use assessment by rheumatologist Follow-up: postintervention, 6 months and 12 months	Multivariate analyses of covariance used analyses of covariance to assess posttreatment between-group differences. With regard to caregivers, no significant differences were noted between groups. With regard to patients, compared with group 3, group 2 had lower levels of pain, psychological disability, and pain behavior; had higher scores on marital adjustment and self-efficacy at postintervention; indicated coping attempts and marital adjustment at 6 months; and noted improvements in physical disability and higher self-efficacy at 12 months. Compared with group 3, group 1 had higher levels of self-efficacy postintervention and at 6 months, marital adjustment at 6 months, and improvements in physical disability at 12 months.	There were no comparisons on racial/cultural factors and no mention of diversity training. There was no control group and all measures were self-reported.

Study	Design	Sample	Intervention	Measures	Results	Comments
van Lankveld et al., 2004	Random assignment to one of two groups. Participant selection from hospital specializing in orthopedics, rheumatology, and rehabilitation medicine	59 RA patients (38 women, 21 men; mean age, 50 years) and their spouses. Group 1: patient cognitive–behavioral self-management program (n = 28). Group 2: dyad cognitive–behavioral self-management program (n = 31)	Patient cognitive-behavioral self-management program: education on treatment of RA focusing on patients' cognitions and behaviors; eight sessions over 4 weeks, each 90 minutes. Dyad cognitive-behavioral self-management program: same protocol as patient cognitive–behavioral condition, but spouses also attended the sessions, and the lessons also focused on the consequences of the disease on the interpersonal relationship. Follow-up: 2 weeks postintervention and at 6 months	Caregiver outcome measures: none reported. Patient self-report pre/post measures: Disease Activity Score, impact of rheumatic diseases on general health and lifestyle to measure physical functioning, psychological functioning, disease stressors, social support, coping with rheumatoid stressors, marital satisfaction of the Maudsley Marital Questionnaire, spousal criticism	With regard to caregivers, additional analyses, not included in the article text, indicated that spouse participation did not improve in any of the psychological variables assessed. With regard to patients, group 2 showed greater improvements in disease-related communication with their spouse postintervention.	There were no comparisons on racial/cultural factors and no mention of diversity training. A usual care control group was lacking.

EDUCATION AND SUPPORT

Study	Design	Sample	Intervention	Measures	Results	Comments
Martire et al., 2003	Random assignment to one of two conditions. Recruitment from two rheumatology clinics	24 OA patients (mean age, 72 years) and their husbands. Group 1: patient education and support (n = 11). Group 2: dyad education and support (n = 13)	Patient education and support: taught etiology and treatment of arthritis, pain management strategies, and effective coping with negative emotions; six weekly sessions, each 2 hours long	Caregiver self-report pre/post measures: caregiving stress rated on a scale from 1 point (not at all) to 4 points (very stressful), caregiving mastery using five-item scale (Lawton et al., 1989), Center for Epidemiological Studies–Depression scale	Two (group)-by-two (time) repeated-measures analyses of variance were conducted for each outcome variable. With regard to caregivers, no significant differences were observed between groups. With regard to patients, compared with group 1, group 2 indicated greater self-efficacy in managing arthritis pain and other symptoms postintervention.	There were no comparisons on racial/cultural factors, no mention of diversity training, no long-term follow-up, and no usual care control group. There was a small number of participants, and all measures were self-reported.

(continued)

Table 8.1. CONTINUED

Author (Year)	Design and Sampling	Subject Characteristics	Methods/Intervention	Data/Measures	Findings/Outcomes	Limitations
			Dyadic education and support: same protocol as patient education condition, but topics were framed as couples' issues; 20-minute supplemental segments at the end of each session targeted couples' issues explicitly Follow-up: postintervention	Patient self-report pre/post measures: Arthritis Impact Measures Scale, Health Assessment Questionnaire, Center for Epidemiological Studies–Depression scale, Arthritis Self-Efficacy scale, satisfaction with spousal assistance rated on a scale from 1 point (not at all) to 4 points (completely satisfied), emotional support (Manne & Zautra, 1989; Revenson et al., 1991) Follow-up: postintervention		
Martire et al., 2007; Martire et al., 2008	Random assignment to one of three groups Recruitment through rheumatology clinics	242 OA patients (177 women, 65 men; mean age, 68 years) and their spouses Group 1: patient education and support (*n* = 89) Group 2: dyad education and support (*n* = 99) Group 3: usual medical care (*n* = 54)	Patient education and support: taught etiology and treatment of arthritis, pain management strategies, the benefits of exercise, communication skills, and effective coping with negative emotions; six weekly sessions, each 2 hours long Dyadic education and support: same protocol as patient education condition, but topics were framed as couples' issues; 20-minute supplemental segments at the end of each session targeted couples' issues explicitly Up to five monthly booster sessions via telephone	Caregiver self-report pre/ post measures: Perceived Stress scale, Center for Epidemiological Studies–Depression scale, caregiver mastery (Lawton et al., 1989), critical attitudes (Stephens et al., 2006), Marital Adjustment Test Patient self-report pre/post measures: Western Ontario and McMaster Universities Osteoarthritis Index, Center for Epidemiological Studies–Depression Scale, Arthritis Self-Efficacy, Marital Adjustment Test Follow-up: postintervention and at 6 months	Repeated-measures analyses of variance were conducted. With regard to caregivers, compared with group 1, group 2 had greater reductions in stress postintervention, greater reductions in depressive symptoms, increases in caregiver mastery for female spouses, and spouses with high marital satisfaction. With regard to patients, compared with group 2, group 1 had greater reductions in reports of spouses' punishing responses (e.g., anger, irritation) postintervention, greater reductions in pain, and improved physical function and spousal support at 6 months.	There were no comparisons of racial/ cultural factors and no mention of diversity training. All measures were self-reported.

COUPLE'S RELATIONSHIP THERAPY

Saarijarvi, 1991; Saarijarvi et al., 1991	Random assignment to one of two groups Recruitment from primary healthcare centers	63 patients with chronic low-back pain (45 women, 39 men; mean age, 45 years) and their spouses Group 1: couple therapy (n = 33) Group 2: usual care (n = 30)	Therapy focused on the couples' relationship and modeling communication (i.e., active questioning and listening) by two therapists Five monthly sessions, each lasting 1 to 2 hours Follow-up: 12 monts	Caregiver self-report pre/post measures: Attitude Scale Patient self-report pre/post measures: Marital Questionnaire, Marital Communication Inventory, Brief Symptom Inventory, Attitude Scale	Multivariate analyses of variance were conducted. With regard to caregivers, there were no significant differences between groups. With regard to patients, group 1 indicated improved marital communication, and decreased psychological distress in male patients.	There were no comparisons of racial/cultural factors and no mention of diversity training. All measures were self-reported.

NOTE: OA, osteoarthritis arthritis; RA, rheumatoid arthritis.

FAMILY-BASED INTERVENTIONS THAT
ASSESS FAMILY MEMBER OUTCOMES

Only a handful of studies have explored whether family-oriented interventions for patients with CMP provide any benefits to the relative. Such studies tend to focus on a singular outcome—most often, spouses' marital adjustment (Keefe et al., 1996, Keefe et al., 1999; Martire et al., 2003; Martire et al., 2007, Martire, Schulz, Keefe, Rudy, & Starz, 2008; van Lankveld et al., 2004), with secondary consideration given to the relative's psychological well-being (Martire et al., 2003; Martire et al., 2007, Martire et al., 2008) or marital communication (Saarijarvi, 1991; Saarijarvi et al., 1991). As shown Table 8.1, these interventions fall into three categories of treatment strategies: cognitive–behavioral or coping skills training (CST) (Keefe et al., 1996; Keefe et al., 1999; van Lankveld et al., 2004), education and support (Martire et al., 2003; Martire et al., 2007; Martire et al., 2008), and couples' relationship therapy (Saarijarvi, 1991; Saarijarvi et al., 1991). Next, we describe the results of these interventions both in the text and in Table 8.1. Because coping skills training and supportive education interventions are the most common approaches, we center the majority of our discussion on these two treatment strategies.

As depicted in Table 8.1, Keefe and colleagues (1996, 1999) used a randomized, controlled design to compare the efficacy of a spouse-assisted cognitive–behavioral CST intervention with a similar CST intervention without spousal involvement, and with a family-oriented educational intervention. Of the 88 patients with OA enrolled in the study, 29 were assigned randomly to the dyad CST. During the course of 10 weekly sessions, couples were taught positive communication strategies for reinforcing coping skills and mutual goal setting. Emphasizing the active participation of patient and spouse, the program required dyadic involvement in behavioral rehearsal of physical (e.g., walking, standing) and emotional (e.g., coping with being late) tasks. While participating in behavioral rehearsal, couples used cognitive coping strategies such as relaxation, imagery, and distraction. A similar protocol was implemented in the patient-only CST condition, but without a focus on couples' communication or mutual goal setting. In contrast, patients and their partners in the education and support control conditions received basic information about OA, and methods of diagnosis and treatment.

Compared with patients in the education control group, patients in the couple-oriented CST condition experienced lower levels of pain, problematic pain behavior, and psychological disability posttreatment. However, in contrast with the authors' expectation, spouse-assisted CST was not significantly more effective than conventional CST in improving patient outcomes. In addition, the dyad CST also provided no advantage in terms of enhancing marital adjustment among patients or their spouses. Although these findings demonstrate the benefit of CST over informational or education meetings for patients' response to treatment, they suggest that spousal involvement may not be essential for improving couples' satisfaction with their relationship.

Another study of 59 patients with RA and their spouses evaluated the effects of a cognitive–behavioral program and found similar results with regard to spousal outcomes (van Lankveld et al., 2004). Patients attended eight sessions over a period of 4 weeks, either with or without a spouse present. The program was aimed specifically at restructuring disease-related cognitions and decreasing passive coping. Although the content covered was similar across conditions, lessons in the couples' condition also focused on the consequences of RA on the patient–spouse relationship. Contrary to prediction, spousal assistance provided no added benefits over the patient-oriented condition in terms of patients' physical or psychological functioning, coping, or marital satisfaction. Although patients in the couple-oriented program reported greater improvement in arthritis-related communication with their spouse, analyses indicated that spouses participating in the treatment did not improve on any of the psychosocial variables assessed (i.e., psychological functioning, coping, or marital satisfaction).

Similar findings have been documented in studies using alternative approaches to behavioral therapy. As delineated in Table 8.1, a study of 63 patients with chronic low-back pain (Saarijarvi, 1991; Saarijarvi et al., 1991) compared the effectiveness of couples-based therapy with usual care. Patients assigned randomly to couples' therapy participated in five monthly sessions, each lasting 1 to 2 hours. Therapists modeled communication through active questioning and feedback. Although patients receiving the intervention showed marked improvements in marital communication compared with those patients receiving usual care, no differences were found for spouses.

The third strategy used in family-based interventions for CMP is that of education and support. In a pilot study of 24 female patients with OA and their husbands, Martire and colleagues (2003) explored whether couple-oriented education and support intervention were more efficacious than a similar patient-oriented intervention. The couples' intervention was adapted from the Arthritis Self-Help Course (ASHC [Lorig, 1995]), which has been used with success in reducing patients' pain severity and depressive symptoms, and in enhancing patients' self-efficacy. The original program included information on improving communication and coping with negative emotions, but was supplemented in the dyadic intervention with 20-minute segments at the end of each weekly session to target couples' issues explicitly. Both interventions were well-received, and patients in the couple-oriented condition reported increased efficacy in managing pain symptoms. However, no treatment effects emerged for spouses in terms of marital satisfaction. Nevertheless, because of the small sample size, the authors concluded that additional research was necessary.

Building on this pilot study, Martire and colleagues (2007) expanded their sample to include 242 older adults with OA and their spouses who were assigned randomly to one of three conditions: patient-oriented education and support, couple-oriented education and support, or usual care. This time, spouses reported greater reductions in stress and less critical attitudes than spouses in the other groups. In particular, moderator analyses revealed that wives of male patients and spouses with high marital satisfaction experienced significantly lower depressive symptoms and greater confidence in their caregiving abilities. Notably, this large-scale study was also successful in showing that dyad education and support not only reduced spouses' punishing responses (e.g., anger, irritation), but also had concrete benefits to the patients' physical symptoms (i.e., reducing pain and improving physical function). Unlike prior educational programs (Keefe et al., 1996; Keefe et al., 1999), this intervention was designed to promote effective communication and strategies for soliciting spousal support and assistance. Moreover, it required active involvement by the spouse, rather than simply attending educational or informational sessions about arthritis.

The interventions just described and outlined in Table 8.1 show varied levels of benefit to patients and family members. More important, the advantages of family involvement may be contingent on the type of intervention delivered (i.e., behavioral vs. educational vs. couple's therapy), as well as the unique clinical problems of individual patients (e.g., behavioral disability and compliance responses) and characteristics of family members (e.g., marital satisfaction, caregiving mastery, proximity to patient). Interventions that address the spouse's role in goal setting and coping directly may have the potential to elicit the strongest benefits that may not be obtained when spouses simply attend an education or instruction program. In general, multicomponent interventions are thought to promote larger (and more long-term) effects for the dyad (Martire et al., 2007). For instance, supplementing education and support interventions with cognitive–behavioral or exercise training may target multiple aspects of the biopsychosocial nature of the pain experience.

EFFORTS TO IMPLEMENT FAMILY-BASED INTERVENTIONS IN THE COMMUNITY

Currently, no efforts have been made to implement family based-interventions for patients with CMP in community settings. However, patient-centered versions have been recommended for dissemination in the public health arena (Brady, Jernick, Hootman, & Sniezek, 2009; Lorig, González, Laurent, Morgan, & Laris, 1998) and have been applied in both national and international contexts. For example, the Arthritis Self-Management Program (ASMP), formerly known as ASHC (Lorig, 1995), has been implemented with success in Hispanic communities (Lorig, Gonzalez, & Ritter, 1999; Wong, Harker, Lau, Shatzel, & Port, 2004). In a randomized controlled trial of Spanish-speakers, participants in the intervention condition demonstrated both short- and long-term benefits over waitlist controls, including improved health status, health behaviors, and self-efficacy (Lorig et al., 1999). The program has since been licensed by Stanford University as the Spanish Arthritis Empowerment Program and was implemented effectively in low-income, indigent, and migrant Hispanic communities (Wong et al., 2004). Given the low cost and versatility of the ASMP, this program has been disseminated in Hong Kong (Siu & Chui, 2004) and Australia (Osborne, Wilson,

Lorig, & McColl, 2007). Participants in both cultures showed long-term gains with regard to self-efficacy and increased health behaviors.

Earlier efforts recommend that cultural adaptations of the ASMP should not be direct translations of the English version, but rather culturally sensitive reflections of the original program content (Lorig et al., 1999; Wong et al., 2004). Accordingly, future translation efforts with family-based programs for CMP should take into account cultural norms and variations in relational exchanges and communication processes while maintaining program fidelity. One strategy used by previous research groups was to draw on feedback from focus groups to develop culturally appropriate content (Lorig et al., 1999). This method would be equally suited for translating family-based programs to diverse communities.

In addition to disseminating the ASMP in culturally diverse settings, the program has also been adapted for arthritis patients who are unable or unwilling to attend the program in person. Both Internet (Lorig, Ritter, Laurent, & Plant, 2008) and mail delivery (Goeppinger et al., 2009) have been deemed viable alternatives to the original, small-group ASMP. Similar modes could be adapted for use with couples. However, given the importance of dyadic communication and interaction in family-based approaches (Martire et al., 2007), this form of delivery would require dyads to cohabit or at least complete the training in person. Last, because the original ASHC has been adapted successfully for use with couples (Martire et al., 2007), it is a promising candidate for further translation and dissemination efforts.

LIMITATIONS OF FAMILY-BASED INTERVENTIONS AND FUTURE RESEARCH

In the intervention literature for patients with CMP and their families, little attention has been given to the benefits of such interventions to family members themselves. Therefore, the need for a larger evidence base is urgent. As is evident from the research described in this chapter, more than half a decade has passed since publication of any novel intervention program for patients with CMP and their partners. Recent meta-analyses (Martire et al., 2010) and review articles (Keefe & Somers, 2010; Martire, 2013) confirm the lag in empirical data, revealing that many of the future directions proposed by earlier studies have yet to be explored.

Although important advances have been made during the past several decades, including examining physical *and* psychosocial variables as well as assessing (to a limited extent) spousal outcomes, several notable gaps and deficiencies remain. Next we describe the strengths and weaknesses of the interventions to date, highlighting the commendable advancements that have been made, as well as several key gaps in the current body of research. After these deficiencies have been addressed, strong efforts are needed to implement family-based interventions for patients with CMP in community settings. As a result of the limited evidence-based research in this area, practitioners should use caution when attempting to translate these findings into practice.

Beyond simply expanding the current evidence base, advancement of intervention research for patients with CMP and their relatives requires addressing certain deficits in study design and methodology, as well as incorporating new program content and delivery methods. For example, mail delivery would be an appropriate method for implementing cognitive–behavioral or educational programs when individuals have difficulty accessing healthcare centers or clinics. Furthermore, assessing multiple outcomes and incorporating a wider range of assessment instruments should be a priority. With the rare exception (Martire et al., 2007; Martire et al., 2008), the majority of intervention studies involving family members measure a singular outcome—most often, spouse's marital adjustment or satisfaction. More important, using a broader spectrum of measures would capture a more nuanced understanding of family members' experiences. For instance, an exemplary study by Martire and colleagues (2007) assessed specific types of marital interactions, such as spouses' emotional support and reactions to patients' pain behavior. In doing so, the authors were able to uncover a fine-grain depiction of couples' relationship function and exchanges. Future studies should capitalize on this strength to replicate and compare these outcomes.

In addition, interventions that incorporate and assess the positive dimensions of caring for individuals with CMP would further contribute to clinical efforts in this area (Zarit, 2012). For example, extending the findings by Martire and colleagues (2003, 2007), program content aimed at enhancing self-efficacy and internal control beliefs could help combat stressors associated with caregiver burden. Likewise, instruction on cognitive reappraisal strategies could aid caregivers in reframing negative experiences during periods of high stress. Scholars have also proposed examining whether spouse-assisted interventions could alter spouses' responses and reactions within specific settings or under particularly stressful circumstances (Keefe et al., 1996); unfortunately, empirical assessments have yet to follow. Because prior interventions have relied almost exclusively on self-reported measures, they may not have detected the full range of spouses' attitudes and behaviors toward the patient. Supplementing self-report with observational methods, although costly, would be a valuable next step.

Another notable deficiency in methodology has been the failure to capture data on treatment fidelity, or even report the extent to which the family member participated in the intervention (e.g., the number of sessions attended, frequency of care provision) (Martire, 2005; Martire, 2013). This information would provide important contextual data for readers to assess the strength of the study design and retention rates of both members of the dyad. In addition, low statistical power and failure to conduct longitudinal assessments have been cited as common limitations. Although earlier studies have advocated for exploring the potential long-term benefits of family involvement (Keefe et al., 1996) as well as the impact of using booster sessions (Riemsma, Taal, & Rasker, 2003), few interventions have done so.

Many of the interventions for patients with CMP and their family members have also been restricted by the homogeneity of their samples. Although CMP conditions affect minorities disproportionately, these groups have been neglected in previous studies (Green et al., 2003). In fact, only three of the interventions described in this chapter mention the racial composition of the study sample (Martire et al., 2007; Martire et al., 2008; Turner et al., 1990), with samples ranging from 90% to 100% white participants. Given the National Institutes of Health emphasis on addressing health disparities (National Institutes of Health, 2012) oversampling of racial and ethnic minorities should be a priority in future interventions.

Another group receiving little attention in family-based interventions has been the adult children of older parents with pain conditions (Riffin et al., 2012). None of the interventions that assess caregiver outcomes have incorporated adult children. Given that adult offspring comprise the largest group of those providing informal assistance to individuals age 65 years or older (Center on Aging Society, 1999), they should not be overlooked in future family-based interventions. A logical next step would be to explore how previously implemented approaches could be modified for use with adult children or friends (Keefe et al., 1996). Differences between spousal and adult child caregivers should also be evaluated to determine how interventions could be tailored for each group. More broadly, studies should explore particular characteristics of caregivers (e.g., gender, relationship to the patient, frequency of contact, relationship quality) and patients (e.g., years lived with pain), and their respective associations with specific intervention outcomes (e.g., caregivers' relational, emotional, and physical well-being).

A particular topic area in need of further investigation is the important role of premorbid and current marital satisfaction. In contrast with empirical evidence documenting marital dissatisfaction within dyads coping with chronic pain (Kerns & Weiss, 1994; Leonard et al., 2006), the samples in the interventions reviewed in this chapter were generally pleased with their marriages and reported high levels of marital satisfaction even before treatment (Keefe et al., 1996; van Lankveld et al., 2004). Interestingly, spouses who were already highly satisfied in their marriage experienced greater treatment gains and better psychological outcomes after participating in a couple-oriented education and support intervention (Martire et al., 2007). Perhaps couples who are already contented in their marriages enjoy the communal style of shared coping and draw more readily on preexisting relational resources necessary to engage in therapy. In future intervention research, an emphasis should be placed on identifying couples who are in unhappy or dysfunctional marriages, and investigating ways to assist these dyads in achieving treatment gains comparable with their well-adjusted counterparts.

Although formalized protocols have yet to emerge, pilot testing is underway to ascertain the feasibility and potential efficacy of an innovative intervention program targeting pain communication between arthritis patients and their relatives (Keefe & Somers, 2010). The authors conjecture that instructing dyads in specific communication and problem-solving skills will confer benefits to both members of the dyad and to the overall relationship. Indeed, recent reviews suggest that couples' communication may play an integral role in marital functioning, especially for those coping with chronic disease (Martire et al., 2010). With regard to empirical assessments, ecological momentary assessment has been proposed as an optimally suited method to capture couple's patterns of communication and interaction (Martire, 2013).

To illustrate the obstacles associated with family-oriented interventions for patients with CMP and their spouses, as well as the salient role of marital satisfaction in moderating intervention effects, we present two case studies of couples enrolled in such programs. A brief discussion follows the case presentations, outlining the challenges and suggestions for improving the care of these patients and their spouses.

Case Study 1: "Successful Outcomes for Spouses Enrolled in a Couple-Oriented Eduation and Support Intervention"

A study investigating the efficacy of a couple-oriented education and support intervention was conducted at the University of Pittsburg. Mrs. G. was referred to the study by her rheumatologist to assist with postsurgical rehabilitation. The written referral indicated that she is 59 years old, white, married, and diagnosed with OA in both knees. Her condition has persisted for the past 9 years, currently affecting her walking ability and preventing her from going up or down stairs. She also reported morning stiffness and reduced range of motion in both knees. Because her condition precluded her from work, Mrs. G. had recently undergone knee replacement surgery. After the operation, her doctor prescribed flurbiprofen (100 mg/day) for short-term relief of her pain symptoms, and recommended the intervention program as an additional recuperative strategy.

Mrs. G.'s primary caregiver was her husband (a 61-year-old white male) of 32 years who also managed multiple health conditions of his own. Because both Mr. and Mrs. G. were unemployed as a result of disability, their income was restricted. With difficulty, they found a provider who took their long-term disability insurance for Mrs. G's surgery. Without a home health aide, Mr. G. took on intense caregiving duties after Mrs. G.'s surgery, including cleaning, driving, preparing meals, coordinating medication, and performing other treatment-related activities (e.g., doctor's visits).

At the baseline assessment, both members of the dyad reported high levels of marital satisfaction and closeness, although Mrs. G. reported low levels of self-efficacy and moderate depressive symptomatology. She also reported high levels of pain and physical dysfunction. Mr. G. scored within the moderate range in confidence in his caregiving abilities and low with regard to critical attitudes. However, he reported high levels of psychological distress, including anxiety, depression, and worry. As is common for spouses scoring high on closeness with their partner, Mr. G. reported significant sleep impairment resulting in extreme fatigue and exhaustion. At the initial intake, he explained that his lack of sleep compromised his ability to carry out physical caregiving tasks as well as maintain a positive outlook on the situation.

The pair attended all six couple-oriented education and support group sessions together. At the end of the first weekly session, when participants were instructed to set a health-related goal for the coming week, she set the goal, "to walk for exercise two times over the next week for 5 minutes each time." Her husband set a related goal to accompany her on both walks. The health-related goal chosen by Mr. and Mrs. G. was manageable for Mrs. G., whose physical condition restricted her physical range of motion, and for Mr. G., who was experiencing significant sleep impairment accompanied by his own physical exhaustion. Moreover, because Mr. G.'s other caregiving duties are time-intensive, efforts were made to minimize additional burdens. Overall, selecting an appropriate goal that considers the needs of both the patient and the caregiver is essential to maintaining success in a couples-oriented program.

Although the education and support group sessions took place at a rheumatology clinic, much of the couples' practice took place in Mr. and Mrs. G.'s home. At the posttreatment assessment, Mrs. G. attributed her ability to maintain her walking regimen to her husband's consistent support during their daily interactions. Mr. G. plotted their walking routes each week, which he managed even through his fatigue. Mrs. G. also described the valuable communication skills she had learned. "I've never been good with words," she said, "but now I know asking for help isn't such a bad thing, after all. Fred's right there with me, willing to give a helping hand—literally!" She noted that she and Mr. G developed nonverbal cues throughout the course of treatment, and cited an example of when she would extend her elbow to Mr. G. when she wanted to request assistance during social situations but didn't want to call attention to her disability. The dyad rehearsed this in their home, then on family visits where descending stairs would have been an inevitable barrier.

Overall, Mrs. G. exhibited significant treatment gains. By the end of the sixth session, Mrs. G. had worked her way up to walking four times a week, 15 minutes at a time. She reported reductions in pain as well as improved physical function. She also scored significantly higher on arthritis self-efficacy than she did at the initial intake. Consistent with daily diary assessments (Martire et al., 2013), Mrs. G.'s pain was predictive of Mr. G.'s sleep patterns and overall feelings of rest. As Mrs. G.'s daily pain decreased, Mr. G.'s sleep quality improved. In addition, Mr. G. reported less anxiety and stress associated with caregiving tasks, as well as enhanced caregiving mastery. Meanwhile, his critical attitudes toward his wife remained low.

Case Study 2: "Challenges to Conducting a Couples-Oriented Education and Support Intervention for Spouses with Low Marital Quality at Baseline"

Mrs. P. is a 62-year-old, overweight, married female with severe OA in her left hip who was referred to a couples-oriented education and support intervention conducted at the University of Pittsburg. She had experienced high levels of pain almost every day for the past 2 years and took tramadol (300 mg/day) for her pain during the past year. Nevertheless, her disease had progressed enough to impair her ability to drive and to complete household tasks. She also had difficulty rising from a sitting position to a standing position, as well as standing for longer than 20 minutes. Her husband, exasperated by her complaints about pain, urged her to ask her doctor about additional treatments. As her condition worsened, she reluctantly agreed to enroll in an intervention study involving couples-oriented education and support.

At the baseline interview, Mrs. P. blamed herself for her condition. "It's all my fault," she lamented, further attributing the disease progression to her lack of exercise and poor diet. This perception was accompanied by a feeling of helplessness, which was reflected in a low score on psychological well-being at the baseline assessment. Mrs. P. scored low on arthritis self-efficacy, including her ability to manage symptoms such as fatigue, and scored high on the Center for Epidemiological Studies–Depression scale for depressive symptomatology. Mr. P. (a 61-year-old white male), her husband of 38 years, was also present at the baseline visit. He reported low levels of depression and perceived stress, but also scored low on caregiving mastery and high on critical attitudes toward his wife. Both members of the pair scored in the low range on marital satisfaction.

During the first session, Mr. P. expressed his frustration with having to take over all the household chores. "I just get fed up because she can't do the things she used to do. She doesn't like cooking because it's too hard for her to stand. She can't iron. Oh! And forget gardening!" At the two following sessions, Mrs. P. seemed more hopeless, noting that she'd "never improve." Mr. P. blamed Mrs. P. for her lack of success in executing the weekly health-related goals. He stated that "if she would just get off the sofa and into the kitchen, that would solve everything." He further explained, "She's become more like a child I need to look after—not like my wife. It's not an equal partnership. I feel more like her father."

Before the fourth session, the therapist received a phone call that Mrs. P. had fallen and would be unable to attend the next session. Because of the 2-week recovery period and Mrs. P.'s inability and unwillingness to come back to the group, she and Mr. P. only made it to four of the six therapy groups.

Mr. and Mrs. P. completed the postintervention measures, but failed to show any gains. At the 6-month follow-up, both individuals reported more depressive symptoms than they had before the treatment. This result is in keeping with the general trend for dyads enrolled in the couples-assisted education and support program, in which individuals who reported low levels of marital satisfaction at baseline became more depressed after participated in the program (Martire et al., 2007).

The case of Mr. and Mrs. P. illustrates several challenges therapists face when attempting to implement education and support interventions with chronic noncancer pain patients and their spouses. The initial challenge involves the dynamic interplay between the patient and spouse. A despairing and despondent attitude exhibited by the patient may be met with a reciprocal, or hostile, response by the spouse. Indeed, couples who initially report low marital satisfaction show marked difficulty throughout the course of the intervention (Martire et al., 2007). On the other hand, supportive couples, such as Mr. and Mrs. G., thrive off of one another's encouragement and appropriate support. They learn to work as a team and embrace the communal style of coping with the pain condition.

In addition to relational discord and marital conflict within the dyad, physical setbacks, such as a fall or sudden increase in pain symptoms, may deter attendance to the program. In turn, a precipitous increase in a patient's pain symptoms or sudden fall may ignite a solicitous or punishing response by the spouse. As in the case of Mr. and Mrs. P., a spouse may then become frustrated and angry with the patient, or deem the patient incapable of doing certain tasks. For the patient, the perilous combination of low self-efficacy in disease management and a physical setback may hinder participation even further, especially when the patient can muster neither the physical nor emotional strength to confront the illness. Similarly, an invasive medical procedure such as joint replacement may exact additional burdens on the caregiver. Surgery necessitates a host of ancillary duties, including coordinating medication and treatment visits for the ailing relative. Without restorative sleep, feelings of fatigue and exhaustion may set in, as they did for Mr. G. Enhancing self-efficacy through the execution of proximal, attainable goals is therefore critical for both the patient and caregiver. Interventions targeting control beliefs and self-management not only hold promise for improving treatment adherence and reducing symptomatology among patients (Gyurcsik et al., 2009; Marks, 2001), but also for preserving feelings of mastery among caregivers (Löckenhoff, Duberstein, Friedman, & Costa, 2011).

Therapists should be aware of these issues at the onset of treatment and attend to couples who have particular difficulty communicating in their marriage. Tailored interventions should maintain an emphasis on helping spouses to recognize their partner's verbal and nonverbal pain expression as well as their own supportive and unsupportive communication. Validating the family member's concerns and experiences may be one way to enhance participation and promote positive outcomes for both members of the dyad.

CONCLUSION

Overall, our review of the literature reveals a clear need for interventions designed specifically to investigate whether family-oriented approaches confer meaningful benefit, rather than burden, to family members with CMP. Assessing caregiver outcomes may provide a window into the mechanisms underlying patient treatment gains, such as spouses' greater compassion or increased knowledge about the condition. Although family-based intervention research for patients with CMP and their family members boasts a promising and growing amount of literature, it is clear that much more research is needed in this area before strong conclusions can be made.

REFERENCES

AGS Panel on Persistent Pain in Older People. (2002). The management of persistent pain in older persons. *Journal of the American Geriatric Society, 50*(6), 205–224.

Bradley, L. A., Young, L. D., Anderson, K. O., Turner, R. A., Agudelo, C. A., McDaniel, L. K., et al. (1987). Effects of psychological therapy on pain behavior of rheumatoid arthritis patients. *Arthritis and Rheumatism, 30*, 1105–1111.

Brady, T. J., Jernick, S. L., Hootman, J. M., & Sniezek, J. E. (2009). Public health interventions for arthritis: Expanding the toolbox of evidence-based interventions. *Journal of Women's Health, 18*(12), 1905–1917.

Center on Aging Society. (1999). *Informal caregiver supplement (ICS) to the 1999 National Longterm Care Survey (NLTCS)*. National Institue on Aging& Duke University Center for Demographic Studies. Retrieved from http://www.nltcs.aas.duke.edu/overview.htm

Fredman, L., Cauley, J. A., Hochberg, M., Ensrud, K. E., & Doros, G. (2010). Mortality associated with caregiving, general stress, and caregiving-related stress in elderly women: Results of caregiver-study of osteoporotic fractures. *Journal of the American Geriatrics Society, 58*(5), 937–943.

Goeppinger, J., Lorig, K. R., Ritter, P. L., Mutatkar, S., Villa, F., & Gizlice, Z. (2009). Mail-delivered arthritis self-management tool kit: A randomized trial and longitudinal follow-up. *Arthritis Care & Research, 61*(7), 867–875.

Green, C. R., Anderson, K. O., Baker, T. A., Campbell, L. C., Decker, S., Fillingim, R. B., et al. (2003). The unequal burden of pain: Confronting racial and ethnic disparities in pain. *Pain Medicine, 4*(3), 277–294.

Gyurcsik, N. C., Brawley, L. R., Spink, K. S., Brittain, D. R., Fuller, D. L., & Chad, K. (2009). Physical activity in women with arthritis: Examining perceived barriers and self-regulatory efficacy to cope. *Arthritis Care & Research, 61*(8), 1087–1094.

Helme, R. D., & Gibson, S. J. (2001). The epidemiology of pain in elderly people. *Clinical Geriatric Medicine, 17*(3), 417–413.

Institute of Medicine. (2011) Relieving pain in America: A blueprint for transforming prevention, care, education, and research. Washington, DC: National Academies Press.

Jakobsson, U., Klevsgard, R., Westergren, A., & Hallberg, I. R. (2003). Old people in pain: A comparative study. *Journal of Pain Symptom Management, 60*(6), 793–797.

Karp, J. F., Reynolds, C. F., 3rd, Butters, M. A., Dew, M. A., Mazumdar, S. Begley, A. E., et al. (2006). The relationship between pain and mental flexibility in older adult pain clinic patients. *Pain Medicine, 7*(5), 444–452.

Keefe, F. J., Blumenthal, J., Baucom, D., Affleck, G., Waugh, R., Caldwell, D. S., et al. (2004). Effects of spouse-assisted coping skills training and exercise training in patients with osteoarthritic knee pain: A randomized controlled study. *Pain, 110*(3), 539–549.

Keefe, F. J., Caldwell, D. S., Baucom, D., Salley, A., Robinson, E., Timmons, K., et al. (1996). Spouse-assisted coping skills training in the management of osteoarthritic knee pain. *Arthritis Care & Research, 9*, 279–291.

Keefe, F. J., Caldwell, D. S., Baucom, D., Salley, A., Robinson, E., Timmons, K., et al. (1999). Spouse-assisted coping skills training in the management of knee pain in osteoarthritis: Longterm follow-up results. *Arthritis Care and Research, 12*, 101–111.

Keefe, F. J., & Somers, T. J. (2010). Psychological approaches to understanding and treating arthritis pain. *Nature Reviews Rheumatology, 6*, 210–216.

Kerns, R. D., & Weiss, L. H. (1994). Family influences on the course of chronic illness: A cognitive–behavioral transactional model. *Annals of Behavioral Medicine, 16*(2), 116–121.

Lawton, M. P., Kleban, M. H., Moss, M., Rovine, M., & Glicksman, A. (1989). Measuring caregiving appraisal. *Journal of Gerontology, 44*(3), 61–71.

Leonard, M. T., Cano, A., & Johansen, A. B. (2006). Chronic pain in a couples context: A review and integration of theoretical models and empirical evidence. *Journal of Pain, 7*(6), 377–390.

Leveille, S. G., Fried, L., & Guralnik, J. M. (2002). Disabling symptoms: What do older women report? *Internal Medicine, 17*(10), 766–773.

Löckenhoff, C. E., Duberstein, P. R., Friedman, B., & Costa, P. T., Jr. (2011). Five-factor personality traits and subjective health among caregivers: The role of caregiver strain and self-efficacy. *Psychology and Aging, 26*(3), 592–604.

Lorig, K. (1995). Arthritis self-help course. *HMO Practice/HMO Group, 9*(2), 60.

Lorig, K., González, V. M., Laurent, D. D., Morgan, L., & Laris, B. A. (1998). Arthritis self-management program variations: Three studies. *Arthritis & Rheumatism, 11*(6), 448–454.

Lorig, K., Gonzalez, V. M., & Ritter, P. (1999). Community-based Spanish language arthritis education program: A randomized trial. *Medical Care, 37*(9), 957–963.

Lorig, K. R., Ritter, P. L., Laurent, D. D., & Plant, K. (2008). The Internet-based Arthritis Self-Management Program: A one-year randomized trial for patients with arthritis or fibromyalgia. *Arthritis Care & Research, 59*(7), 1009–1017.

Manne, S. L., & Zautra, A. J. (1989). Spouse criticism and support: their association with coping and psychological adjustment among women with rheumatoid arthritis. *Journal of personality and social psychology, 56*(4), 608–617.

Marks, R. (2001). Efficacy theory and its utility in arthritis rehabilitation: Review and recommendations. *Disability & Rehabilitation, 23*(7), 271–280.

Martire, L. M. (2005). The "relative" efficacy of involving family in psychosocial interventions for chronic illness: Are there added benefits to patients and family members? *Families, Systems, & Health, 23*(3), 312–328.

Martire, L. M. (2013). Couple-oriented interventions for chronic illness: Where do we go from here? *Journal of Social and Personal Relationships, 30*(2), 207–214.

Martire, L. M., Keefe, F. J., Schulz, R., Parris Stephens, M. A., & Mogle, J. A. (2013). The impact of daily arthritis pain on spouse sleep. *Pain, 154*(9), 1725–1731.

Martire, L. M., Lustig, A. P., Schulz, R., Miller, G. E., & Helgeson, V. S. (2004). Is it beneficial to involve a family member? A meta-analysis of psychosocial interventions for chronic illness. *Health Psychology, 23*(6), 599–611.

Martire, L. M., Schulz, R., Helgeson, V. S., & Small, B. J. (2010). Review and meta-analysis of couple-oriented interventions for chronic illness. *Annals of Behavioral Medicine, 40*(3), 325–342.

Martire, L. M., Schulz, R., Keefe, F. J., Rudy, T. E., & Starz, T. W. (2007). Couple-oriented education and support intervention: Effects on individuals with osteoarthritis and their spouses. *Rehabilitation Psychology, 52*(2), 121–132.

Martire, L. M., Schulz, R., Keefe, F. J., Rudy, T. E., & Starz, T. W. (2008). Couple-oriented education and support intervention for osteoarthritis: Effects on spouses' support and responses to patient pain. *Families, Systems, & Health, 26*(2), 185–295.

Martire, L. M., Schulz, R., Keefe, F. J., Starz, T. W., Osial, T. A., Dew, M. A., et al. (2003). Feasibility of a dyadic intervention for management of osteoarthritis: A pilot study with older patients and their spousal caregivers. *Aging and Mental Health, 7*(1), 53–60.

Matheson, L., Harcourt D., & Hewlett, S. (2010). "Your whole life, your whole world, it changes": Partners' experiences of living with rheumatoid arthritis. *Musculoskeletal Care, 8*, 46–54.

National Center for Chronic Disease Prevention and Health Promotion. (2000). *Chronic diseases and their risk factors: The nation's leading causes of death, 1999.* Bethesda, MD:Department of Health & Human Services.

Line, A. (2010). *NIAMS long-range plan: Fiscal years 2010–2014.* National Institute of Arthritis and Musculoskeletal and Skin Diseases. Retrieved from http://www.niams.nih.gov/about_Us/Mission_and_Purpose/long_range.asp

National Institutes of Health. (2012). *Science of eliminating health disparities summit.* National Harbor, MD: National Institute on MInority Health and Health Disparities.

Osborne, R. H., Wilson, T., Lorig, K. R., & McColl, G. J. (2007). Does self-management lead to sustainable health benefits in people with arthritis? A 2-year transition study of 452 Australians. *The Journal of Rheumatology, 34*(5), 1112–1117.

Parmelee, P. A., Katz, I. R., & Lawton, M. P. (1991). The relation of pain to depression among institutionalized aged. *Journals of Gerontology, 46*, P15–P21.

Radojevic, V., Nicassio, P. M., & Weisman, M. H. (1992). Behavioral intervention with and without family support for rheumatoid arthritis. *Behavior Therapy, 23*, 13–20.

Reid, M. C., Williams, C. S., & Gill, T. M. (2005). Back pain and decline in lower extremity physical function among community-dwelling older persons. *Journals of Gerontology: Medical Sciences, 60*(6), 793–797.

Revenson, T. A., Schiaffino, K. M., Majerovitz, S. D., & Gibofsky, A. (1991). Social support as a double-edged sword: The relation of positive and problematic support to depression among rheumatoid arthritis patients. *Social Science & Medicine, 33*(7), 807–813.

Riemsma, R. P., Taal, E., & Rasker, J. J. (2003). Group education for patients with rheumatoid arthritis and their partners. *Arthritis & Rheumatism, 49*, 556–566.

Riffin, C., Suitor, J. J., Reid, M. C., & Pillemer, K. (2012). Chronic pain and parent–child relations in later life: An important, but understudied issue. *Family Science, 3*(2), 75–85.

Rosland, A. M., Heisler, M., & Piette, J. D. (2012). The impact of family behaviors and communication patterns on chronic illness outcomes: A systematic review. *Journal of Behavioral Medicine, 35*(2), 221–239.

Saarijarvi, S. (1991). A controlled study of couple therapy in chronic low back pain patients: Effects on marital satisfaction, psychological distress and health attitudes. *Journal of Psychosomatic Research, 35*, 265–272.

Saarijärvi, S., Rytökoski, U., & Alanen, E. (1991). A controlled study of couple therapy in chronic low back pain patients. No improvement of disability. *Journal of psychosomatic research, 35*(6), 671–677.

Siu, A. M., & Chui, D. Y. (2004). Evaluation of a community rehabilitation service for people with rheumatoid arthritis. *Patient Education and Counseling, 55*(1), 62–69.

Sperry, L. (2009). *Treatment of chronic medical conditions: Cognitive–behavioral therapy strategies and integrative treatment protocols.* Washington DC: American Psychological Association.

Stephens, M. A. P., Martire, L. M., Cremeans-Smith, J. K., Druley, J. A., & Wojno, W. C. (2006). Older women with osteoarthritis and their caregiving husbands: Effects of patients' pain and pain expression. *Rehabilitation Psychology, 51*, 3–12.

Stephenson, E., DeLongis, A., Esdaile, J. M., & Lehman, A. J. (2013). Depressive symptoms and rheumatoid arthritis: Spouse empathic responding as a buffer. *Arthritis Care & Research, 66*, 532–541.

Tan, G., Jensen, M. P., Thornby, J., & Sloan, P. A. (2008). Negative emotions, pain and functioning. *Psychological Services, 5*(1), 26–35.

Turk, D. C., Flor, H., & Rudy, T. E. (1987). Pain and families: I. Etiology, maintenance, and psychosocial impact. *Pain, 30*, 3–27.

Turner, J. A., Clancy, S., McQuade, K. J., & Cardenas, D. D. (1990). Effectiveness of behavioral therapy for chronic low back pain: A component analysis. *Journal of Consulting and Clinical Psychology, 58*, 573–579.

van Lankveld, W., van Helmond, T., Naring, G., de Rooij, D. J., & van den Hoogen, F. (2004). Partner participation in cognitive–behavioral self-management group treatment for patients with rheumatoid arthritis. *Journal of Rheumatology, 31*, 1738–1745.

Walsh, J. D., Blanchard, E. B., Kremer, J. M., & Blanchard, C. G. (1999). The psychosocial effects of rheumatoid arthritis on the patient and the well partner. *Behaviour Research and Therapy, 37*, 259–271.

Wilson, S. J., Martire, L. M., Keefe, F. J., Mogle, J. A., Stephens, M. A. P., & Schulz, R. (2013). Daily verbal and nonverbal expression of osteoarthritis pain and spouse responses. *Pain, 154*, 2045–2063.

Wolfe, F., & Michaud, K. (2009). Predicting depression in rheumatoid arthritis: The signal importance of pain extent and fatigue, and comorbidity. *Arthritis & Rheumatism, 61*, 667–673.

Wong, A., Harker, J. O., Lau, V. P., Shatzel, S., & Port, L. H. (2004). Spanish Arthritis Empowerment Program: A dissemination and effectiveness study. *Arthritis & Rheumatism, 51*, 332–336.

Zarit, S. H. (2012). Positive aspects of caregiving: More than looking on the bright side, *Aging & Mental Health, 16*(6), 673–674,

Zhu, K., Devine, A., Dick, I. M., & Prince, R. L. (2007). Association of back pain frequency with mortality, coronary heart events, mobility, and quality of life in elderly women. *Spine, 32*(18), 2012–2018.

9

Heart Failure and Debilitating Cardiovascular Problems

SUSAN J. PRESSLER, MIYEON JUNG, AND JAMES FRIEDMAN ■

Cardiovascular syndromes and diseases are prevalent and debilitating. In 2010, approximately 83.6 million persons in the United States suffered from cardiovascular syndromes and diseases, making them some of the most common problems among older adults (Go et al., 2013). Estimates are that by 2030 40% of the United States population will have some form of cardiovascular disease.

During the past 30 years, tremendous improvements have been achieved in the treatment of persons with cardiovascular conditions. During this same period of time, chronic heart failure has become much more prevalent, with people living longer with more severe symptoms. Heart failure has become widely recognized as the "final common pathway" for multiple cardiovascular conditions, including hypertension and coronary artery disease (Bonow, Mann, Zipes, & Libby, 2011). Many cardiovascular diseases are preventable or can be delayed with lifestyle choices, including regular exercise, healthy diet, weight management (Aggarwal, Liao, Christian, & Mosca, 2008), abstinence from tobacco smoking, and early treatment of hypertension and hypercholesteremia. As we age, maintaining such a regimen may be commensurate with preserving life quality and delaying disease progression. Often, family members are integral to helping older persons with debilitating cardiovascular conditions maintain such regimens.

Caregivers who are involved substantially in the welfare of loved ones with heart failure or its precipitating disease states may also be at increased risk for heart disease themselves. Recent research suggests that caregiving is an independent risk factor for cardiovascular illness and even death. In addition, family caregivers often experience depression, obesity, anxiety, and emotional distress (Aggarwal et al., 2008; Hartmann, Bazner, Wild, Eisler, & Herzog, 2010). Furthermore, research findings suggest that caregiving is associated with poor social support and poor family support. As a result, family caregivers may not be able to meet their own needs for healthy lifestyle choices themselves. Finding ways to empower healthy lifestyle choices is important for families living with the influence of heart disease and heart failure, and is considered a crucial research area (Aggarwal et al., 2008).

A number of previous studies have been conducted among patients who have a chronic disease and family members to improve education and care after these events. Reviews of these studies, including meta-analyses, demonstrate that interventions that engage family caregivers and the individual living with a chronic disease such as heart failure experience reciprocal benefit from specific interventions aimed at improving outcomes and preventing myriad comorbid conditions (Hartmann et al., 2010; Martire, Schulz, Helgeson, Small, & Saghafi, 2010). Although the effects of such interventions are small to modest (0.35 for family member health), such effects are broad, significant, and stable over long follow-up intervals (Hartmann et al., 2010). The purpose of this chapter is to review and synthesize available interventions for family caregivers of older adults with cardiovascular conditions—specifically, chronic heart failure.

BACKGROUND

One of the most severe cardiovascular conditions, chronic heart failure has received a great deal of attention from healthcare providers and researchers during the past two decades because of its prevalence and severity. Heart failure is recognized as the "final common pathway" for multiple cardiovascular conditions, including hypertension and coronary heart disease (Bonow et al., 2011). More than 5.1 million Americans have heart failure, and 670,000 new cases are reported annually (Roger et al., 2012). Heart failure is a life-limiting illness with a 12-month mortality rate of 29.6%; approximately 70% of patients will survive longer than 12 months (Chen, Normand, Wang, & Krumholz, 2011). The burden of heart failure to patients and families is tremendous. Most patients with heart failure are required to follow a complex medication and dietary regimen, and to monitor symptoms indicating sodium and fluid volume excess to prevent major complications, unnecessary hospitalizations, and death (Riegel et al., 2009).

During the past two decades, high-tech therapeutic interventions (e.g., implantable cardioverter defibrillators, vascular assistive devices) have become increasingly common in heart failure, contributing further to the complexity of care required by these patients (Yancy et al., 2013). Family caregivers are responsible for providing daily care associated with these life-saving technologies. The most frequent daily tasks reported by 63 family caregivers of heart failure patients were providing transportation (81%), seeking information (81%), monitoring symptoms (70%), and completing tasks outside the home (68%) (Pressler et al., 2012).

As anticipated, caregivers of patients with more severe heart failure had significantly more perceived time and difficulty with tasks, greater anxiety, and poorer physical health. The tasks on which caregivers reported spending most time daily were providing emotional support (mean, 10.7 hours; median, 3.5 hours), monitoring symptoms (mean, 10.7 hours; median, 4 hours), and helping patients communicate (mean, 6.7 hours; median, 1 hour). The tasks on which caregivers reported spending the most time weekly were household tasks (mean, 7.5 hours; median, 3 hours), providing emotional support (mean, 4.7 hours; median, 2 hours), managing dietary needs (mean, 4.4 hours; median, 3 hours), and providing transportation (mean, 4.4 hours; median, 3 hours). Caregivers of patients with advanced heart failure who have ventricular assistive devices implanted require additional training to learn skills to maintain proper functioning of such devices and to troubleshoot problems. More frequent healthcare visits are usually indicated for assessment of device functioning, contributing further to family caregivers' demands.

The care needs of patients with heart failure are well described (Riegel et al., 2009). As heart failure progresses, patients experience diminished quality of life because of dyspnea, fatigue, cognitive dysfunction, edema, depression, anxiety, and sleep disturbances. Frequent exacerbations are common, necessitating intermittent, unplanned hospitalizations. Patients' conditions have been shown to deteriorate with each hospitalization (Gheorghiade & Pang, 2009). The high symptom burden of heart failure, which is frequently exacerbated after hospitalizations, makes the condition of heart failure particularly challenging for family caregivers to manage effectively (Murray, Kendall, Boyd, & Sheikh, 2005; Pressler et al., 2009). Specifically, the shrinking length of hospital stays and affordable presence of professional support means family members must function as primary caregivers for relatives who experience progressive burdens of chronic disease (Shewchuk & Elliott, 2000). Often, such responsibilities include the provision of nursing-like care, including equipment monitoring, discharge coordination after hospital visits, and administration of medications. These activities, coupled with the provision of care to address activity of daily living dependencies common in older adults with heart failure, strongly emphasize the potential emotional and psychological distress for which family caregivers of older adults with debilitating cardiovascular conditions are at risk. Molloy and colleagues summarize several studies that describe these challenges further in terms of poor adherence to interventional regimens and lack of understanding in recognizing and managing emergent circumstances or worsening symptoms that may propagate rehospitalizations (Molloy, Johnston, Gao, & Witham, 2004). In addition, they found that lack of knowledge or misconceptions about heart failure, relationship intimacy, and sexuality contribute to increasing caregiver stress and symptoms of depression. Molloy and colleagues suggest that deficits in information may influence care management negatively, and may influence both patient and caregiver quality of life negatively (Molloy et al., 2004).

The 2009 National Alliance of Caregiving/American Association of Retired Persons report on family caregiving in the United States found that 5% of all caregivers were assisting someone with heart disease (National Alliance of Caregiving/American Association of Retired Persons, 2009). The majority (40%–75%) of family caregivers of patients with heart failure are spouses (Ågren, Evangelista, Hjelm, & Strömberg, 2012; Chiang, Chen, Dai, & Ho, 2012; Hwang, Fleischmann, Howie-Esquivel, Stotts, & Dracup, 2011; Leff et al., 2006; Molloy et al., 2006; Sebern & Woda, 2012), who may themselves have chronic health conditions (e.g., hypertension, diabetes). Thus, caregivers may be managing their own health conditions as well as their spouses' heart failure, and this may increase caregiver stress and burden even further. Family caregivers providing care to a relative living with heart failure generally report their lives change for the worse as a result of care responsibilities (Bakas, Pressler, Johnson, Nauser, & Shaneyfelt, 2006). Furthermore, Bakas and colleagues found that 57% of caregivers rated their emotional well-being as worsening as a result of caring for someone with heart failure, and 48% of these caregivers reported change for the worse in terms of their future outlook, level of energy, time for social activities, and their financial wellness (Bakas et al., 2006). Another 48% reported a change for the worse with regard to their physical health, and one third reported worsening of their general overall health.

Case Study 1: "I Have a Husband and Children To Care For, a Job to Make a Living, and Mom to Care For"

Multiple Demands and Financial Losses

Forty-one-year-old S. M. is the primary caregiver for her mother who is 78 years old and was diagnosed with heart failure 3 years previously. They do not live together; her mother lives in a nearby assisted-living facility. S. M. has been a caregiver for a long time, not only for her mother, but also for her father. Her father, who died 2 years earlier, had dementia for more than a decade. Before she got married 5 years earlier, S. M. had helped her mother take care of her father while living in the same home. When her mother developed heart failure, S. M. became the adult child who provided most of the care for both parents. Her brother was not close to the parents and now he is on active duty in the military. S. M. feels exhausted mentally and physically. After being a caregiver for her father and now her mother, it feels like she has been a caregiver forever.

In addition to caring for her mother, S. M. has a very busy life, with two young children and her job. Her husband has helped and is very supportive, but her multiple responsibilities remain. She has to hire a sitter to care for her children when she is caring for her mother. The cost of the sitter and the extra expenses for her mother's health care make it difficult for S. M. to take time off from work. Fortunately, her work schedule is flexible. However, she has to be careful about time away from work and can only take her mother to doctor appointments when there is a real need, because her time is limited and one appointment may take the entire afternoon. She hopes that caregiving will get easier, but it seems doubtful.

Possible Intervention

Few interventions are available to assist adult children caring for aging parents who are balancing multiple roles. In the case of S. M., she could consider working fewer hours, but this would cause financial hardship for her family. Hiring more help to care for her mother would also add to her family's financial hardship. One possible intervention is for S. M. to talk with her healthcare providers to determine whether her mother is eligible for coverage of home healthcare aides to assist with her care. Another option is for S. M. to hire a home healthcare aide for a limited time, such as one evening a week, to provide some more time for her husband and children. Another intervention could be for S. M.'s mother to move in with S. M. so it would be easier to provide her care and could ease some financial burden.

REVIEW OF LITERATURE ON CAREGIVERS OF PATIENTS WITH HEART FAILURE

Results of the review of literature about caregivers of patients with heart failure are presented below. The search strategies are first presented, followed by studies obtained and a critique of the studies.

Search Strategies

In three separate literature reviews of published articles spanning January 1990 to December 2012, 199 publications about family caregiving in heart failure were found (Bakas et al., 2006; Pressler et al., 2012). Databases searched were Medline, Cumulative Index to Nursing and Allied Health Literature, and PsycInfo. Keywords used in the searches were *caregivers, caregiving, heart failure—congestive, heart failure, heart transplantation, heart transplant*, and *cardiac transplant*. In the search from 1990 to 2004, 79 publications were found and reviewed. Family caregivers reported increased stress and decreased physical and emotional health (Bakas et al., 2006). In the search from 2004 through 2011, an additional 83 publications were found (Pressler et al., 2012). This search was expanded from 2011 through December 2012, and another 37 publications were identified, for a total of 120 publications from 2004 to 2012. The abstract of each publication was reviewed. In cases when the abstract was not available or was insufficient to categorize the publication, the full publication was reviewed. The 120 publications were categorized as follows: did not address family caregivers although matched by keywords ($n = 18$, 15%), included data from patients about their caregivers but not data from family caregivers ($n = 1$, 1%), commentary ($n = 6$, 5%), review ($n = 9$, 8%), clinical care ($n = 6$, 5%), ethical issues ($n = 3$, 3%), and data-based study ($n = 77$, 64%; Figure 9.1). The 77 data-based publications were categorized by study design as follows: nonexperimental quantitative ($n = 38$), qualitative ($n = 22$), methodological/psychometric ($n = 9$), experimental or quasi-experimental ($n = 7$), and focus group ($n = 1$). The focus of the following synthesis is on experimental or quasi-experimental studies ($n = 7$). Table 8.1 features key extracted information from included reviews and individual studies.

Results of Experimental and Quasi-experimental Studies

Seven of the 120 publications reported results of tests of interventions, with three studies using experimental designs (Ågren et al., 2012; Molloy et al., 2006; Schwarz, Mion, Hudock, & Litman, 2008) and four using quasi-experimental designs (Chiang et al., 2012; Leff et al., 2006; Piette et al., 2008; Sebern & Woda, 2012). An additional randomized controlled trial was also found. These eight interventions are summarized in Table 9.1.

STUDY CHARACTERISTICS

Types of interventions delivered included nurse-led education and support classes (Agren et al., 2012), telehealth monitoring with nurse follow-up and discharge planning (Chiang et al., 2012), physician and nurse visits for patients receiving acute hospital care at home (Leff et al., 2006), an exercise intervention for patients (Molloy et al., 2006), an automated intervention to assist caregivers in managing patients' health (Piette et al., 2008), classes to improved shared decision making with regard to patients' health (Sebern & Woda, 2012), electronic health monitoring with support from advanced practice nurses to improve patients' health (Schwarz et al., 2008), and telehealth counseling to improve family caregivers' own heart health. The most common type of intervention modalities were care management ($n = 3$) and self-care/counseling approaches ($n = 2$).

Although all studies included measures completed by caregivers, the interventions tested were targeted primarily at improving patients' health rather than being focused on caregivers' health. The study by Sebern and Woda (2012) did incorporate shared decision making between patients and their caregivers. Designs of the studies varied. Two studies were reported as feasibility studies (Piette et al., 2008; Sebern & Woda, 2012) and one as a pilot study (Schwarz et al., 2008). Three studies reported that dyads or family caregivers were randomized to treatment and control groups (Ågren et al., 2012; Schwarz et al., 2008), and one reported that patients were randomized to groups (Molloy et al., 2006).

EDUCATIONAL AND TRANSITIONAL CARE

Chiang and colleagues (2012) tested an educational intervention that was based on Meleis' transition theory (Chick & Meleis, 1986; Schumacher & Meleis, 1994) and included discharge planning and telehealth education delivered by

Table 9.1. Intervention Studies for Family Caregivers of Patients with Heart Failure (2004–2012, $N = 7$)

Author (Year)	Design/Sampling	Subject Characteristics	Methods/Interventions	Data/Measures	Findings/Outcomes	Limitations
Ågren et al., 2012	Experimental/ random assignment to intervention or control groups Recruitment by invitation to eligible dyad from two hospitals in Sweden	155 caregiver–patient with heart failure dyads; 71 intervention, 84 control Intervention group: caregiver mean age, 67 years; 69.1% women; patient mean age, 69 years; 69.1% men Control group: caregiver mean age, 70 years; 80.9% women; patient mean age, 73 years; 80.9% men	Theoretical background: shared care Intervention: usual care plus integrated dyad care including psychosocial support, three sessions (each session ≥60 minutes) through nurse-led face-to-face counseling, computer- based education, and written teaching materials at 2, 6, and 12 weeks after hospital discharge Control: usual care of patient education (caregivers were excluded in this usual care) Follow-up at 3 and 12 months after baseline assessment	Pre/post measures: Medical Outcomes Study Short Form-36 (patient + caregiver) Beck Depression Inventory (patient + caregiver) Control Attitude Scale (patient + caregiver) European Heart Failure Self-Care Behavior Scale (patient only) Caregiver Burden Scale (caregiver only)	*t*-Tests and chi-square tests were conducted. Patients' perceived control over the cardiac condition increased more in the intervention group compared with the control group after 3 months ($p < .05$) but not after 12 months. No effect was seen for caregivers. No group differences were noted in dyads' health- related quality of life, depressive symptoms, patients' self-care behaviors, and caregivers' experiences of caregiver burden.	No detailed information about caregivers was included except age, gender, and comorbidity. Race and ethnicity were not reported. No description of cultural aspects was included.

| Chiang et al., 2012 | Quasi-experimental, no randomization Dyads chose either intervention or control group as a result of intervention cost for telehealth device and service fee Recruitment from a heart failure center in Taiwan | 60 caregiver–patient with heart failure dyads; 30 intervention, 30 control Intervention group: caregiver: relationship, 46.7% spouse; 66.7% female; 86.7% older than 40 years; 56.7% with chronic disease; patient: 66.7% female, 100% older than 40 years, 66.7% more than two comorbidities Control group: caregiver: 76.6% female; 80.0% older than 40 years; relationship, 50% spouse; 50% with chronic disease; patient: 66.7% female, 100% older than 40 years, 76.7% more than two comorbidities | Theoretical background: Meleis' transition theory Intervention: discharge planning and telehealth care by a team of physicians and nurses; telenursing specialist educated family caregiver to measure patients' physiological changes and to upload data through telehealth device, which monitored 24/7 and was connected to the hospital Control: traditional discharge planning by a care manager Follow-up at 30 days after baseline. | Pre/post measures: (caregiver only for all outcome variables) Chinese version of Caregiver Burden Inventory Mastery of Stress Scale Chinese version of Feetham Family Functioning Survey | Mixed-model analyses were conducted. Baseline equivalency was confirmed except for greater developmental burden among caregivers in the intervention group. Overall caregiver burden decreased in the intervention group compared with the control group at 30 days follow-up ($1F = 11.4333$, $p < .001$). Mastery of stress and family functioning were improved in the intervention group over the control group at 30 days ($F = -22.733$, $p < .001$; $F = -5.767$, $p < .001$). | No randomization occurred in this study. Patients in the telehealth intervention group were required to pay for the telehealth system. Race and ethnicity were not reported and there was no description of cultural aspects. |

(continued)

Table 9.1. CONTINUED

Author (Year)	Design/Sampling	Subject Characteristics	Methods/Interventions	Data/Measures	Findings/Outcomes	Limitations
Leff, 2006	Quasi-experimental, no randomization (only intervention-phase data were used for this study); patients offered Hospital at Home care, refused, or not offered because of service time (6 a.m.–10 p.m.) Recruitment from four hospitals in United States	141 patients (congestive heart failure, chronic obstructive pulmonary disease, pneumonia, or cellulitis) and caregiver dyads; 84 intervention, 57 control Intervention group: caregiver mean age, 59.0 years; 18% men; relationship, 36% spouse; 69% living with patient; patient mean age, 76.6 years; 67% men; primary diagnosis, congestive heart failure (22%), chronic obstructive pulmonary disease (33%), pneumonia (24%), cellulitis (21%) Control group: caregiver mean age, 61.8 years; 17% men; relationship, 49% spouse; 62% living with patient; patient mean age, 77.1 years; 74% men; primary diagnosis congestive heart failure (20%), chronic obstructive pulmonary disease (17%), pneumonia (39%), cellulitis (24%)	Intervention: Hospital at Home care, which provides daily physician visits and nursing supervision for initial period of event, and intermittent nursing visits Control: acute care hospital admission with usual care	Post measures: Patient and caregiver satisfaction were measured 2 weeks after acute care hospital or Hospital at Home admission via telephone interviews A satisfaction survey developed from the Picker Commonwealth Scale for this study (patient and caregiver)	Chi-square test, Fisher's exact test, and logistic regression analyses were conducted. Patient and caregiver characteristics were similar except for patients' instrumental activities of daily living (more limitation in intervention group). Patient satisfaction with physicians ($p = .007$), comfort and convenience of care ($p = .0003$), admission procedures ($p = .0003$), and overall satisfaction ($p = .034$) were greater in the intervention group than in the control group, but no significant differences were found in satisfaction with nurse, pain control, safety, or discharge procedure. Caregiver satisfaction was similar to patient satisfaction, but caregivers using Hospital Home care were satisfied with nurses ($p = .013$) and the discharge procedure ($p = .0003$), but not the admission procedure.	A theoretical background was not described and there was no randomization. The study targeted patients primarily. Race and ethnicity were not reported and there was no description of cultural aspects.

| Molloy et al., 2006 | Experimental/random assignment of patients to intervention or control groups Recruitment by invitation to caregivers identified from patients in Scotland, UK | 60 caregivers of 82 patients with heart failure; 30 intervention, 30 control. Intervention group: caregiver mean age, 65.0 years; 13 men; relationship, 14 spouses; patient mean age, 79.7 years; 21 men; NYHA class II, $n = 16$; NYHA class III, $n = 14$ Control group: caregiver mean age, 61.6 years; 8 men; relationship, 10 spouses; patient mean age, 80.8 years; 19 men; NYHA class II ($n = 14$), NYHA class III ($n = 16$) | Intervention: 12-week, twice-a-week, hospital-based exercise followed by home-based exercise program for patients with heart failure; caregiver attendance voluntary Control: no exercise Follow-up at 3 months and 6 months after baseline | Pre/post measures (caregiver only for all outcome variables): Care Work Strain Scale Hospital Anxiety and Depression Scale | Analyses of variance were conducted. Baseline equivalency was confirmed. Caregiver burden among caregivers of exercise intervention group was greater than control group caregivers at 6 months of follow-up ($F = 4.29, p = .045$), possibly because of increased supervision for home exercise. Caregiver burden at baseline and the 3-month follow-up indicated that anxiety and depression throughout the study were not significantly different between groups. Anxiety and depression levels were greater in the caregivers compared with healthy people. | The theoretical background was not described and the intervention targeted patients only. Race and ethnicity were not reported and there was no description of cultural aspects. |

(continued)

Table 9.1. CONTINUED

Author (Year)	Design/Sampling	Subject Characteristics	Methods/Interventions	Data/Measures	Findings/Outcomes	Limitations
Piette et al., 2008	Quasi-experimental, one group pre/post (feasibility study) Recruitment by invitation to eligible dyads from two hospitals in United States	52 caregiver–patient with heart failure dyads for intervention Caregiver: mean age, 42.3 years; 58% women; relationship, 75% adult children. Patient: mean age, 65.9 years; 11% women; 50% NYHA class III, other NYHA classes not reported	Intervention: CarePartner program, which provided automated weekly assessment phone calls measuring patients' perceived health status, shortness of breath, sodium intake, weight, and medication supply Immediate feedback for the assessment was asked for each call, and the caregiver and care manager (nurse) received report for patients' weekly assessment results. Mean duration of intervention 12 weeks	Pre/post measures: Structured interview about health and self-care problems by weekly phone calls (patient only) Feedback survey about the program (patient and caregiver)	Frequency and chi-square analyses were conducted. At the 6-week follow-up, caregivers did not report increased burden with more engagement in patient's self-care and weekly e-mail reports. Patients and caregivers believed the program was important and helpful (77% and 84%, respectively). Sixty-eight percent of caregivers reported they contacted patients more often, and 92% reported no increase in stress because of more attention to patients.	The theoretical background was not described and there was no randomization and no control group. Race and ethnicity of patient and caregiver were not reported, and there was no description of cultural aspects.

12-month randomized trial Recruitment via advertisement, and flyers distributed to patients and family at and around the University of Ottawa Heart Institute, Canada Siblings, children, and spouses of patients with coronary artery disease who had at least one modifiable risk factor were eligible	426 participants, 211 family heart-health intervention; 215 control. Intervention: mean age ± SD, 52 ± 11.9 years; 128 females, 201 white, 79 with BMI ≥30 Control: mean age ± SD, 51.1 ± 11.3 years; 133 female; 205 white; 87 with BMI ≥30	Intervention: Feedback about risk factors, assistance with goal setting and counseling from health educators for 12 months Coordination also provided to primary care providers of caregivers whose lipid levels and blood pressure exceeded thresholds All participants received printed materials about health promotion	Primary outcomes: Ratio of total cholesterol to high-density lipoprotein cholesterol Physical activity Fruit and vegetable consumption All assessments at 3 months and 12 months	Time effects using mixed-models analyses were conducted, with the baseline values as covariates. No effect of the intervention on the ratio of total cholesterol to high-density lipoprotein cholesterol was noted. Participants in the intervention group reported consuming more fruit and vegetables (1.2 servings per day more after 3 months and 0.8 serving at 12 mo; $p < 0.001$) and increased physical activity ($p = 0.03$). At 3 months, those in the intervention group reported 65.8 more minutes of physical activity per week. At 12 months, participants in the intervention group reported 23.9 more minutes each week.	A theoretical model was lacking, and race and ethnicity subgroup effects were not reported.

(continued)

Table 9.1. CONTINUED

Author (Year)	Design/Sampling	Subject Characteristics	Methods/Interventions	Data/Measures	Findings/Outcomes	Limitations
Sebern & Woda, 2012	Quasi- experimental, one group pre/post (feasibility study) Recruitment by invitation to eligible dyads from a home care agency in United States	11 caregiver–patient with heart failure dyads for intervention Caregiver: mean age, 61 years; 10 women; 5 white, 6 black; relationship, 4 spouses Patient: mean age, 80 years; 5 women; 5 white, 6 black; NYHA class III ($n = 6$), NYHA class IV, 3 = I and II, 2 unknown	Theoretical background: shared care conceptual model Intervention: SCDI consisted of seven sessions (60–120 minutes each) of structured one-on-one and dyadic interventions over 10 weeks; patient and caregiver taught about heart failure self-care and goal setting	Pre/post measures: self-care of Heart Failure Index (patient only) Preparedness subscale from Home Care Effectiveness Scale (caregiver only) Dyadic Relationship Scale (patient and caregiver) Kansas City Cardiomyopathy Questionnaire (patient only) Rand Medical Outcomes Study Short Form-36 (caregiver only)	A nonparametric Wilcoxon's test was conducted. After SCDI, self-care maintenance, management, and confidence improved among six, three, and four patients, respectively. Patients' clinical status improved overall (6.4 points), along with their quality of life (4.9 points among 5 patients). Caregivers were satisfied with the intervention (6.3 points out of 7 points), and there were improvements in caregivers' readiness to take part in care, family relationships, and quality of life.	There was no randomization and no control group. Ethnicity was not reported, nor was there a description of cultural aspects.

Citation	Design	Sample	Intervention	Measures	Analysis/Results	Comments
Schwarz, Mion, Hudock, & Litman, 2008	Experimental pilot study Random assignment to intervention or control groups Recruitment by invitation to eligible dyads in a hospital in United States	102 caregiver–patient with heart failure dyads (51 dyads for each/84 dyads completed); 44 intervention, 40 control. Intervention group: caregiver mean age, 63.9 years; 64% spouse; patient mean age, 77.1 years; 43% women, 82% white; NYHA class II, 24%; NYHA class III, 45%; NYHA class IV, 31%; comorbidity, 4.2 Control group: caregiver mean age, 63.0 years; 43% spouse; patient mean age, 79.1 years; 61% women; NYHA class II, 18%; NYHA class III, 51%; NYHA class IV, 31%; comorbidity, 4.9	Intervention: usual care plus Cardiocom EHM system, which measured weight daily and transferred the data to the advanced practice nurse responsible for monitoring daily body weight and contacting the caregiver-patient dyad and the primary physician for further evaluation as needed; 90-day posthospital discharge intervention delivered Control: usual care	Pre/post Measures: Center for Epidemiological Studies–Depression scale (patient only) Minnesota Living with Heart Failure Questionnaire (patient only) Philadelphia Geriatric Center Caregiving Appraisal Scale (caregiver only) Modified Inventory of Socially Supportive Behaviors Scale (caregiver only) Hospital readmission Emergency department visits Costs of care	Intention-to-treat analyses and survival analyses with Cox proportional hazard modeling were conducted. The baseline equivalency was confirmed. No significant differences were noted between groups at the 90-day follow-up on all outcome variables: hospital readmission, days to readmission, emergency department visits, costs, depressive symptoms, quality of life, and caregiver mastery.	The theoretical background not described and the ethnicity of patients and caregivers was not reported. The race of caregivers was not reported, nor was there a description of cultural aspects.

NOTE: BMI, body mass index; EHM, electronic home monitoring; NYHA, New York Heart Association; SCDI, Shared Care Dyadic Intervention; SD, standard deviation.

a team of physicians and nurses after hospitalization in a quasi-experimental study without random assignment. The sample included 60 patients with heart failure and their family caregivers in Taiwan. Patients and family caregiver dyads in the control group received traditional discharge planning by a care manager. Follow-up data were collected 30 days after baseline. Caregiver burden decreased significantly compared with the control group ($F = 11.43$, $p < .001$). In addition, mastery of stress ($F = -22.73$, $p < .001$) and family function ($F = -5.77$, $p < .001$) improved in the intervention group compared with the control group.

Care Management

Leff and colleagues (2006) tested in a quasi-experimental study without random assignment an intervention called Hospital at Home that included provision of daily physician visits and nursing supervision, followed by intermittent nurse visits for ill patients in place of hospitalization. The sample included 141 patients with heart failure, chronic obstructive pulmonary disease, pneumonia, or cellulitis and their family caregivers in the United States. Patient and caregiver satisfaction were measured 2 weeks after the receipt of Hospital at Home services or after hospitalization. Caregivers in the Hospital at Home group reported more satisfaction with nurses ($p = .013$) and discharge procedures ($p = .0003$) than caregivers in the hospital group. Caregiver satisfaction with admission procedure did not vary across the two groups.

Piette and colleagues (2008) tested a 12-week CarePartner program intervention that provided automated weekly assessment phone calls measuring patients' perceived health status, shortness of breath, sodium intake, weight, and medication supply in a quasi-experimental one-group pre- and posttest feasibility study. The sample was 52 patients with heart failure and family caregiver dyads in the United States. Follow-up data collection occurred 6 weeks after intervention delivery. Caregivers did not report increased burden with the additional engagement in patients' self-care and weekly e-mail reports. Patients (77%) and caregivers (84%) believed the program was important and helpful. Most caregivers (92%) reported no increase in stress because of the increased attention to patients.

Schwarz and colleagues (2008) tested an intervention that included usual heart failure care plus the Cardiocom Electronic Home Monitoring system to assess daily weight and to transfer data to advanced practice nurses for referral back to patient–caregiver dyads or physicians for further intervention. The study was a randomized pilot study conducted in the United States. Patients in the control group received usual care. The sample included 102 patients with heart failure after hospital discharge and family caregiver dyads. Follow-up data collection occurred 90 days after hospital discharge. No significant differences were found between the groups on any patient outcome (i.e., hospital readmission, days to readmission, emergency department visits, costs, depressive symptoms, and quality of life) or caregiver mastery.

Exercise

Molloy and colleagues (2006) tested a 12-week, twice-per-week hospital-based exercise intervention followed by a home-based exercise intervention in a randomized controlled study in Scotland. The sample included 82 patients with heart failure; 60 caregivers were also invited to attend the sessions. The control group received no exercise intervention. Follow-up data collection occurred 3 months and 6 months after baseline. Compared with caregivers of patients in the control group, caregiving burden increased among caregivers of patients in the intervention group at the 6-month follow-up ($F = 4.29$, $p = .045$). Caregiver anxiety and depression did not differ between the two groups. This study is important in highlighting that interventions to improve patient outcomes may have negative consequences for family caregivers. It is critical when designing patient interventions not to increase caregiver burden further and to consider clinical components that can minimize or ameliorate caregiver burden.

Self-management Counseling

Sebern and Woda (2012) tested a shared care dyadic intervention that consisted of seven sessions, 60 to 120 minutes each, of structured one-on-one and dyadic interventions in which patients with heart failure and caregivers were taught about heart failure self-care and goal setting. The intervention was delivered over 10 weeks in a single-group, pre-/posttest feasibility study. The small sample included 11 heart failure patient–caregiver dyads in the United States. Caregivers were satisfied with the intervention ($M = 6.3$ points on a 7-point scale) and reported improvements in their readiness to provide care, family relationships, and quality of life.

Multicomponent

Ågren and colleagues (2012) tested a multicomponent intervention based on a shared care model that included psychosocial support in three 60-minute sessions, nurse-led communication, and computer-delivered and written education in a randomized study. The sample included 155 patients with heart failure and their family caregivers in Sweden. Dyads assigned to the control group received usual patient education; caregivers were excluded from the control group. Follow-up measures were administered at 3 months and 12 months after baseline. Patients' perceived control over their heart failure increased significantly in the intervention group at 3 months ($p < .05$) but not at 12 months. No differences were found post-intervention in dyads' health-related quality of life, depressive symptoms, patients' self-care behaviors, and caregivers' experience of burden.

Case Study 2: "I Am a Patient Who Is Taking Care of a Patient"

M. J. is a 55-year-old woman who has taken care of her husband with heart failure for 9 years. Her husband, L. J., is 61 years old and he has become increasingly short of breath as his heart failure has worsened during the past year, at which point M. J. quit her job to care for her husband. She did not want him to be alone for fear that he might die while she was working at the office. After his first heart attack 10 years earlier, L. J. was hospitalized several times over 3 months. M. J. has her own health problems; she has diabetes mellitus and her blood glucose levels are not well controlled. She believes the uncontrolled glucose levels are the result of stress from caring for a sick husband and not taking care of her own health. However, M. J.'s priority is her husband's care because she believes that he is at risk for death.

M. J. attended two discharge education classes that provided information about what she needs to do every day to care for L. J., such as preparing low-sodium meals and monitoring his weight. Although she now devotes much of her time to her husband's care and says "there is nothing new to know; I feel like I know everything about heart failure care," she admits that she wonders if what she is doing is right. She expresses guilt about her husband's repeated admissions to the hospital. She has done her best in caring for him, but when he was readmitted to the hospital a week after being discharged, she felt like it was her fault. Searching the Internet for information does not help anymore because she knows what is available. She does not want to make phone calls to the nurses or doctors because it may cost more money. Therefore, her questions about caring for L. J. have not been answered fully. For example, when L. J. has increased shortness of breath, she wonders whether to call 911 for an ambulance, call the doctor's office, or watch L. J. and hope his breathing gets better.

During the past year, M. J.'s life has changed a great deal because her husband's heart failure has become more severe. She feels depressed about their future. M. J. was able to follow her required diabetic diet and routine exercise until the past year, but now that is more difficult to do. She used to spend time with friends taking exercise classes, bowling, and going to the movies, but she has stopped these activities. M. J. says that now her whole life is focused on L. J.'s heart failure care. M. J. feels she is on duty to watch L. J. 24 hours a day, 7 days a week. For example, she even watches him breathe at night when he sleeps.

Her friends suggested that M. J. hire somebody to help with L. J. so she has time to do the things she needs to do for her own health. Hiring a regular caregiver would cost more than this couple can afford on their limited budget. Their children live in other states and the couple has no close friends in town. At times, M. J. thinks that she wants to retire from this kind of family caregiving duty.

Possible Interventions

M. J. sounds as though she is doing moderately well with caregiving, but it is taking a toll on her own health and well-being. There are a number of potential interventions that could be recommended to improve this family's situation. One intervention is the addition to the healthcare team of an advanced practice nurse with expertise in care coordination (Sochalski et al., 2009). These nurses are effective in improving the complex care required by patients with heart failure by performing activities such as streamlining medication regimens, teaching patients and families to monitor symptoms, and helping manage the transitions from hospital to home.

To reduce the stress and sense of loss of her previous life that M. J. reports, stress management and cognitive restructuring interventions could be completed. She should be evaluated for depression and, if indicated, medications should be prescribed. The high level of vigilance that M. J. reports is common in caregivers. An assessment of whether such a level is necessary on a daily basis needs to be completed, and M. J. may need to be taught that high levels of vigilance are unnecessary. Providing clear direction about what to do in emergency situations can be incorporated as part of the plan of care and taught to M. J. Although their adult children live in different states, they can be involved in the family caregiving team through planned activities and use of modern technologies. Perhaps the adult children would be able to pay for a housekeeper or a companion to stay with L. J. while M. J. goes out to do routine tasks (e.g., grocery shopping) or one or two weekly social activities.

One area that requires focused attention and intervention is M. J.'s physical health and control of her diabetes. Nurses and social workers working with M. J. could develop a detailed plan for her that would allow her to have time for her own daily diabetes care, including physical activity. Modification of the home environment may be possible (such as purchasing home exercise equipment) to allow her to have daily exercise without leaving home. Other strategies for social activities on a routine ongoing basis need to be developed along with strategies for how M. J. can do them without feeling guilt. Helping her to understand that caring for oneself is essential to being a caregiver may be useful in reducing guilt.

Last, because heart failure is a progressively worsening condition, providers will want to assess the caregiving experience of M. J. periodically to ensure she receives additional assistance if L. J.'s health deteriorates further. Palliative care services are best provided in heart failure before patients become highly symptomatic, but are especially needed for patients with symptoms unresponsive to therapies.

Theoretical/Conceptual Frameworks in Existing Interventions

Theories that guided existing interventions were not well explicated. Two studies used a framework of shared care (Ågren et al., 2012; Sebern & Woda, 2012). Shared care is an information process that is based on the idea that each participant affects and is affected by the other. Shared commitment and shared goals provide the essentials of the information process (Ågren et al., 2012). Shared care is a dynamic partnership of three relational interactions: communication, decision making, and reciprocity. Conceptually, shared care is linked to social support because relationships and their processes are the context for support expression and receipt as well as a source for individualized meaning (Sebern & Woda, 2012). In both studies presented here, didactic partnerships were forged between clinical staff, patients with heart failure, and their family members, and success of the interventions was measured through several surveillance tools or surveys.

Chiang and colleagues (2012) used Meleis' transition theory (Chick & Meleis, 1986; Schumacher & Meleis, 1994) to frame their educational intervention. Health changes and disease status of individuals bring about transitions, and those in transition tend to be more vulnerable to the risks and perils that influence their health and that of their families even further. Transition theory is defined as the movement from the status quo to a different life experience. Often, this transition requires the acquisition of new knowledge or behavioral changes that bring about an evolution of self. Indicators of successful transitions include individualized perceptions of wellness, relationship wellness, and mastery of the new role. In the evaluation by Chiang and colleagues (2012), education provided about the transition to heart failure was expected to result in family caregivers' improved well-being and less burden (which, as summarized earlier, occurred).

Leff and colleagues (2006) reported using the Hospital at Home care model that was developed to provide acute care in patients' homes rather than in hospitals, but an actual theoretical model was not described. The remaining four publications did not mention use of a theoretical framework to guide their interventions. All four engaged in clinician-led educational interventions through engaging with patients and family caregivers to achieve improved outcomes of patients on behalf of the dyad.

Cultural Variations

Cultural differences among caregivers of patients with heart failure are a critically important but understudied dimension of research. Cultural norms for family care and roles and responsibilities vary widely among cultures. Development of interventions should incorporate these norms. For example, caregivers are expected to assist patients with heart failure when adhering to a low-sodium diet, but food preparation and intake in different cultures influence dietary sodium during preparation and may interfere with performance of interventions.

Demographic and clinical characteristics were reported for samples that included patients with heart failure, although data were limited by infrequent reports about clinical status (e.g., ejection fraction, New York Heart Association class) that are necessary when characterizing the sample and comparing results across studies. Characteristics reported about family caregivers were limited to demographics; in three studies, comorbidity of caregivers (Agren et al., 2012; Chiang et al., 2012; Sebern & Woda, 2012) and, in one study, general health status and physical function of caregivers (Leff et al., 2006) were described. No studies addressed ways that race, ethnicity, gender, or cultural background of participants may have influenced the reported results.

CONCLUSION

As the results of available findings suggest, interventions for family caregivers of persons with heart failure are underdeveloped when compared with family caregiving interventions in other chronic disease contexts. It is unclear why this is the case; as noted earlier and in several descriptive studies, family caregivers of persons with heart failure are at considerable risk for stress as a result of patients' medical management needs and long-term symptomatology, which are the result of debilitating cardiovascular conditions. Much like other areas of caregiving intervention that are highlighted in this volume, a number of scientific steps could help to address this gap, including the following:

- *Longitudinal descriptive studies*: The longitudinal implications of heart failure for family caregivers and how various health transitions influence family caregivers and their emotional, psychological, and physical health outcomes are needed. Various candidate transitions could include diagnosis/onset, hospital admission, discharge from hospital to home, and perhaps how heart failure may trigger the onset of other comorbid chronic conditions (e.g., dementia), which may further complicate the family caregiving experience. Examining such phenomena in culturally and racially diverse contexts would also advance the state-of-the-art.
- *Incorporation of more robust theoretical and conceptual models*: A culmination of descriptive research, particularly long-term cohort studies, could better refine existing or result in new theoretical and conceptual models of heart failure family caregiving. More appropriate theoretical frameworks and conceptual models would result in improved measurement and assessment of family caregiver domains that are relevant to heart failure, and would better inform the development of subsequent clinical interventions to alleviate family caregiver distress and potentially enhance family caregivers' health as well.

In general, results of existing intervention studies are modest or unclear at this stage, and interventions did not improve caregivers' measured outcomes. This result is not surprising, given the lack of theoretically based interventions to guide existing studies, few randomized control trials, and the lack of adequate sample sizes. In addition, given the chronic nature of heart failure symptoms, most existing caregiver interventions in this context consider fairly short follow-up intervals. Given the long-term nature of family caregiving for heart failure, constructing interventions that offer similarly long-lasting clinical services and evaluating the long-term effects of such services is warranted. Particularly noteworthy is that interventions were targeted at the patients' health in most cases and it may not be possible to change caregivers' outcomes with an intervention targeted to patients' health. Furthermore, interventions for patients may increase caregivers' burden in terms of the time and tasks required, such as providing transportation (e.g., Molloy et al., 2006). Heart failure is a serious debilitating condition known to be associated with severe symptoms, decreased functioning, and frequent use of healthcare resources. Even interventions that improve patients' health in the short term may not benefit caregivers who have been in the caregiving role for many years (Pressler et al., 2012). A holistic approach might be needed when intervening with patients with heart failure, and additional considerations for caregivers is likely required because an improved heart failure condition does not guarantee decreased burden for caregiving (ongoing vigilance on the part of the family caregiver to maintain the health of the heart failure patient is often needed).

The literature supporting that caregivers of patients with heart failure experience poor physical and emotional health is extensive, and theoretically based interventions targeted at improving caregivers' health and outcomes are urgently needed. Efficacious interventions that improve family caregivers' health in other major chronic conditions are available and could be adapted for heart failure (Bakas, Austin, Buelow, & Williams, 2010; Burgio et al., 2009; Garand et al., 2002; Northouse et al., 2012). Randomized controlled trials of head-to-head comparisons of theoretically based, efficacious interventions have potential for advancing the science of caregiving in heart failure more quickly, although until single interventions prove efficacious such strategies are premature.

Testing interventions that can be "scaled up" and translated into practice more rapidly is needed for the large population of caregivers of patients with heart failure. Recruiting large samples of caregivers is important to allow for evaluation of variables that influence intervention response (e.g., age, gender, race, ethnicity, culture). It is also important to note that many existing intervention efforts that target family caregiver outcomes may include caregivers of patients with heart failure as well as other chronic diseases, and more attention to how these intervention models influence subsamples of family caregivers according to a relative's condition may further determine how families of persons with heart failure can be best supported. Pertinent to scalability, several of these efforts are currently in translation. For example, several care coordination models have received attention for their potential to reduce patient care costs and, to a lesser extent, improve family caregiver outcomes (Gaugler, 2015). Two of the most prominent examples include the transitional care model and the Care Transitions Program. The transitional care model involves transitional care nurses in conducting patient assessments before discharge, engaging in care planning with other care providers, and visiting the patient and family caregiver at home 1 to 2 days after discharge and on a weekly basis up to 3 months after discharge. The Care Transitions Program uses "transition coaches" to monitor patients and family members from hospital to home or subacute care and focuses on family education and self-care over a 14-day period. Both models draw heavily on existing theoretical or conceptual frameworks, and existing randomized controlled trials have revealed improved outcomes for patients and family caregivers as well as cost savings (Coleman, Parry, Chalmers, & Min, 2006; Levine, Halper, Peist, & Gould, 2010; Naylor et al., 1999; Naylor et al., 2004). Given the length of time and resources necessary to build an evidence base that better describes the longitudinal ramification of family caregiving for persons with heart failure as well as test interventions tailored to this population, translational efforts that rely on these now widely disseminated models may be advisable.

Overall, the lack of guiding theoretical frameworks and limitations of study designs and samples hinder the ability to make decisions about efficacy or effectiveness about studies of family caregivers of patients with heart failure. The intervention studies do provide a base for future larger trials to demonstrate efficacy, but stronger integration of theory-guided interventions, more advanced designs, and larger as well as more diverse samples are warranted.

DISCLOSURE

The two case studies were developed using qualitative descriptive data obtained from the study Family Caregiver Outcomes in Heart Failure (supported by Research Investment Funds, Indiana University School of Nursing; Barron Quality of Life Research Award, Center for Enhancing Quality of Life in Chronic Illness, at Indiana University School of Nursing; and in part by National Institute of Nursing Research grants R01 NR08147 and R01 NR009280).

REFERENCES

Aggarwal, B., Liao, M., Christian, A., & Mosca, L. (2008). Influence of caregiving on lifestyle and psychosocial risk factors among family members of patients hospitalized with cardiovascular disease. *Journal of General Internal Medicine*, 24(1), 93–98.

Ågren, S., Evangelista, L. S., Hjelm, C., & Strömberg, A. (2012). Dyads affected by chronic heart failure: A randomized study evaluating effects of education and psychosocial support to patients with heart failure and their partners. *Journal of Cardiac Failure*, 18(5), 359–366.

Bakas, T., Austin, J., Buelow, J. M., & Williams, L. S. (2010). Preliminary efficacy of a stroke caregiver intervention program for reducing depressive symptoms. *Stroke*, 40(4), e138.

Bakas, T., Pressler, S. J., Johnson, E. A., Nauser, J. A., & Shaneyfelt, T. (2006). Family caregiving in heart failure. *Nursing Research*, 55(3), 180–188.

Bonow, R. O., Mann, D. L., Zipes, D. P., & Libby, P. (2011). *Braunwald's heart disease: A textbook of cardiovascular medicine*. Elsevier Health Sciences.

Burgio, L. D., Collins, I. B., Schmid, B., Wharton, T., McCallum, D., & DeCoster, J. (2009). Translating the REACH caregiver intervention for use by area agency on aging personnel: The REACH OUT program. *The Gerontologist, 49*(1), 103–116.

Chen, J., Normand, S.- L. T., Wang, Y., & Krumholz, H. M. (2011). National and regional trends in heart failure hospitalization and mortality rates for Medicare beneficiaries, 1998–2008. *Journal of the American Medical Association, 306*(15), 1669–1678.

Chiang, L., Chen, W., Dai, Y., & Ho, Y. (2012). The effectiveness of telehealth care on caregiver burden, mastery of stress, and family function among family caregivers of heart failure patients: A quasi-experimental study. *International Journal of Nursing Studies, 49*(10), 1230–1242.

Chick, N., & Meleis A. I. (1986). Transitions: A nursing concern. In: Chinn, P. L. (Ed.), *Nursing research methodology: Issues and implementation* (pp. 237–257). Aspen, Rockville.

Coleman, E. A., Parry, C., Chalmers, S., & Min, S. J. (2006). The care transitions intervention: Results of a randomized controlled trial. *Archives of Internal Medicine, 166*, 1822–1828.

Garand, L., Buckwalter, K. C., Lubaroff, D., Tripp-Reimer, T., Frantz, R. A., & Ansley, T. N. (2002). A pilot study of immune and mood outcomes of a community-based intervention for dementia caregivers: The PLST intervention. *Archives of Psychiatric Nursing, 16*(4), 156–167.

Gaugler, J. E. (2015). Innovations in long-term care. In L. George & K. Ferraro (Eds.), *Handbook of aging and the social sciences* (8th ed.). London: Elsevier.

Gheorghiade, M., & Pang, P. S. (2009). Acute heart failure syndromes. *Journal of the American College of Cardiology, 53*(7), 557–573.

Go, A. S., Mozaffarian, D., Roger, V. L., Benjamin, E. J., Berry, J. D., Borden, W. B., et al. (2013). Heart disease and stroke statistics: 2013 update: A report from the American Heart Association. *Circulation, 127*(1), e6–e245.

Hartmann, M., Bazner, E., Wild, B., Eisler, I, & Herzog W. (2010). Effects of interventions involving the family in the treatment of adult patients with chronic physical diseases: A meta-analysis. *Psychotherapy and Psychosomatics, 79*, 136–148.

Hwang, B., Fleischmann, K. E., Howie-Esquivel, J., Stotts, N. A., & Dracup, K. (2011). Caregiving for patients with heart failure: Impact on patients' families. *American Journal of Critical Care, 20*(6), 431–442.

Leff, B., Burton, L., Mader, S., Naughton, B. Burl, J., Clark, R., et al. (2006). Satisfaction with hospital at home care. *Journal of the American Geriatrics Society, 54*(9), 1355–1363.

Levine, C., Halper, D., Peist, A., & Gould, D. A. (2010). Bridging troubled waters: Family caregivers, transitions, and long-term care. *Health Affairs, 29*, 116–124.

Martire, L. M., Schulz, R., Helgeson, V. S., Small, B. J., & Saghafi, E. M. (2010). Review and meta-analysis of couple-oriented interventions for chronic illness. *Annals of Behavioral Medicine, 40*, 325–342.

Molloy, G. J., Johnston, D. W., Gao, C., & Witham, M. D. (2004). Family caregiving and congestive heart failure: A review and analysis. *European Journal of Heart Failure, 7*(2005), 592–603.

Molloy, G. J., Johnston, D. W., Gao, C., Witham, M. D., Gray, J. M., Argo, I. S., et al. (2006). Effects of an exercise intervention for older heart failure patients on caregiving burden and emotional distress. *European Journal of Cardiovascular Prevention and Rehabilitation, 13*(3), 381–387.

Murray, S. A., Kendall, M., Boyd, K., & Sheikh, A. (2005). Illness trajectories and palliative care. *British Medical Journal, 330*(7498), 1007–1011.

National Alliance of Caregiving/American Association of Retired Persons, 2009

Naylor, M. D., Brooten, D., Campbell, R., Jacobsen, B. S., Mezey, M. D., Pauly, M. V., et al. (1999). Comprehensive discharge planning and home follow-up of hospitalized elders: A randomized clinical trial. *Journal of the American Medical Association, 281*, 613–620.

Naylor, M. D., Brooten, D. A., Campbell, R. L., Maislin, G., McCauley, K. M., & Schwartz, J. S. (2004). Transitional care of older adults hospitalized with heart failure: A randomized, controlled trial. *Journal of the American Geriatrics Society, 52*, 675–684.

Northouse, L. L., Mood, D. W., Schafenacker, A., Kalemkerian, G., Zalupski, M., LoRusso, P., et al. (2012). Randomized clinical trial of a brief and extensive dyadic intervention for advanced cancer patients and their family caregivers. *Psycho-Oncology, 22*(3), 555–563.

Piette, J. D., Gregor, M. A., Share, D., Heisler, M., Bernstein, S. J., Koelling, T., et al. (2008). Improving heart failure self-management support by actively engaging out-of-home caregivers: Results of a feasibility study. *Congestive Heart Failure, 14*, 12–18.

Pressler, S. J., Gradus-Pizlo, I., Chubinski, S. D., Smith, G., Wheeler, S., Sloan, R., et al. (2013). Family caregivers of patients with heart failure. *Journal of Cardiovascular Nursing, 28*(5), 417–428.

Pressler, S. J., Gradus-Pizlo, I., Chubinski, S. D., Smith, G., Wheeler, S., Wu, J., et al. (2009). Family caregiver outcomes in heart failure. *American Journal of Critical Care, 18*(2), 149–159.

Riegel, B., Moser, D. K., Anker, S. D., Appel, L. J., Dunbar, S. B., Grady, K. L., et al. (2009). State of the science: Promoting self-care in persons with heart failure: A scientific statement from the American Heart Association. *Circulation, 120*(12), 1141–1163.

Roger, V. L., Go, A. S., Lloyd-Jones, D. M., Benjamin, E. J., Berry, J. D., Borden, W. B., et al. (2012). Heart disease and stroke statistics: 2012 update: A report from the American Heart Association. *Circulation, 125*(1), e2–e220.

Schumacher, K. L., & Meleis, A. I. (1994). Transitions: A central concept in nursing. *Image: Journal of Nursing Scholarship, 26*, 119–127.

Schwarz, K. A., Mion, L. C., Hudock, D., & Litman, G. (2008) Telemonitoring of heart failure patients and their caregivers: A pilot randomized controlled trial. *Progress in Cardiovascular Nursing, 23*(1), 18–26.

Sebern, M., & Woda, A. (2012) Shared care dyadic intervention: Outcome patterns for heart failure care partners. *Western Journal of Nursing Research, 34*(3), 289–316.

Shewchuk, R., & Elliott, T. (2000). Family caregiving in chronic disease and disability. In R. G. Frank & T. Elliott (Eds.), *Handbook of rehabilitation psychology* (pp. 553–563). Washington, DC: American Psychological Association.

Sochalski, J., Jaarsma, T., Krumholz, H. M., Laramee, A., McMurray, J. J., Naylor, M. D., Rich, M. W. Riegel, B., & Stewart, S. (2009). What works in chronic care management: the case of heart failure. *Health Affairs, 28*(1), 179–189.

Yancy, C. W., Jessup, M., Bozkurt, B., Butler, J., Casey, D. E., Drazner, M. H., et al. (2013). 2013 ACCF/AHA guideline for the management of heart failure: A report of the American College of Cardiology Foundation/American Heart Association Task Force on Practice Guidelines. *Circulation, 128*, e240–e327.

10

Caregiving for the Chronically Ill: State of the Science and Future Directions

LOUIS D. BURGIO AND JOSEPH E. GAUGLER ■

This final chapter is divided into three sections. In the first two sections we summarize the state of the science on caregivers and the caregiving role, and evidence-based interventions for reducing caregiver stress and burden included in this book. In the final section we discuss the most relevant challenges and barriers faced by today's caregivers and caregiver advocates. We also take a peek into the future of caregiving for the chronically ill, discuss emerging issues, and offer some suggestions for averting what can become the "perfect storm" (Gaugler & Kane, 2015) if the status quo remains just that.

CAREGIVERS AND THE CAREGIVING ROLE

To the extent there are similarities in the number and types of demands placed on caregivers of different chronic conditions, research findings should apply across chronic conditions, and some duplication of research effort may be avoided. For this purpose, we first examine the relatively small amount of literature that compares caregivers of different chronic conditions directly.

The Comparison Studies

Two studies compared caregivers of a specific chronic illness with a combined group of individuals providing care for various other chronic conditions (Magliano et al., 2005; Ory, Hoffman, Yee, Tennstedt, & Schulz, 1999), and two studies made direct comparisons among caregivers of specific chronic illnesses (Clipp & George, 1993; Kim & Schultz, 2008). Regardless of these procedural differences, the major conclusions of these studies converge. After adjusting for between-group demographic differences, number of hours dedicated to caregiving, intensity of caregiving, and other relevant variables, there are differences in the nature and impact of different caregiving experiences.

Clipp and George (1993) compared cancer and dementia caregiving on a number of dimensions. The authors report that dementia caregivers experience the greatest impact across all dimensions of well-being. In this early study, the authors hypothesize that the differences may have to do with caring for an individual with cognitive impairment as opposed to a lucid care recipients. In a more recent study, Kim and Schulz (2008) reported that dementia and cancer caregivers showed significantly more stress and burden then caregivers of individuals with diabetes or physical frailty. These authors also conclude that caring for individuals with cognitive impairments likely creates unique challenges for caregivers. However, these authors add that both conditions are typically characterized by overt psychological and physical suffering that are likely to be major contributors to caregiver distress. (This theory is developed further in an article by Monin and Schulz [2009]).

Continuing with the theme that caring for individuals with cognitive impairment presents unique challenges, Magliano et al. (2005) compared caregivers of individuals with schizophrenia and other "brain disorders" with a combined group of caregivers of patients with other chronic conditions. In that study, both objective and subjective burden were reported to be greatest in the schizophrenia/brain disorder caregiving group. The authors note there are similarities between schizophrenia and other brain disorders (e.g., dementia), in that they all manifest several cognitive and behavioral symptoms, and that both symptoms are strong predictors of anxiety and depression in caregivers. Last, Ory et al. (1999) analyzed data from more than 1,500 family caregivers from a 1996 national caregiver survey. Two groups were formed: dementia caregivers and nondementia caregivers (i.e., caregivers of other chronic conditions). Results showed that caregiving had greater effects on dementia caregivers than nondementia caregivers in a variety of important domains. Dementia caregivers are more involved in caregiving in terms of hours per week that they spend on caregiving tasks as well as a number of activity of daily living and instrumental activity of daily living tasks with which they assist. They are affected more negatively in terms of employment complications, caregiver strain, mental and physical health problems, and amount of time available for leisure. Again, after controlling for social demographics, level of caregiving involvement, and a number of other variables, dementia caregivers continued to show differences in caregiving strain.

The authors present three possible conclusions for their findings. These are worth discussing because they should apply to caregiving for individuals with any chronic condition that presents with similar symptoms. First, conditions in which patients display a high frequency of problem behaviors appear to be particularly stressful for caregivers (Williamson et al., 2005). Second, the authors suggest that another contributing factor may be caregiver experiences when there is anticipation that things will only get worse and that this will happen in an unpredictable and uncontrolled manner (e.g., dementia and some forms of cancer). Last, chronic conditions that are accompanied by progressive cognitive impairment often result in the loss of personhood or identity of the care recipient. The authors suggest that this loss of personhood may be a source of strain that is particularly damaging to caregivers.

Factors That Can Affect the Caregiving Experience

There are a number of factors, both intrinsic and external to the caregiving experience, that can affect the influence of the stressors and burdens of caring for an individual with a chronic illness. Technically, these variables are categorized as either mediators or moderators (see Baron and Kenny [1986] for a discussion). For the purpose of this chapter, we are not using this distinction in our discussion. There are a several articles that discuss these factors in detail (Pinquart & Sörensen, 2005; Shoemaker, Buntinx, & Delepeleire, 2010; Wolfs et al., 2012). Here, we discuss only those factors that we believe have the greatest overall impact on the caregiving experience. As we see in the evidence-based intervention section of this chapter, some of these factors have implications for the design of interventions for reducing caregiver burden.

COPING STYLES

In Chapter 1 we examined the stress process model by Pearlin and colleagues, in which caregivers use coping strategies to buffer against objective stressors in their environment (Pearlin, Mullan, Semple, & Skaff, 1990). This theoretical model posits that caregivers differ in the way they cope with these stressors, and that different coping styles or strategies can lead to positive or negative effects on caregiver physical health and emotional well-being. Li and colleagues identified three classifications of coping strategies. The first, *solution–focus* coping, includes strategies such as planful problem solving of issues common to the caregiving experience (Li, Cooper, Austin, & Livingston, 2012). The second, *emotional support and acceptance-based* coping strategies, include activities such as reappraising various challenges positively by trying to see the positive side of the situation (affective regulation), as well as "active cognition," such as praying for guidance and strength. Li and colleagues labeled the third classification *dysfunctional coping*, which includes blaming oneself for the caregiving situation or avoiding caregiving duties altogether, to name a few.

Research suggests that a general tendency toward problem solving and the acceptance styles of coping is likely to be advantageous to caregivers of individuals with chronic illnesses (Kneebone & Martin, 2003). Conversely, researchers report that caregivers who engage in escape, avoidance coping, and self-blame are more likely to experience health problems, depression, and anxiety (Neundorfer, 1991; Pett, Caserta, Hutton, & Lund, 1988).

Although spirituality/religiosity and focusing on the positive aspects of caregiving (PAC) can be subsumed under classification of coping styles by Li and colleagues (2012), extensive research has been conducted on these factors and has found that each transcends the confines of a coping style or strategy. Consequently, these factors are discussed separately.

SPIRITUALITY/RELIGIOSITY

For the majority of people in every culture, belief in a divine or transcendent reality is an important fact of daily life. Breakey (2001) defines spirituality as that which gives meaning to life and draws one to transcendence, to whatever is larger than or goes beyond the limits of the individual human lifetime. People who do not espouse any religion can be quite spiritual. On the other hand, religiosity is defined in terms of adherence to a system of spiritual beliefs and/or participation in a community of faith and practice.

In their review of the literature on mental health and religiosity, Koenig and Larson (2001) report that individuals with a greater sense of spirituality and/ or religiosity are less likely to manifest affect disorders and substance abuse. They also found that religious involvement is, in general, associated with greater well-being, less depression, and greater social support.

Caregiving researchers such as Chang and colleagues have found data that support the hypothesis that religious and spiritual coping influences caregiver distress indirectly through the quality of the relationship between caregivers and care recipients (Chang, Noonan, & Tennstedt, 1998). Specifically, caregivers who use religious or spiritual beliefs to cope with caregiving had a better relationship with care recipients, which was associated with lower levels of depression. Others (Rabinowitz, Hartlaub, Saenz, Thompson, & Gallagher-Thompson, 2009) have differentiated between negative and positive religious coping. Positive religious coping is associated with endorsement of items such as "trying to find a lesson from God in this," and "looking to God for strength support and guidance in this." Negative religious coping is associated with endorsement of survey items such as "wondered whether God had abandoned us," and "felt that my relatives' dementia was God's way of punishing me for my sins or lack of spirituality." Findings revealed that negative religious coping was associated significantly with increased cumulative health risk, whereas positive religious coping was predictive of decreased cumulative health risk. Thus, although the mechanism of action is unknown at this time, caregiver religiosity and spirituality are potent factors that can exert mostly a positive effect on the caregiver's sense of stress and burden.

POSITIVE ASPECTS OF CAREGIVING

The stress process model by Pearlin and colleagues (1990), probably the dominant theoretical model guiding caregiving research, focuses on the stressors and burden experienced by caregivers. Similarly, the majority of research on caregiving for chronic illness focuses on the causes and mediators of stress and burden in the caregiving role. However, in 1989, a pioneering article was published by

Kinney and Stephens in which the authors discussed events that were experienced by caregivers as positive. This was followed by an article by Lawton and colleagues that discussed positive and negative appraisals of events in the caregiver's life, and explored the appraisals' differential association with positive and negative affect (Lawton, Moss, Kleban, Glicksman, & Rovin, 1991). Pearlin and colleagues proffered the constructs of "gain" and "competence," which, they hypothesized, might have beneficial effects on the health and well-being of caregivers. However, these were hypothetical constructs and did not result in a revision of their stress process model.

Based on her work with HIV/AIDS caregivers, Folkman (1997, 2008) revised her stress process model to include adaptive coping mechanisms and positive emotions that resulted from favorable resolution of problems in caregiving situations (see Chapter 1 for a discussion of caregiving models). Folkman (2008) reported finding that positive and negative emotions can occur at the same time during periods of high stress. Subsequent research has found that positive and negative aspects of caregiving are not opposite ends of the same continuum. Correlations between the two are low (Rapp & Chao, 2000), and predictors of positive and negative aspects have little overlap (Pinquart & Sörensen, 2005).

During the past decade, researchers have paid increasing attention to this area of research, known generically as *positive aspects of caregiving* (Lawton, Kleban, Moss, Rovine, & Glicksman, 1989; Zarit, 2012). PAC has been conceptualized differently across studies to include phenomena such as how caregiving impacts caregiver self-evaluations (e.g., self-esteem, self-efficacy), positive appraisal of various events that occur during the caregiving experience, and the presence of enjoyable moments in daily experience (Carbonneau, Caron, & Desrosiers, 2010). Considering this broad range of phenomena, it is challenging to provide a definition of PAC. However, Zarit (2012) provides a reasonable working definition of PAC by describing it as "the positive dimensions of caregiving, including experiences, appraisals, emotions, and the strengths and resources that caregivers can call upon in managing the challenges they face" (p. 673).

Because of the importance of PAC in understanding the caregiving experience, and its implications for developing effective interventions (described later), several researchers have proposed theoretical models to gain a better understanding of the construct (Carbonneau et al, 2010; Lloyd, Patterson, & Muers, 2015). Very briefly stated, Carbonneau and colleagues (2010) hypothesize three domains of PAC: (1) quality of the caregiver/care recipient's premorbid and daily relationship, (2) the feeling of accomplishment, and (3) the meaning of the caregiver's role in daily life. Two factors are identified that facilitate or limit the manifestation of these domains: enrichment events in daily life and the caregiver's sense of self-efficacy. The predictive validity of the theoretical model by Carbonneau and colleagues is unknown at this time. However, the elements in the model are themes that one encounters throughout the PAC literature.

There is considerable variability in the literature on how PAC has been measured by researchers. Investigators have used semistructured interviews in which caregivers are simply asked whether there are positive aspects associated with their role (Hudson, 2004). A similar, but somewhat more quantitative strategy was used by Cohen and colleagues in a study of PAC with caregivers of various chronic conditions (Cohen, Colantonio, & Vernich, 2002). These researchers interviewed caregivers who were presented with a list of PAC. Although the researchers did not identify the number of PAC on the list, the number of items endorsed by the caregiver was recorded. Caregivers were also asked to rank their caregiving experience in general on a 7-point Likert-type scale representing very positive to very negative. Last, researchers have developed more traditional measures of PAC with known psychometric qualities. One measure, developed by the Resources for Advancing Caregiver Health (REACH) consortium (Roff et al., 2004) contains nine items that assess caregivers' subjectively perceived gains from, desirable aspects of, or positive affective returns from providing care for their family member. Caregivers are asked to rate, on a 5-point Likert-type scale, the extent to which they agree or disagree with statements such as "made me feel appreciated" and "enable me to appreciate life more."

Regardless of how PAC has been measured, the construct has been related to many positive outcomes. Although far from an exhaustive list, researchers have consistently reported that the presence of PAC increases caregiver's well-being (Cartwright, Archbold, Stewart, & Limandri, 1994; Cohen et al., 2002), decreases depressive symptoms (Pinquart & Sörensen, 2004), and reduces the level of burden associated with the caregiving role (Gold et al., 1995). Although it would be an error to glorify the caregiving experience, the absence of information about the positive dimensions of caregiving would limit both researchers and clinicians from gaining a thorough understanding of the caregiving role.

Caregiving and Race/Ethnicity

A large body of research has examined ethnic differences in stressors, resources, and psychological outcomes of the family caregiving experience. Pinquart and Sörensen (2005) published an exhaustive meta-analysis of the 116 empirical studies available at that time. Paraphrasing the findings of this meta-analysis, the authors stated that ethnic minority caregivers had a lower socioeconomic status, were younger, were less likely to be a spouse, and were more likely to receive informal support. They provided more care than white caregivers and had stronger filial obligation beliefs than white caregivers. Furthermore, Asian American caregivers, but not black or Hispanic caregivers, use less formal support than non-Hispanic white caregivers. Black caregivers had lower levels of caregiver burden and depression than white caregivers; Hispanic and Asian American caregivers were more depressed than their white non-Hispanic peers. Last, all groups of ethnic minority caregivers reported worse physical health than whites. These findings are relatively consistent across studies.

However, even before the publication by Pinquart and Sörensen (2005), literature reviews on ethnicity and caregiving emphasized the need to measure and assess explicitly the impact that cultural values have on caregiving experiences instead of simply using group membership to examine ethnic differences in caregiving (Dilworth-Anderson, Goodwin, & Williams, 2004; Janevic &

Connell. 2001). To explore this notion further, Aranda and Knight (1997) proposed the sociocultural stress and coping model based on the stress and coping model proposed earlier by Lazarus and Folkman (1984). This coping model added an emphasis on "ethnicity as culture." More specifically, this model proposed that individuals—or in this case, ethnic groups—with a greater sense of the importance of family ("familism") would perceive caregiving stresses as less burdensome.

Although this model offered a tremendous amount of appeal, Knight and Sayegh (2009) published an article that summarized a rather large body of research on "familism" that had appeared since the sociocultural stress and coping model had been introduced. In this now seminal paper, the authors concluded (1) the differences among diverse ethnic groups are built around a shared common core model in which caregiving stressors lead to the appraisal of caregiving as burdensome and thus to poor health outcomes; (2) familism is multidimensional and complex, and its influence in the caregiving experience is not as positive as had been expected; and (3) cultural values, including familism, operate through influences on coping resources such as social support and coping styles (discussed earlier) rather than through caregivers' appraisals of burden. In short, race/ethnicity is epiphenomenal; cultural values associated with race/ethnicity affect the caregiving experience because of their influence on social support and coping styles, which in turn affect the appraisal of stress.

EVIDENCE-BASED INTERVENTIONS FOR REDUCING CAREGIVER STRESS AND BURDEN

In this section we discuss some important dimensions of interventions designed to ease the burdens of caregiving for the chronically ill. We explore whether there are commonalities among effective treatments, and examine briefly some methodological limitations of intervention research. We also discuss what we don't know about caregiver interventions today. Last, we discuss the importance of efforts to translate evidence-based interventions for use in clinical and community settings, where they will be accessible to caregivers seeking assistance. This section does not include a compendium of caregiver interventions. Various types of interventions are described in Chapters 3 through 9. A section of *additional resources* is located at the end of this book that includes links to a number of sites where readers can find compendia of caregiver interventions that provide descriptions in considerable detail.

Some Dimensions of Caregiver Interventions

Caregiver interventions can be organized along a number of dimensions. Intended outcome, therapeutic focus, and mode of delivery are three often selected when discussing interventions. Other important characteristics of interventions include mode of delivery (e.g., clinic based, in home), dosage, and duration of treatment. A major factor determining where an intervention falls along these dimensions is the type of problems encountered while providing care to a chronically ill individual. Another factor is the intensity of caregiving burden associated with providing care. For example, it would appear that chronic illnesses characterized by cognitive decline and behavioral disturbances result in a high degree of caregiver burden. Thus, interventions developed for dementia and stroke caregivers tend to be intensive and include multiple treatment components that include instruction in multiple skill sets. Caregivers of individuals with cardiovascular problems and early-stage cancer require information about the disease and disease course, and interpreting and managing symptoms, monitoring nutrition, and providing emotional, spiritual, and social support. Caregivers of individuals with chronic musculoskeletal pain (CMP) are faced with a very different set of problems. CMP is characterized by uncertainty in diagnosis and unpredictability in course, and leads to significant impairments in individual and family functioning. Consequently, couples and family therapy is most efficacious in addressing the problems encountered by these caregiver–care recipient dyads.

We have organized our discussion of evidence-based interventions around the dimension of Therapeutic Focus. Other dimensions, such as mode of delivery, will be found in the discussions of treatment categories; however, they will not be emphasized. The reader can find complete descriptions of all interventions in the "Additional Resources" section at the end of the book.

Therapeutic Focus

When discussing the therapeutic focus of an intervention, we are examining the activities that occur during intervention sessions. We describe five categories of activities that one is most likely to find during caregiver interventions sessions. It should be noted that (1) authors use intervention terminology loosely; thus, our descriptions below might not necessarily correspond to their use in any particular article; and (2) although "pure" examples can be found for each of the first four categories, one often finds these activities combined into a multicomponent treatment package (the fifth category).

INFORMATION AND SKILL BUILDING
Information is provided about the chronic illness, course of the disease, and the caregiving experience. In addition, instruction is provided on various caregiving skills. Skills are targeted based on the needs of the caregivers. For cancer caregivers, skills may include interpreting and managing symptoms, monitoring nutrition, and providing emotional support. For dementia and stroke caregivers, the targeted skills often include managing problematic behaviors and improving caregiver coping skills.

Psychotherapy/Counseling

Psychotherapy/counseling involves a series of one-on-one meetings between a therapist or counselor and the caregiver or caregiving dyad. If other family members are involved in the caregiving role, they would be included in some or all of the sessions. Typically, a trusting relationship would first be established between the therapist and individual(s) involved in therapy. Through this trusting relationship, the therapist assists the caregiver in identifying dysfunctional beliefs and behaviors surrounding the caregiving experience. If successful, these beliefs are replaced by more adaptive beliefs and the development of a new behavioral repertoire to deal with caregiving demands. Although there are numerous therapeutic strategies, a number of studies have used cognitive behavior therapy for the treatment of depression in caregivers (Butler, Chapman, Forman, & Beck, 2006). Other examples include the use of family therapy for dementia caregiving (Joling et al., 2012; Mittelman et al., 1995;) and couples therapy for various chronic conditions (Martire, Schulz, Helgeson, Small, & Saghafi, 2010).

Strength/Emotion-Based Interventions

These interventions stand in stark contrast to traditional caregiver interventions that focus on reducing stressors in the caregiving experience that can result in burden and depression. Most researchers in this area acknowledge the influence of Folkman's revised stress process model (Folkman, 1997), which noted that HIV/AIDS caregivers reported positive cognitions and emotions as often as negative ones. The goal of these interventions is to help caregivers reframe negative experiences in positive terms, and/or to assist caregivers in identifying PAC and refocusing their attention on these PAC in their daily lives. One example is the Legacy Program of Allen and colleagues used with palliative care patients and their caregivers living at home (Allen et al., 2008) The dyad was asked to focus on a time in the patient's life that could represent adequately in one tangible project (e.g., a scrapbook) the patient's values and achievements in life. The purpose of working on this project together and reviewing these materials regularly was to increase attention on positive events in the past that would produce positive emotions in the present. Working with dementia caregivers, Cheng and colleagues used a benefit-finding intervention in which caregivers were taught cognitive restructuring techniques and means of reframing negative experiences in positive terms (Cheng, Lau, Mak, Ng, & Lam, 2014). The interventions described in these studies rely almost exclusively on teaching strength-based techniques. A more typical application combines strength-based techniques with more traditional skills training components that focus on reducing stress and burden (Hebert et al., 2003).

Technology and Web-Based Support

A comprehensive review of the use of technology-based interventions to assist caregivers of chronically ill patients was published by Chi and Demiris (2015). Thirty-three articles focused on family caregivers of adult and older patients. The review covered various chronic illnesses, including dementia, cancer, stroke, cardiovascular disease, severe mental illness, and end-of-life care. The most common technology used was video-conferencing with healthcare providers who delivered various cognitive–behavioral or educational interventions to the caregivers. The authors stated that more than 95% of studies reported significant improvements in caregiver outcomes, and that caregivers were satisfied and comfortable with technological interventions. However, it should be noted that 25% of the studies included in this review used nonexperimental designs. Moreover, the authors combined various forms of technology, and studies with very different outcomes in forming their conclusions. Last, there is a paucity of studies that compare technology-based interventions with more traditional caregiver interventions (Davis, Burgio, Buckwalter, & Weaver, 2004). Still, this review showed that technological interventions can affect chronic disease care positively. Although there is little doubt that technology will play an increasing role in supporting caregivers of chronically ill patients, more research is needed to ascertain how it can best be used to achieve positive outcomes.

MULTICOMPONENT INTERVENTIONS

Multicomponent interventions have been defined to include "two or more conceptually different approaches that have been woven into one intervention package" (Gallagher-Thompson & Coon, 2007, p. 38). An example of this type of intervention is the REACH II intervention for dementia caregivers (Belle et al., 2006). The authors hypothesized that caregiver stress and burden came from multiple sources in the caregiving experience. Consequently, the intervention involved a range of treatment strategies: provision of information, didactic instruction, role playing, problem solving, skills training, stress management techniques, and telephone support groups to reduce risk in five frequent problem areas by providing caregivers with education, skills to manage troublesome care recipient behaviors, social support, cognitive strategies for reframing negative emotional responses, and strategies for enhancing healthy behaviors and managing stress.

Which Caregiver Interventions Are Most Efficacious?

A number of reviews and meta-analyses have concluded that multicomponent interventions are the most efficacious among all categories of interventions discussed thus far (Brodaty & Arasaratnam, 2012; Pinquart & Sörensen, 2006; Zarit & Femia, 2008). In addition to using multicomponent interventions, there is emerging consensus among researchers on other commonalities of efficacious interventions. Specifically, although gaining new knowledge is necessary, to render the knowledge effective caregivers must engage actively with the interventionist by practicing new skills, receiving feedback, and developing plans to implement these skills in the types of situations they encounter (Gitlin, 2013). Also, it would appear that interventions that are designed to be flexible by providing different dosages of treatment components in response to dyad needs, allowing the interventionists in partnership with the caregiver to tailor treatment to the specific needs of the caregiving dyad, are superior to boilerplate, one-size-fits-all interventions (Zarit & Reamy, 2012). Last, interventions that provide more treatment (greater dosage) generally have better outcomes (Pinquart & Sörensen, 2006). More specifically, in their review, Brodaty and Arasaratnam (2012) suggested that delivering 9 to 12 sessions over a 3- to 6-month period seemed ideal for caregiving efforts associated with marked stress and burden.

Yet, these statements must be tempered by *what we don't know* about caregiver interventions. The results of the various intervention studies in this book indicate that there are many promising interventions for caregiving in most chronic illnesses. However, treatment effect sizes found in meta-analyses of these intervention studies are more sobering. Pinquart and Sörensen (2006) examined the outcomes of 127 caregiver intervention studies using randomized controlled trials, and rated the studies for quality. The meta-analysis included a variety of types of interventions, including both group and face-to-face interventions, interventions that were primarily psychoeducational, and more complex multicomponent interventions that taught skills that could assist caregivers in coping with various forms of everyday stressors. Their results estimated small to moderate positive effect sizes (range, 0.14–0.40) on measures of caregiver strain (e.g., caregiver burden, depressive symptoms, subjective well-being, perceived ability). More recent meta-analyses have reported more promising results. For example, in their meta-analysis published in 2012, Brodaty and Arasaratnam found that "nonpharmacological" interventions were effective in reducing behavioral and psychological symptoms, with an overall effect size of 0.34 (range, 0.20–0.48). Nevertheless, these results suggest there is still much that we need to learn while developing interventions for caregivers of the chronically ill.

What else don't we know? At the time of this writing (February 2015), none of the published research studies has included a component analysis to ascertain which of the individual treatment components in a treatment package contribute most to positive outcomes or add significant marginal value (Collins, Murphy, Nair, & Strecher, 2005; Jacobson et al., 1996). Without this knowledge, developing efficient interventions remains a matter of guesswork. Another strategy for addressing efficiency is to compare the effectiveness of caregiver interventions directly. Currently only one small-scale study using a comparative effectiveness design has been published (Chodosh et al., 2015). That study compared a care management protocol using two different formats. To our knowledge, only one large-scale study has been funded to examine which of two established dementia caregiver interventions is most effective for which type of caregiver (Luchsinger, Burgio & Mittelman, manuscript in preparation, Patient Centered Outcomes Research Institute (PCORI). Last, and perhaps most important, few caregiving interventions, developed through traditional randomized clinical trials, have been adapted for use in community settings, despite the fact that they were intended to be applied in the real world.

EMERGING ISSUES/FUTURE OF CAREGIVING

There is little doubt that a number of sociodemographic, chronic illness, and political trends are converging to threaten the status quo of family caregiving in the United States (Gaugler & Kane, 2015). There are currently 36 million family caregivers of older adults in the United States (Giovannetti & Wolff, 2010) that provide assistant valued at $234 billion in 2011 (Wolff & Jacobs, 2015). Clearly, the prominence of family caregivers in the care of adults with chronic illness demonstrates they are the primary source of long-term care in this country. However, this overreliance on family caregivers may be threatened by a number of factors. During the upcoming decades there will be fewer family caregivers available to care for chronically disabled older persons as a result of a declining fertility rate, delayed marriage in younger cohorts, increased participation of women in the workforce, less adherence to traditional gender roles in family care responsibilities, and rapidly declining nuclear family structures. These sociodemographic trends are colliding with concomitant chronic illness trends; older adults with chronic diseases (often co-occurring) will need support in the upcoming decades, and there is the possibility that fewer informal/unpaid supports will be available to offer long-term, needed help resulting from obesity and diabetes in younger candidate family caregiver cohorts.

Unfortunately, a shortage in geriatric care providers may mean that formal care simply will not substitute for family care in upcoming decades. The long-term care workforce is aging, and the supply of specialists such as geriatricians or licensed geriatric social workers is far outstripped by the current and future demand for such services (Institute of Medicine, 2008; Stone, 2015). This is the result, in part, of poor pay compared with other healthcare specialties; a work environment that is challenging because of the chronic, progressive nature of the disorders that many older persons experience (as opposed to acute diseases that can be "cured" in other healthcare settings and patient populations); and a lack of training and education that could better prepare the long-term care workforce to manage the challenges associated with chronic diseases. There is little evidence that the geriatric workforce situation is improving (Stone, 2015).

An ongoing issue as it relates to family caregiving in general as well as intervention research is that it is unclear whether the provision of "improved" family care (often a goal of family caregiver interventions, at least indirectly) results in improved health outcomes for care recipients. Because these outcomes are potentially reimbursable by third-party payers, a lack of clarity regarding whether caregiver interventions influence patient outcomes may explain why these protocols are not integrated routinely into standard healthcare delivery models. Specifically, payers are not convinced that psychoeducation, support groups, or therapy for family caregivers warrants reimbursement to care providers because the evidence that such interventions actually reduce harm to the care recipient or reduce health care expenditures remains mixed at best.

Although this is a challenge, it can also be seen as a great opportunity for family caregiver intervention advocates and researchers; healthcare reform is rapidly emphasizing pay for performance models based on patient outcomes. Future or existing caregiver intervention protocols that strongly demonstrate their effects on care recipient outcomes that are aligned with payer imperatives could facilitate their implementation as standard, routine components of chronic disease care. As it stands now, the literature has not made a convincing argument in favor of caregiving interventions occupying such positions.

Related to this point is the need for caregiver interventions, particularly those that have demonstrated efficacy over time, and ideally across settings and samples, to generate evidence of cost savings or cost-effectiveness. For example, in the dementia caregiving literature (see Chapter 2), there is some suggestion that multicomponent dementia caregiver intervention models delay residential long-term care placement of older persons with Alzheimer's disease or a related dementia. Although some cost-savings analyses have been conducted that suggest benefits, these studies are either rare or beset by assumptions that likely do not hold in actual translation/implementation efforts (Gitlin, Hodgson, Jutkowitz, & Pizzi, 2010; Long, Moriarty, Mittelman, & Foldes, 2014; Mittelman & Bartels, 2014; Nichols et al., 2008). When considering the future of caregiving intervention in various chronic disease contexts, it is clear the need for more refined cost data is necessary to elevate these approaches further as part of the "healthcare crisis solution."

Additional challenges relate to the economic status of many families, particularly Baby Boomers and younger cohorts, as they begin to grapple with the likelihood of providing family care to an older, chronically ill relative (Van Houtven, 2015). The "boom-and-bust" economic cycles that members of the Baby Boom generation have experienced throughout their life course has greatly influenced their ability to save, and thus pay for, long-term care expenses. Thus, many aging Baby Boomers will not have the financial resources at their disposal simply to pay for long-term care in the absence of available family members, which is compounded by the low percentage of older adults who currently have long-term care insurance in the United States. The public security net of Medicare and Medicaid is threatened further as a result of impending insolvency in upcoming decades.

Clearly, the convergence of sociodemographic, chronic illness, and economic trends will challenge the current reliance on family caregivers in the United States. Has current policy addressed these concerns? In light of the 2008 recession, it could be argued that policymakers have avoided this pressing issue (Lipson, 2015). Expansion of publicly funded programs to support caregivers (e.g., payment vouchers to family members who provide help to older adults in need) is viewed as unpalatable in the current political environment (Simon-Rusinowitz et al., 2010).

Will healthcare reform efforts help family caregivers? Some argue that, in fact, the responsibilities of family caregivers will expand, not shrink, with an emphasis on reducing admissions or readmissions to hospitals. Families may be required to shoulder not only more care, but also perhaps more complex care tasks (e.g., care coordination across transitions [Levine, Halper, Peist, & Gould, 2010]). In general, as healthcare strives to become more efficient, it often does not mean that more or better care is provided to chronically ill adults; instead, it means that families often shoulder at least some of the care provision that is reduced or eliminated from the service portfolio of formal healthcare organizations.

Although there have been policy successes in the past two decades, such as the Family Caregiver Support Program and state-level efforts to "rebalance" long-term care services and supports away from institutional care and toward home and community-based services (some of which could be of help to family caregivers, such as in-home help and adult day services), the polarized nature of many state and the federal branches of government do not augur well for family caregiver support via political means or compromise. As Debra Lipson, a long-term care policy expert notes, the recent 2013 Commission on Long-Term Care's (http://ltccommission.org/) recommendations were illustrative of this dynamic (Lipson, 2015). Although the Commission recognized family caregivers' pivotal role in long-term care, its lack of support for either public or privately financed solutions reflected the current state of policy developments for family caregivers.

As noted in Chapter 1, chronic disease models such as the model proposed by Wagner (1998) (see Figure 1.2 and http://www.improvingchroniccare.org/) suggest a framework for how to deliver optimal chronic disease care and to integrate family caregivers in such efforts fully. However, the U.S. healthcare system remains dominated by acute care philosophies and practices, which result in misalignment with chronic disease care principles. This lack of coordination leads to poor care quality, resulting in greater, more complex responsibilities and challenges for family caregivers.

Into this complex environment comes the suggestive evidence, and in some cases, translation, of family caregiver interventions. As noted throughout this book, there are many caregiver intervention protocols that have demonstrated significant efficacy in various disease contexts. Although there is much more empirical work to be done, cost studies seem to suggest that caregiving interventions are potentially low cost as well as cost-effective. For some chronic diseases such as Alzheimer's disease, it has been argued that caregiving interventions are at least as, if not more, effective in managing symptoms of dementia than pharmacological therapies (Brodaty & Arasaratnam 2012; Covinsky & Johnston, 2006). Taken together, the advances seen in family caregiving science supports the dissemination and implementation of these programs to settings that serve family caregivers on a day-to-day basis. However, as caregiver interventions may have considerable benefit in the overall treatment regimen of older adults or others with chronic diseases, why have they not been implemented successfully to a greater extent? One reason is the challenge in translating many caregiver interventions into real-world settings, and another is the lack of comparative effectiveness research that compares the benefits of one evidence-based intervention with another in a real-world setting (Wethington & Burgio, 2015). Family caregivers themselves are often not engaged in either the original development, testing, and evaluation of caregiver interventions, and because of this a gap exists between the generation and dissemination of scientific evidence, and the feasibility of implementing an evidence-based intervention into a clinic, community organization, or program in which it was not originally tested. Creating strategies and best practices to overcome these barriers to translation would greatly advance the "reach" of efficacious caregiving interventions.

Clearly, research evidence supporting caregiving interventions requires ongoing refinement and development, but for many protocols sufficient evidence exists to support the translation in community and clinical settings, and some interventions have undergone such translation. Several tools and resources could facilitate the successful implementation of caregiver interventions further. First, organizations or providers who are primed to translate interventions often require better information and decision-making tools to do so (Maslow, 2012). Information on training requirements, flexibility in modification, expectations of benefits for a given organization's client base, reimbursement potential, and similar data can help the eventual "translators" of caregiver interventions select the given protocol that is right for them. Without such decision-making tools, caregiving interventions are not likely to reach those individuals they are meant to reach as a result of barriers in translation and implementation.

As Gitlin and Hodgson note, several other advances in caregiving science could greatly facilitate the translation of caregiver interventions (Gitlin et al., 2015). For example, more easily administered measures that are rapid and brief could be of great appeal to care providers in the position to translate caregiving interventions. These interventions could identify family members at risk as well as inform the targeting of specific interventions (Czaja et al., 2009), such as caregiver measures that could be included in the Patient Reported Outcome Measurement Information System (or PROMIS, www.nihpromis.org) or developed using more advanced, modern measurement theory (iterative individualized response). Such strategies could help to advance caregiving intervention science and practice.

As opposed to relying on highly controlled settings or limited samples, pragmatic, embedded trials that test a given intervention in the intended real-world setting would help to expedite the oft-cited delay between evidence testing and implementation. Using more novel designs that allow for intervention component modification in terms of content, duration, and timing to match the context more completely in which the intervention is implemented (e.g., cultural, racial, geographic context) would also help to shorten the pipeline greatly between caregiving intervention and successful translation. More effective and efficient modes of interventionist training (as opposed to costly, intensive, in-person training sessions) would also aid in the implementation process. Often, with the advent of successful evidence of a given intervention, the inventors or champions of that given intervention position it as a "one-size-fits-all" solution, when in fact a given organization likely should have at its disposal the tools to modify or deliver various intervention components that best meet the needs, disease stage,

disease type, and caregiving context of a given client or client base
Potter, & Pruinelli, 2014).

CONCLUSION

The information provided in Chapters 2 through 9 has shown us that caregivers are a diverse group. Caregiving experiences range from those that are relatively easy to manage to those that are burdensome to the extent that many caregivers experience significant physical, emotional, and economic hardship. Caregivers of family members with dementia, stroke, and cancer—particularly in the later stages of these chronic diseases—face the greatest demands as a result of the behavioral deficits their loved ones display across instrumental and functional activities of daily living. In addition, caregivers of chronic illnesses that affect both cognitive and physical functioning (e.g., stroke and dementia) often encounter behavioral excesses such as agitation and physical aggression. Not surprisingly, research on the caregiving role, supportive interventions, and translation/implementation have reached a greater level of sophistication in chronic illnesses associated with greater burden. Still, as we surmised in the early days of our caregiving workgroup (see Preface) researchers even in these more developed areas of caregiving have worked predominantly from within academic silos, rarely referencing work done outside the confines of their chronic disease focus area. Our hope is that by offering caregiving researchers and clinicians a view into an array of "research silos," perhaps this book can play a role in advancing the field as a whole, bringing us closer to a necessary synthesis of knowledge about caregiving for individuals with chronic conditions.

REFERENCES

Allen, R. S., Hilgeman, M. M., Ege, M. A., Shuster, J. L., Jr., & Burgio, L. D. (2008). Legacy activities as interventions approaching the end of life. *Journal of Palliative Medicine, 7*(11), 1029–1038.

Aranda, M. P., & Knight, B. G. (1997). The influence of ethnicity and culture on the caregiver stress and coping process: A sociocultural review and analysis. *The Gerontologist, 37*(3), 342–354.

Baron, R. M., & Kenny, D. A. (1986). The moderator–mediator variable distinction in social psychological research: Conceptual, strategic, and statistical considerations. *Journal of Personality and Social Psychology, 51*, 1173–1182.

Belle SH, Burgio L, Burns R, Coon, D., Czaja, S. J., Gallagher-Thompson, D. et al. (2006). Enhancing the quality of life of dementia caregivers from different racial/ethnic groups: A randomized, controlled trial. *Annals of Internal Medicine, 145*, 727–738.

Breakey, W. R. (2001). Psychiatry, spirituality and religion. *International Review of Psychiatry, 13*, 61–66.

Brodaty, H., & Arasaratnam, C. (2012). Meta-analysis of nonpharmacological interventions for neuropsychiatric symptoms of dementia. *American Journal of Psychiatry*, *169*, 946–953.

Butler, A. C., Chapman, J. E., Forman, E. M., & Beck, A. T. (2006). The empirical status of cognitive–behavioral therapy: A review of meta-analyses. *Clinical Psychology Review*, *26*(1), 17–31.

Carbonneau, H., Caron, C., & Desrosiers, J. (2010). Development of conceptual framework of positive aspects of caregiving in dementia. *Dementia*, *9*(3), 327–353.

Cartwright, J. C., Archbold, P. C., Stewart, B. J., & Limandri, B. (1994). Enrichment processes in family caregiving to frail elders. *Advances of Nursing Science*, *77*(1), 31–43.

Chang, B., Noonan, A. E., & Tennstedt, S. L. (1998). The role of religion/spirituality in coping with caregiving for disabled elders. *The Gerontologist*, *38*(4), 463–470.

Cheng, S. T., Lau, R. W. L., Mak, E. P. M., Ng, N. S. S., & Lam, L. C. W. (2014). Benefit-finding intervention for Alzheimer caregivers: Conceptual framework, implementation issues, and preliminary efficacy *The Gerontologist*, *54*(6), 1049–1058.

Chi, N. C., & Demiris, G. (2015). A systematic review of telehealth tools and interventions to support family caregivers. *Journal of Telemedicine and Telecare*, *21*(1), 37–44.

Chodosh, J., Colaiaco, B. A., Connor, K. I., Cope, D. W., Liu, H., Ganz, D. A., et al. (2015). Dementia care management in an underserved community the comparative effectiveness of two different approaches. *Journal of Aging and Health*. [online] http://jah.sagepub.com.libdata.lib.ua.edu/content/early/2015/02/03/0898264315569454.full.pdf+html

Clipp, E. C., & George, L. K. (1993). Dementia and cancer: A comparison of spouse caregivers. *The Gerontologist*, *33*(4), 534–541.

Cohen, C., Colantonio, A., & Vernich, L. (2002). Positive aspects of caregiving: Rounding out the caregiving experience. *International Journal of Geriatric Psychiatry*, *17*, 184–188.

Collins, L. M., Murphy, S. A., Nair, V. N., & Strecher, V. J. (2005). A strategy for optimizing and evaluating behavioral interventions. *Annals of Behavioral Medicine*, *30*(1), 65–73.

Covinsky, K. E, & Johnston, C. B. (2006). Envisioning better approaches for dementia care. *Annals of Internal Medicine*, *145*(10), 780–781.

Czaja, S. J., Gitlin, L. N., Schulz, R., Zhang, S., Burgio, L. D., Stevens, A. B., et al. (2009). Development of the Risk Appraisal Measure: A brief screen to identify risk areas and guide interventions for dementia caregivers. *Journal of the American Geriatrics Society*, *57*, 1064–1072.

Davis, L., Burgio, L., Buckwalter, K., & Weaver, M. (2004). A comparison of in-home and telephone-based skill training interventions with caregivers of persons with dementia. *Journal of Mental Health & Aging*, *10*(1), 31–44.

Dilworth-Anderson, P., Goodwin, P. Y., & Williams, S. W. (2004). Can culture help explain the physical health effects of caregiving over time among African American caregivers? *Journals of Gerontology, Series B, Psychological Sciences and Social Sciences*, *59B*, S138–S145.

Folkman S. (1997). Positive psychological states and coping with severe stress. *Social Science and Medicine*. *45*, 1207–1221.

Folkman S. (2008). The case for positive emotions in the stress process. *Anxiety Stress Coping*, *21*(1), 3–14.

Gallagher-Thompson, D., & Coon, D. W. (2007). Evidence-based psychological treatments for distress in family caregivers of older adults. *Psychology and Aging, 22*(1), 37.

Gaugler, J. E., & Kane, R. L. (2015). The perfect storm? The future of family caregiving. In J. E. Gaugler & R. L. Kane (Eds.), *Family caregiving in the new normal* (pp. 357–377). San Diego, CA: Academic Press.

Gaugler, J. E., Potter, T., & Pruinelli, L. (2014). Partnering with caregivers. *Clinics in Geriatric Medicine, 30*, 493–515.

Giovannetti, E. R., & Wolff, J. L. (2010). Cross-survey differences in national estimates of numbers of caregivers of disabled older adults. *Milbank Quarterly, 88*, 310–349.

Gitlin, L. N. (2013). Introducing a new intervention: An overview of research phases and common challenges. *American Journal of Occupational Therapy, 67*(2), 177–184.

Gitlin, L. N., Hodgson, N., Jutkowitz, E., & Pizzi, L. (2010). The cost-effectiveness of a nonpharmacologic intervention for individuals with dementia and family caregivers: The Tailored Activity Program. *American Journal of Geriatric Psychiatry, 18*, 510–519.

Gitlin, L. N., Marx, K., & Stanley, I. H. (2015). Translating Evidence-Based Dementia Caregiving Interventions into Practice: State-of-the-Science and Next Steps. *The Gerontologist*, 1–17. doi:10.1093/geront/gnu123

Gold, D. P., Cohen, C., Shulman, K., Zucchero, C., Andres, D., & Etezadi, J. (1995). Caregiving and dementia: Predicting negative and positive outcomes for caregivers. *The International Journal of Aging and Human Development, 41*(3), 183–201.

Hebert, R., Levesue, L., Vezina, J., Lavoie, J. P., Ducharme, F., Gendron, C., et al. (2003). Efficacy of a psychoeducative group program for caregivers of demented persons living at home: A randomized control trial. *Journal of Gerontology, 58B*(1), S58–S67.

Hudson, P. (2004) Positive aspects and challenges associated with caring for a dying relative at home. *International Journal of Palliative Nursing, 10*(2), 58–65.

Institute of Medicine. (2008). *Retooling for an aging America: Building the health care workforce*. Washington, DC: National Academies Press.

Jacobson, N. S., Dobson, K. S., Truax, P. A., Addis, M. E., Koerner, K., Gollan, J. K., et al. (1996). A component analysis of cognitive–behavioral treatment for depression. *Journal of Consulting and Clinical Psychology, 64*(2), 295–304.

Janevic, M. R., & Connell, C. M. (2001). Racial, ethnic, and cultural differences in the dementia caregiving experience recent findings. *The Gerontologist, 41*(3), 334–347.

Joling, K. J., van Marwijk, H. W. J., Smit, F., van der Horst, H. E., Scheltens, P., van de Ven, P. M., et al. (2012). Does a family meetings intervention prevent depression and anxiety in family caregivers of dementia patients? A randomized trial. *PLoS One, 7*(1), e30936.

Kim, Y., & Schultz, R. (2008). Family caregivers' strains: Comparative analysis of cancer caregiving with dementia, diabetes, and frail elderly caregiving. *Journal of Aging and Health, 20*(5), 483–503.

Kinney, J. M., & Stephens, M. A. P. (1989). Hassles and uplifts of giving care to a family member with dementia. *Psychology and Aging, 4*(4), 402–408.

Kneebone, I. I., & Martin, P. R. (2003). Coping and caregivers of people with dementia. *British Journal of Health Psychology, 8*, 1–17.

Knight, B. G., & Sayegh, P. (2009). Cultural values and caregiving: The updated sociocultural stress and coping model. *The Journals of Gerontology, Series B, Psychological Sciences and Social Sciences*, 1–9.

Koenig, H. G., & Larson, D. B. (2001). Religion and mental health: Evidence for an association. *International Review of Psychiatry, 13*, 67–78.

Lawton, M. P., Kleban, M. H., Moss, M., Rovine, M., & Glicksman, A. (1989). Measuring caregiving appraisal. *Journal of Gerontology, 44*(3), P61–P71.

Lawton, M. P., Moss, M., Kleban, M. H., Glicksman, A., & Rovine, M. (1991). A two-factor model of caregiving appraisal and psychological well-being. *Journal of Gerontology, 46*(4), P181–P189.

Lazarus, R. S., & Folkman, S. (1984). *Stress, appraisal, and coping.* New York: Springer.

Levine, C., Halper, D., Peist, A., & Gould, D. A. (2010). Bridging troubled waters: Family caregivers, transitions, and long-term care. *Health Affairs, 29*, 116–124.

Li, R., Cooper, C., Austin, A., & Livingston, G. (2012) Do changes in coping style explain the effectiveness of interventions for psychological morbidity in family carers of people with dementia? A systematic review and meta-analysis. *International Psychogeriatrics, 25*(2), 204–214.

Lipson, D. J. (2015). The policy and political environment of family caregiving: A glass half-full. In J. E. Gaugler & R. L. Kane (Eds.), *Family caregiving is the New Normal* (pp. 137–152). San Diego, CA: Academic Press.

Lloyd, J., Patterson, T., & Muers, J. (2015). The positive aspects of caregiving in dementia: A critical review of the qualitative literature. *Dementia.*

Long, K. H., Moriarty, J. P., Mittelman, M. S., & Foldes, S. S. (2014). Estimating the potential cost savings from the New York University Caregiver Intervention in Minnesota. *Health Affairs, 33*, 596–604.

Magliano, L., Fiorillo, A., De Rosa, C., Malangone, C., Maj, M., & National Mental Health Project Working Group. (2005). Family burden in long-term diseases: A comparative study in schizophrenia vs. physical disorders. *Social Science & Medicine, 61*(2), 313–322.

Martire, L. M., Schulz, R., Helgeson, V. S., Small, B. J., & Saghafi, E. M. (2010). Review and meta-analysis of couple-oriented interventions for chronic illness. *The Society for Behavioral Medicine, 40*, 325–342.

Maslow, K. (2012). *Translating innovation to impact: Evidence-based interventions to support people with Alzheimer's disease and their caregiver at home and in the community.* Washington, DC: Administration on Aging.

Mittelman, M. S., & Bartels, S. J. (2014). Translating research into practice: Case study of a community-based dementia caregiver intervention. *Health Affairs, 33*, 587–595.

Mittelman, M. S., Ferris, S. H., Shulman, E., Steinberg, G., Ambinder, A., Mackell, J. A., et al. (1995). A comprehensive support program: Effect on depression in spouse-caregivers of AD patients. *The Gerontologist, 35*(6), 792–802.

Monin, J. K., & Schulz, R. (2009). Personal effects of suffering in older adult caregiving relationships. *Psychology and Aging, 24*(3), 681–695.

Neundorfer, M. M. (1991). Coping and health outcomes in spouse caregivers of persons with dementia. *Nursing Research, 40*, 260–265.

Nichols, L. O., Chang, C., Lummus, A., Burns, R., Martindale-Adams, J., Graney, M. J., et al. (2008). The cost-effectiveness of a behavior intervention with caregivers of patients with Alzheimer's disease. *Journal of the American Geriatrics Society, 56*, 413–420.

Ory, M. G., Hoffman, R. R., 3rd, Yee, J. L., Tennstedt, S., & Schulz, R. (1999). Prevalence and impact of caregiving: A detailed comparison between dementia and nondementia caregivers. *The Gerontologist, 39*(2), 177–185.

Pearlin, L. I., Mullan, J. T., Semple, S. J., & Skaff, M. M. (1990). Caregiving and the stress process: An overview of concepts and their measures. *The Gerontologist, 30*(5), 583–594.

Pett, M. A., Caserta, M. S., Hutton, A. P., & Lund, D. A. (1988). Intergenerational conflict: Middle-aged women caring for demented older relatives. *American Journal of Orthopsychiatry, 58*(3), 405–417.

Pinquart, M., & Sörensen, S. (2005). Ethic differences in stressors, resources, and psychological outcomes of family caregiving: A meta-analysis. *The Gerontologist, 45*(1), 90–106.

Pinquart, M., & Sörensen, S. (2006). Helping caregivers of persons with dementia: Which interventions work and how large are their effects? *International Psychogeriatrics, 18*(4), 577–595.

Rabinowitz, Y. G., Hartlaub, M. G., Saenz, E. C., Thompson, L. W. & Gallagher-Thompson, D. (2009). Is religion coping associated with cumulative health risk? An examination of religious coping styles and health behavior patterns in Alzheimer's dementia caregivers. *Journal of Religion and Health, 49*, 498–512.

Rapp, S. R., & Chao, D. (2000). Appraisals of strain and of gain: Effects on psychological wellbeing of caregivers of dementia patients. *Aging & Mental Health, 4*(2), 142–147.

Roff, L. L., Burgio, L. D., Gitlin, L., Nichols, L., Chaplin, W., & Hardin, J. M. (2004). Positive aspects of Alzheimer's caregiving: The role of race. *Journal of Gerontology, 59B*(4), P185–P190.

Shoemaker, B., Buntinx, F., & Delepeleire, J. (2010). Factors determining the impact of care-giving on caregivers of elderly patients with dementia: A systematic literature review. *Maturitas, 66*, 191–200.

Simon-Rusinowitz, L., Garcia, G. M., Martin, D., Sadler, M. D., Tilly, J., Marks, L. N., et al. (2010). Hiring relatives as caregivers in two states: Developing an education and research agenda for policy makers. *Social Work in Public Health, 25*, 17–41. doi:10.1080/19371910802678970

Stone, R. I. (in press). Factors affecting the future of family caregiving in the United States. In J. E. Gaugler & R. L. Kane (Eds.), *Family caregiving and the new normal* (pp. 57–78). San Diego, CA: Academic Press.

Van Houtven, C. H. (2015). Informal care and economic stressors. In J. E. Gaugler & R. L. Kane (Eds.), *Family caregiving in the new normal* (pp. 105–136). San Diego, CA: Academic Press.

Wagner, E. H. (1998). Chronic disease management: What will it take to improve care for chronic illness? *Effective Clinical Practice, 1*, 1–4.

Wethington, E., & Burgio, L. D. (2015). Translational research on caregiving: Missing links in the translation process. In J. E. Gaugler & R. L. Kane (Eds.), *Family caregiving in the new normal* (pp. 193–210). San Diego, CA: Academic press.

Williamson, G. M., Martin-Cook, K., Weiner, M. F., Svetlik, D. A., Saine, K., Hynan, L. S., et al. (2005). Caregiver resentment: Explaining why care recipients exhibit problem behavior. *Rehabilitation Psychology, 50*(3), 215–223.

Wolff, J. L., & Jacobs, B. J. (2015). Chronic illness trends and challenges of the family caregivers: Organizational and health system barriers. In J. E. Gaugler & R. L. Kane (Eds.), *Family caregiving in the new normal* (pp. 79–104). San Diego, CA: Academic Press.

Wolfs, C. A. G., Kessels, A., Severens, J. L., Brouwer, W., de Vugt, M. E., Verhey, F. R. J., et al. (2012). Predictive factors for the objective burden of informal care in people with dementia: A systematic review. *Alzheimer Disease and Associated Disorders, 14*(3), 197–204.

Zarit, S. (2012). Positive aspects of caregiving: More than looking on the bright side. *Aging and Mental Health, 16*(6), 673–674.

Zarit, S., & Femia, E. (2008). Behavioral and psychosocial interventions for family caregivers. *The American Journal of Nursing, 108*(9), 47–53.

Zarit, S. H., & Reamy, A. M. (2012). Future directions in family and professional caregiving for the elderly. *Gerontology, 59*(2), 152–158.

ADDITIONAL RESOURCES ON CAREGIVING AND INTERVENTIONS

GENERAL CAREGIVING

Administration on Aging (AOA)—U.S. Department of Health & Human Services: AOA National Family Caregiver Support Program Resource Room (http://www.acl.gov/Get_Help/Help_Caregivers/Index.aspx): Established to promote community living and carry out the Older Americans Act of 1965, which in part describes the distribution of funds to states for supporting older individuals with services

Aging and Disability Resource Center (ADRC)—U.S. Department of Health & Human Services (http://adrctae.org/tiki-searchresults.php?highlight=caregiver&where=files&search=go): Searchable resources page for researchers and practitioners

American Association of Retired Persons (AARP) Caregiving Resource Center (www.aarp.org/caregiving): Content pages and articles across a variety of domains, including planning and resources, benefits and insurance, legal and money matters, care for yourself, providing care, senior housing, end-of-life care, and grief and loss

American Psychological Association (APA): Resources on depression, capacity assessment, memory, elder abuse, psychotherapy, dementia, and integrated health care

Family Caregivers Briefcase (http://www.apa.org/pi/about/publications/caregivers/index.aspx)

Psychological Practice with Caregivers (http://www.apa.org/pi/about/publications/caregivers/practice-settings/index.aspx)

APA Office on Aging (http://www.apa.org/pi/aging/)

American Red Cross (http://www.redcross.org/take-a-class/Learn-About-Our-Programs): Family caregiver skills training programs; available in some locations

Area Agencies on Aging (http://www.n4a.org/): Staff identified as family caregiver support specialists available at every Area Agencies on Aging in the United States as part of the National Family Caregiver Support Program; searchable local resources area available through the national website

Caregiver Assessment: Voices and Views from the Field (https://caregiver.org/sites/caregiver.org/files/pdfs/v2_consensus.pdf): Report from a national consensus development conference amendment

Caregiver Tip Sheet (www.aoa.gov/prof/aoaprog/caregiver/overview/docs/CaregiverTipSheet.pdf)

Caregivers Count Too! An Online Toolkit to Help Practitioners Assess the Needs of Family Caregivers (www.caregiver.org/caregiver/jsp/content_node.jsp?nodeid=1695): Recommendations for assessing caregivers, including established measures for use by practitioners

Caring.com (https://www.caring.com/caregiver-wellness): Website designed to provide resources for family caregivers, including a resource listing for senior care services; content ranges across multiple domains, including cancer, shingles, memory disorders, online support groups, financial information, depression, retirement communities and supportive housing options, sleep, diabetes, fibromyalgia, irritable bowel syndrome, oral health, vision health, and more

Elder Care Locator (http://www.eldercare.gov/Eldercare.NET/Public/Index.aspx)

Extension—America's Research-Based Learning Network, Family Caregiving Website (http://www.extension.org/family_caregiving): Content and resources (including webinars) for a broad array of caregiving topics and populations ranging from military family caregiving to grandparents raising grandchildren to mental health caregiving

Family Caregiver Alliance, National Center on Caregiving: (www.caregiver.org/): Content and resources on topics including preparing for caregiving, new to caregiving, daily or in-home caregiving, long-distance caregiving, caregiving and advanced illness, and postcaregiving

GeroCentral: Caregiving (http://gerocentral.org/clinical-toolbox/clinical-issues/caregiving/): Research articles and other resources for professionals and researchers on caregiving

Mayo Clinic—Healthy Lifestyle Caregivers (http://www.mayoclinic.org/healthy-living/caregivers/basics/aging-parents/hlv-20049441)

Medicare Caregiver Information (http://www.medicare.gov/campaigns/caregiver/caregiver.html): PDF content links and podcasts on what Medicare covers, planning for the future, caregiver support by location, caregiver resources, and more

National Alliance for Caregiving (www.caregiving.org): Publications and resources for professionals and family caregivers, including ratings and reviews of websites, books, and other materials on caregiving; research; and advocacy

National Conference of State Legislatures: Family Caregiver Support—State Facts at a Glance (http://www.nasuad.org/documentation/tasc/FamilyCaregiverSupport_StateFactsataGlance.pdf): A collection of information about family caregivers of older Americans and the state-level programs that serve them

Ottawa Hospital Research Institute—Decision Making Tools (http://decisionaid.ohri.ca/): A collection of decisional tools that guide families through critical decisions associated with a variety of chronic illness conditions

Rosalyn Carter Institute on Caregiving's Evidence-Based Caregiver Intervention Resource Center (http://www.rosalynncarter.org/caregiver_intervention_database/): A drop-down menu and search function for different categories of chronic conditions (e.g., stroke, cancer, dementia)

World Health Organization—Caregiver Booklet (http://applications.emro.who.int/aiecf/IMAI_Caregiver_en.pdf): Educational tool for patients and caregivers developed by Hospice Africa in Uganda

SELECTED DISEASE-SPECIFIC RESOURCES FOR CAREGIVERS

Aging and Disability Resource Center (ADRC)—U.S. Department of Health & Human Services (http://adrctae.org/tiki-searchresults.php?highlight=disease&where=file s&search=go): Compendium of evidence-based Alzheimer's disease interventions, two volumes

Alzheimer's Association—Alzheimer's and Dementia Caregiver Center (http://www. alz.org/care): Extensive caregiver resources, customizable tools, educational materials, community message boards, information on clinical trials, and 24-hour helpline

Alzheimer's Foundation of America (AFA) Education and Care, Caregiving Tips (http://www.alzfdn.org/EducationandCare/strategiesforsuccess.html): Caregiver tips, educational materials, safety information, and other resources

American Cancer Society—Caregivers and Family (http://www.cancer.org/treatment/ caregivers/): Resources and content for families caring for someone with cancer, including information on Family and Medical Leave Act, insurance issues, and more

American Heart Association (http://www.heart.org/HEARTORG/Caregiver/ Caregiver_ UCM_001103_SubHomePage.jsp# and http://www.heart.org/HEARTORG/ Caregiver/Resources/ResourcesIntroduction/Caregiver-Resources-Introduction_ UCM_301850_Article.jsp): Printable resources for caregivers (e.g., caregiver burnout, caregiver rights, caregiver guide to strokes, monthly e-newsletters, healthy living tips, and self-care for caregivers

American Psychological Association

When the Care Recipient Is Someone with a Mental Health Disorder (http://www. apa.org/pi/about/publications/caregivers/faq/family.aspx)

Interventions for Caregivers of Those with Substance Abuse Disorders (http:// www.apa.org/pi/about/publications/caregivers/practice-settings/intervention/ substance-abuse.aspx)

American Stroke Association (http://www.strokeassociation.org/STROKEORG/#)

ARCH National Respite Network's Fact Sheet: Respite for Caregivers of Adults with Mental Disorders (http://archrespite.org/images/docs/Factsheets/FinalRespite_for_ Caregivers_of_Adults_with_Mental_Disorders_TP_edits_dle_edits_Oct_4.pdf)

Arthritis Foundation—Caregiving Resources (http://www.arthritis.org/ and http://www.arthritistoday.org/what-you-can-do/everyday-solutions/caregiv-ing/): Resources and content from the *Arthritis Today Magazine*, ranging from long-distance caregiving to parenting with arthritis to hiring the right caregiver

Caregiver Stress Check (www.alz.org/stresscheck/overview.asp): Eight-item quiz designed to help family caregivers of individuals with dementia identify symptoms of stress and related resources

National Institute on Aging—Alzheimer's Disease Education and Referral Site (http:// www.nia.nih.gov/alzheimers): Free resources for patients and families that are also well-suited for healthcare providers' offices, links to online information, and support communities

Savvy Caregiver Program DVDs—Health Care Interactive (http://www.hcinterac-tive.com/440 and http://www.hcinteractive.com/SavvyCaregiver): Savvy caregiver educational program for families of individuals with dementia; four DVDs or online content modules based on an evidence-based intervention program covering introduction to dementia and caregiving, minimizing confusion and taking charge, activities and loss of abilities, and providing structure and support.

TOOLS FOR TRANSLATION AND INTERVENTION RESEARCH

CDC Action Guides

  Assuring Healthy Caregivers: A Public Health Approach to Translating Research into Practice: The RE-AIM Framework (http://www.cdc.gov/aging/caregiving/assuring.htm)

  Implementing a Community-Based Program for Dementia Caregivers: An Action Guide Using REACH OUT (https://c.ymcdn.com/sites/chronicdisease.site-ym.com/resource/resmgr/Healthy_Aging_Critical_Issues_Brief/ReachOutActionGuide.pdf)

  Translation and Caregiving (http://www.nrepp.samhsa.gov/AboutGlossary.aspx): Evidence based, evidence informed, promising practice, and emerging program and practices

National Center for Advancing Translational Sciences—National Institutes of Health & US Department of Health & Human Services (http://www.ncats.nih.gov/research/cts/cts.html): Tools for researchers, clinical trial information, scientific publications, and more

Ohio Department of Job and Family Services—Ohio Children's Trust Fund (https://jfs.ohio.gov/OCTF/Evidence_Based_Evidence_Informed_Promising_Practice_and_Emer.pdf)

Substance Abuse and Mental Health Services Administration (SAMHSA)'s National Registry of Evidence-Based Programs and Practices (NREPP) (http://www.nrepp.samhsa.gov/AboutGlossary.aspx)

CAREGIVING AND INTERVENTION-FOCUSED GLOSSARIES OF TERMS

California Evidence-Based Clearinghouse for Child Welfare (http://www.cebc4cw.org/glossary/): Intervention and study design glossary

Disabled World Caregiver Glossary of Terms (http://www.disabled-world.com/definitions/caregivers-definitions.php): International online resource page for individuals with disabilities

University of Missouri–Kansas City's Center on Aging Studies without Walls (http://cas.umkc.edu/casww/glossary.htm): Caregiver glossary

AUTHOR INDEX

SUBJECT INDEX

CPSIA information can be obtained
at www.ICGtesting.com
Printed in the USA
BVHW082058041219
565568BV00003B/9/P